Antenatal Consults

A Guide for Neonatologists and Paediatricians

Antenatal Consults

A Guide for Neonatologists and Paediatricians

Mark Davies
MB BS PhD FRACP DCH

Garry Inglis
MB BS FRACP

Luke Jardine
MBBS MClinEpid FRACP

Pieter Koorts
MB ChB FCP FRACP Cert Neonatology

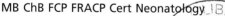

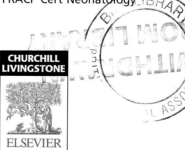

CHURCHILL
LIVINGSTONE

ELSEVIER

Sydney   Edinburgh   London   New York   Philadelphia   St Louis   Toronto

ELSEVIER

Churchill Livingstone
is an imprint of Elsevier

Elsevier Australia. ACN 001 002 357
(a division of Reed International Books Australia Pty Ltd)
Tower 1, 475 Victoria Avenue, Chatswood, NSW 2067

National Library of Australia Cataloguing-in-Publication Data

Title: Antenatal consults : a guide for neonatologists and paediatricians /
         Mark Davies … [et al.].

ISBN: 9780729541084 (pbk.)

Subjects: Prenatal diagnosis. Pregnancy—Complications.

Other Authors/Contributors: Davies, Mark. Garry Inglis, Luke Jardine, Pieter Koorts.

Dewey Number: 618.32075

Publishing Director: Luisa Cecotti
Developmental Editor: Neli Bryant
Project Coordinators: Geraldine Minto and Nayagi Athmanathan
Proofread by Tim Learner
Cover and internal design by Lisa Petroff
Index by Robert Swanson
Typeset by Toppan Best-set Premedia Limited
Printed in China by 1010 Printing Int'l Ltd.

CONTENTS

FOREWORD

When I started looking after sick babies over 40 years ago there were no antenatal diagnoses except for multiple pregnancies and small for dates babies and even that was hit and miss. So we did not have to think about antenatal consultation except for imminent preterm deliveries and that was more a comment of "we will do our best but the outcome is usually poor" because we knew little about caring for such babies and did not have any respiratory support. I was told not to resuscitate any baby born weighing less than 1500 g because their outcome was so bad.

Even when I became a consultant paediatrician in the 1980s antenatal diagnosis was unusual. As the years went by and antenatal ultrasound diagnoses, and other techniques, became more accurate, we started being asked to talk to parents about their baby's condition and what the future might hold. We had two problems: firstly was the diagnosis accurate, and secondly we knew very little about the outcome of babies with antenatal diagnoses. I remember one baby that I was asked to see because it had been diagnosed on ultrasound as having an encephalocoele. Discussing the management and outcome was made worse by the fact that the parents were friends of mine. I duly attended the caesarean section only to be presented with a baby who had a cystic hygroma on its neck!

I always had a sinking feeling when asked to talk to parents about a relatively rare condition I was unfamiliar with let alone tell them about the prognosis. What did I say to parents whose baby was diagnosed with "bright kidneys", "asymmetric hydrocephalus" or "possibly short arms"? I was ignorant about the outcome of many of these things. The problem was that there was little good information published to help me. In addition, I came to realise that the prognosis of a baby with an antenatal diagnosis might be very different from one made after birth.

Now we are in an age of detailed antenatal diagnoses leading to frequent calls for paediatric consultations and multi-discipline clinics to advise the parents and plan for the baby's care. The key role of the people involved is to ensure that the diagnosis and prognosis are accurate. This has meant that obstetricians and neonatologists have been on a steep learning curve to become informed about the details of diagnosis, management and particularly prognosis of rare conditions they previously knew little about and which may have a lot of interpatient variation.

For several years I have wanted those who were providing antenatal advice to keep a database about all their patients and particularly get good follow-up so that the prognosis was based on evidence rather than experience. Such a database could then be continuously updated so that it could be used to inform any obstetrician, paediatrician or surgeon who was asked to advise parents in the future.

As perinatologists, an important part of the work is to talk to parents who may deliver a very preterm baby and give them some accurate information about the treatment and management of their baby. One of the problems with this is to ensure that the many different people who are asked to give advice have a similar understanding about the management and outcomes of babies at different gestational ages otherwise the parents can become very confused.

Mark Davies, the editor, is an organised and hardworking neonatologist from Brisbane. He has gathered a large number of local, national and international co-authors with expertise in a wide variety of antenatally diagnosed problems.

I am delighted that this very practical book by Mark Davies and his colleagues is going to provide such information about very preterm babies and others with different abnormalities, for the increasing numbers of perinatologists who need to acquire a good understanding of antenatal problems. I am sure it will help improve the accuracy of communication with the parents. When I mentioned it to a Dutch neonatologist he said, "We need that book". I certainly wish I had it when I was giving such advice.

Colin Morley MB, BChir, MA, DCH, MD, FRCPCH, FRACP
Retired Professor of Neonatal Medicine
The Royal Women's Hospital, Melbourne, Victoria, Australia

LIST OF AUTHORS

Dr Mark W Davies MB BS PhD FRACP DCH
Senior Staff Specialist in Neonatology, Grantley Stable Neonatal Unit,
Royal Brisbane & Women's Hospital, Brisbane, Queensland, Australia
Associate Professor of Neonatology, Department of Paediatrics & Child
Health, The University of Queensland, Brisbane, Queensland, Australia

Dr Garry DT Inglis MB BS FRACP
Staff Specialist in Neonatology, Grantley Stable Neonatal Unit, Royal
Brisbane & Women's Hospital, Brisbane, Queensland, Australia
Senior Lecturer in Neonatology, Department of Paediatrics & Child
Health, The University of Queensland, Brisbane, Queensland, Australia

Dr Luke A Jardine MBBS MClinEpid FRACP
Neonatologist, Division of Neonatology, Mater Mother's Hospital, Brisbane,
Queensland, Australia
Honorary Researcher, Mater Medical Research Institute, Brisbane,
Queensland, Australia
Senior Lecturer, Department of Paediatrics & Child Health, The University
of Queensland, Brisbane, Queensland, Australia

Dr Pieter J Koorts MB ChB FCP FRACP Cert Neonatology
Deputy Director of Neonatology, Grantley Stable Neonatal Unit, Royal
Brisbane & Women's Hospital, Brisbane, Queensland, Australia
Senior Lecturer of Neonatology, Department of Paediatrics & Child Health,
The University of Queensland, Brisbane, Queensland, Australia

LIST OF CONTRIBUTORS

Benjamin W Anderson MBBS FRACP
Paediatric Cardiologist, Queensland Paediatric Cardiac Service, Mater
Children's Hospital, Queensland, Australia

Catherine Bagley B Phty MAPA
Clinical Physiotherapist Consultant, Mater Mother's/Children's Hospital,
Queensland, Australia

Dirk Bassler MD MSc
Neonatologist and Director of the Center for Pediatric Clinical Studies,
University Children's Hospital, Tuebingen, Germany

Ulrike Brandenburg MD FRACP
Staff Neonatologist, Kingswood, Nepean Hospital, New South Wales,
Australia

Tammy Brinsmead MBBS (Hons) FRACP
Senior Staff Specialist, Monash Medical Centre, Clayton, Victoria, Australia

Christopher Burke MB BS FRACP FRCPath
Neurologist, Royal Children's Hospital, Brisbane, Australia

Anita Cairns MBBS FRACP
Paediatric Neurologist, Royal Children's Hospital, Brisbane, Australia

Robert Cincotta MBBS FRANZCOG DDU CMFM
Visiting Staff Specialist in MFM, Mater Mothers Hospital, Queensland,
Australia
Associate Professor, Department of Obstetrics and Gynaecology, University
of Queensland, Queensland, Australia

Timothy Colen MBBS FRACP
Clinical Research Fellow in Echocardiography, Division of Paediatric
Cardiology, Stollery Children's Hospital, Edmonton, Alberta, Canada

Lucy Cooke MBBS FRACP
Senior Staff Specialist, Mater Mothers' Hospital, Queensland, Australia

Lisa Copeland MBBS FRACP FAFRM
Paediatric Rehabilitation Specialist, Royal Children's Hospital, Queensland, Australia

Jonathan W Davis MB BCh BAO MRCPCH
Consultant in Neonatal Medicine, St Michael's Hospital, Bristol, United Kingdom

Peter Davis MD FRACP
Professor/Director of Neonatal Medicine, Melbourne, Victoria, Australia

Maureen Dingwall MBChB DCH FRACP
Neonatal Staff Specialist, Mater Mothers' Hospital, Queensland, Australia
Senior Lecturer, University of Queensland, Queensland, Australia

Kelly-Marie Dixon MBBCh DCH
Neonatology Senior Registrar, Grantley Stable Neonatal Unit, Royal Brisbane & Women's Hospital, Queensland, Australia

Greg Duncombe MBBS FRANZCOG DDU CMFM
Staff Specialist, Royal Brisbane & Women's Hospital, Qld, Australia
Director, Queensland Ultrasound for Women, Queensland, Australia
Senior Lecturer, Department of Obstetrics and Gynaecology, University of Queensland, Queensland, Australia

Glenn J Gardener MBBS FRANZCOG CMFM
Director, Mater Centre for Maternal Fetal Medicine, Mater Health Services, Queensland, Australia

Peter H Gray MD FRCPI FRACP
Associate Professor, Department of Paediatrics and Child Health, University of Queensland, Queensland, Australia
Honorary Professorial Research Fellow, Mater Medical Research Institute, South Brisbane, Queensland, Australia
Eminent Staff Specialist, Newborn Services, Mater Mothers' Hospital, South Brisbane, Queensland, Australia

Anthony Herbert MBBS FRACP FAChPM B Med Sci
Staff Specialist, Paediatric Palliative Care Service, Royal Children's Hospital, Brisbane, Queensland, Australia

Adam B Hoellering MB BCh (Hons) Bsc (Hons) FRACP
Staff Specialist, Grantley Stable Neonatal Nursery, Royal Brisbane &
Women's Hospital, Brisbane, Queensland, Australia

David Hou MBChB FRACP
Neonatologist, Middlemore Hospital, Auckland, New Zealand

Judy Hough BHMS BPhty MPhty PhD
Physiotherapist, Mater Mother's and Children's Hospitals, Queensland,
Australia
Honorary Researcher, Mater Medical Research Institute, Queensland,
Australia
Senior Lecturer, School of Physiotherapy, Australian Catholic University,
Queensland, Australia

Elizabeth Hurrion MB ChB FRACP
Senior Staff Neonatologist, Mater Mothers' Hospital, Queensland, Australia

Fiona Hutchinson MBBS DCH(London)
Senior Registrar, Royal Brisbane & Women's Hospital, Brisbane,
Queensland, Australia

Ian Jones AM MB ChM M Ed Studies MHA PhD FRCOG FRANZCOG
Executive Director, Women's and Newborn Services, Royal Brisbane &
Women's Hospital, Brisbane, Queensland, Australia

Zsuzsoka Kecskes Dr Med FRACP PhD
Clinical Director and Senior Staff Specialist, Canberra Hospital, Australian
Capital Territory, Australia

**Professor Roy M Kimble MD(Research UQ) MBChB FRCS FRACS
(Paed Surg)**
Consultant Paediatric Surgeon & Urologist, Queensland Children's Medical
Research Institute, University of Queensland Department of Paediatrics &
Child Health, Royal Children's Hospital, Brisbane, Queensland, Australia

Melissa M Lai MBBS
Neonatology Advanced Trainee, Queensland, Australia

Karin Lust MBBS FRACP
General & Obstetric Physician, Clinical Director of Obstetric Medicine,
Royal Brisbane & Women's Hospital, Queensland, Australia
Senior Lecturer, University of Queensland, Queensland, Australia

Meryta May MBBS BMedSci FRACP FRCPA
Clinical Microbiologist, Sullivan Nicolaides Pathology, Brisbane,
Queensland, Australia
Visiting Paediatric Infectious Diseases Physician, Mater Children's Hospital,
Brisbane, Queensland, Australia

Craig A McBride BHB MBChB FRACS
Staff Specialist Paediatric Surgeon, Royal Children's Hospital, Queensland,
Australia
Visiting Paediatric Surgeon, Mater Children's Hospital, Queensland,
Australia
Senior Lecturer, University of Queensland, Queensland, Australia

Julie McGaughran BSc (Hons) MB ChB (Hons) MD FRCP FRACP
Director of Genetic Health Queensland, Royal Brisbane and Women's
Hospital, Queensland, Australia
School of Medicine, University of Queensland, Brisbane, Queensland,
Australia

Linda McLaughlin MBBS BSc
Neonatal Registrar, Royal Brisbane and Women's Hospital, Queensland,
Australia

Sarah Kate McMahon MBBS (Hons) PhD FRACP
Staff Specialist, Royal Children's Hospital, Queensland, Australia

Steven McTaggart MBBS FRACP PhD
Paediatric Nephrologist, Royal Children's and Mater Children's Hospitals,
Queensland, Australia

Linda Mellick MBBS BSc/LLB
Paediatric Fellow, Royal Children's Hospital, Queensland, Australia

Lindsay Mildenhall MBChB FRACP
Consultant Neonatologist, Middlemore Hospital, Auckland, New Zealand

David Millar MB MRCP FRCPCH
Consultant Neonatologist, Royal Jubilee Maternity Service, Belfast, United
Kingdom

Charlotte Mooring MBChB MRANZCOG
Senior Registrar, Royal Brisbane & Women's Hospital, Queensland,
Australia

Richard Muir MBBS FRACP
Paediatric Gastroenterologist, VMO, Mater Children's Hospital, Queensland, Australia

Michael Nissen BMedSc MBBS FRACP FRCPA FFS(RCPA)
Director, Infection Management & Prevention Service, Royal Children's Hospital, Queensland, Australia

Clare Nourse BA MB Bch BAO DCH MRCPI FRACP MD
Director, Paediatric Infection Management Service, Mater Health Services, Associate Professor, University of Queensland, Queensland, Australia

Colm O'Donnell MB MRCPI MRCPCH FRACP FJFICMI PhD
Consultant Neonatologist, The National Maternity Hospital & Our Lady's Children's Hospital, Dublin, Ireland
Director of Clinical Research, National Children's Research Centre, Dublin, Ireland
Senior Clinical Lecturer, School of Medicine & Medical Science, University College Dublin, Dublin, Ireland

Scott G Petersen MBBS BMedSci FRANZCOG CMFM
Staff Specialist, Mater Mother's Hospital, Queensland, Australia

Carol Portmann MBBS FRANZCOG CMFM MSc
Acting Clinical Director, Maternal Fetal Medicine, Royal Brisbane & Women's Hospital, Queensland, Australia

Benjamin Reeves MBBS FRACP
Paediatric Cardiologist, Cairns Base Hospital, Cairns, Queensland, Australia

Jeremy Robertson MBBS FRACP FRCPA
Paediatric Haematologist, Royal Children's Hospital, Queensland, Australia

Kate Sinclair MBBS MRCPCH FRACP
Staff Specialist in Child Neurology, Royal Brisbane & Women's Hospital, Royal Children's Hospital, Queensland Australia

Alice Stewart BSc MBBS GCHlthSc FRACP
Monash Newborn, Monash Medical Centre, Melbourne, Victoria, Australia

Rachel Susman MBBS MRCP FRACP
Clinical Geneticist, Genetic Health Queensland, Royal Brisbane & Women's Hospital, Brisbane, Queensland, Australia

Dr Joseph Thomas MBBS MD(O&G) FRANZCOG DDU C MFM
Staff Specialist Maternal Fetal Medicine and Obstetrics, Mater Mothers Hospital, Queensland, Australia
Associate Senior Lecturer, Department of Obstetrics & Gynaecology, School of Medicine, University of Queensland, Queensland, Australia

Bronwyn Williams MBBS FRACP FRCP FASCP
Senior Staff Specialist, Pathology Queensland/Royal Children's Hospital, Herston, Queensland, Australia

Judith Williams MBBS QLD FRACP PSM
Staff Paediatrician, Bundaberg Hospital, Queensland, Australia

Paul Woodgate MBBS B Med Sc FRACP
Associate Professor, Griffith Medical School, Queensland, Australia
Senior Staff Specialist, Mater Mother's Hospital, Brisbane, Queensland

Andreas Zankl MD FMH FRACP
Head, Bone Dysplasia Research Group, UQ Centre for Clinical Research, The University of Queensland, Queensland, Australia
Associate Professor, Pediatrics and Child Health, The University of Queensland, Queensland, Australia

Angelika Zankl FMH FRACP
Staff Specialist, Mater Mother's Hospital, Brisbane, Queensland, Australia

LIST OF REVIEWERS

Patricia Green RN, RM, B Hlth Sc, M Clin Prac
Assistant Professor Faculty of Health Sciences and Medicine, Bond University, Gold Coast, Queensland, Australia

Jane Morrow RN, RM, B Hth Sci (Nursing)
MHealth Management, Grad Dip Teaching and Learning, PhD candidate, Midwifery Courses Co-ordinator, Australian Catholic University, Melbourne, Victoria, Australia

Colleen Rolls PhD, RN, RM
Senior Lecturer, Australian Catholic University, Melbourne, Victoria, Australia

The aim of the book is to provide information to neonatal and paediatric staff who need to counsel parents expecting a fetus at risk.

Expectant parents are managed by a multidisciplinary team including maternity staff, obstetricians and materno-fetal medicine specialists who look after the pregnant mother and her fetus. However any problems with the pregnancy and/or the fetus will have implications for the baby when it is born. Neonatal and paediatric staff are often asked to speak to expectant parents under these circumstances. This consultation is known as an "antenatal consult".

The information expectant parents want includes: What is the diagnosis? What problems will baby have when it is born? Where should baby be born? What treatment will be needed after birth? What are the long-term prospects for my child?

A single, handy, concise source of information can be invaluable. This book provides a very useful guide to those who have been asked to provide parents with the information they seek and does so in a single succinct resource.

Our aim in producing this small handbook was to cover the 50 or so most common (or most important) reasons for an antenatal consultation. This will range from the baby that is threatening to deliver prematurely or is severely growth restricted, to those with significant abnormalities such as congenital heart disease, spina bifida or gastroschisis.

This book is also useful for trainees: not only trainee neonatologists and paediatricians but trainee obstetricians and materno-fetal specialists; and any nursing or allied health staff who care for mothers and babies.

Mark Davies
Garry Inglis
Luke Jardine
Pieter Koorts

Section 1
General Principles

CHAPTER 1

The Antenatal Consult

Mark W Davies, Garry DT Inglis, Alice E Stewart, Luke A Jardine

Neonatologists and paediatricians are often asked to speak to the parents of a fetus who is at significant risk of problems. The request for a paediatric antenatal consultation should come from members of the obstetric team or maternal fetal specialists caring for the mother. Such requests are essential for those facing extreme prematurity or a serious congenital anomaly.

Neonatologists and/or paediatricians should be involved in the decision making process with parents and obstetricians or maternal fetal medicine specialists around the timing and place of delivery for these high risk fetuses.

THE NATURE OF ANTENATAL CONSULTATIONS

The consultation with the parents will usually fall into two broad groups: a case conference involving the many specialists who will be involved in the care of the mother or baby and the parents; or a talk involving the neonatologist/paediatrician and the parents alone. In either case, the expertise of the paediatric specialists is required to provide information on the care of the baby that will eventually be delivered.

Often other paediatric specialists will talk to the parents, either in addition to the neonatologist or as the sole paediatric antenatal involvement. This is common in cases such as congenital heart disease, where the parents may only be seen by a paediatric cardiologist, and other congenital anomalies where paediatric surgeons, neurologists and spinal specialists etc. would be more appropriate than a neonatologist alone. Nevertheless, the input of the medical team that will care for the baby in the delivery room and the neonatal nursery can be very valuable to the parents.

Many of the problems for which an antenatal consult is requested are detected following routine antenatal screening tests. The nature and timing of these tests are summarised in Table 1.1.

Data on the frequency of occurrence of various problems for which a paediatric antenatal consult is required is sparse. We have examined the data from the Centre for Fetal Diagnosis and Treatment at the Royal

Table 1.1 Routine antenatal tests	
Timing	**Screening Tests**
At booking-in or first visit (after 12 weeks)	Blood group and antibodies Rubella titre Syphilis serology Hepatitis B serology Hepatitis C serology* Human Immunodeficiency Virus (HIV) serology*
10–14 weeks	Chorionic villus sampling (CVS) for karyotype*
11–13 weeks	Ultrasound for fetal nuchal translucency*
16–18 weeks	Triple test* (alpha-fetoprotein, unconjugated oestriol and human chorionic gonadotrophin) for Down Syndrome risk
16 weeks	Amniocentesis for karyotype*
18–20 weeks	Ultrasound for fetal morphology
26–28 weeks	Screening for gestational diabetes—glucose challenge test Blood group and antibodies screen for Rhesus negative women

These tests may not be routine for all pregnancies.

Brisbane and Women's Hospital for the year of 2007 (Table 1.2). While not all of these problems would have required a paediatric antenatal consult, they do give an idea of the scope of problems that are likely to. The data are consistent with our experience; the most common problem faced is that of impending prematurity and giving parents information on the likely consequences of preterm birth at various gestations for a variety of reasons (including spontaneous preterm labour, ruptured membranes, intrauterine growth restriction and multiple pregnancy). The other common problems dealt with include chromosomal abnormalities and congenital anomalies of the heart, kidneys and central nervous system. Others include cleft lip and/or palate, abdominal wall defects, diaphragmatic hernia, skeletal problems and fetal infections. Less common but regular problems include chest masses, neck or sacrococcygeal teratoma, talipes, cystic hygroma, bowel obstruction and non-immune hydrops.

Not all discussions with parents will be concerned with informing them of the likely clinical course for their baby once it is born. Sometimes the parents will be deciding whether to continue with or terminate the pregnancy and the information that paediatric specialists provide, especially with regard to survival and the likelihood of disability, will help them make that decision.

The antenatal consult will not only provide information for the parents but will also provide information to the obstetric and maternal fetal medicine specialists and others caring for the mother. This may be especially useful when the timing and location of delivery is being planned.

Table 1.2 Fetal problems presenting to the Centre for Fetal Diagnosis and Treatment at the Royal Brisbane and Women's Hospital in 2007 (there were 4830 births at this hospital in 2007)

Problem	Number
Chromosomal abnormality (including aneuploidy)	46
Cardiac abnormality	42
Kidney or renal tract abnormality	36
Brain abnormality (excluding isolated ventriculomegaly)	35
Threatened preterm delivery (excluding Premature prelabour rupture of membranes (PPROM), multiples)	26
Cleft lip/palate	18
Spina bifida	16
Isolated ventriculomegaly	16
Maternal medical problem	15
Monochorionic diamniotic twins	13
Dichorionic diamniotic twins	12
Intrauterine growth restriction	12
Gastroschisis	11
Skeletal dysplasia	11
Confirmed TORCH infection	10
Congenital diaphragmatic hernia	9
Echogenic bowel	9
Talipes	9
Cystic hygroma	7
Multiple severe abnormalities	7
Premature prelabour rupture of membranes (PPROM)	6
Hydrops fetalis	6
Oligohydramnios	6
Abdominal mass (including liver cyst)	5
Triplets	5
Chest mass (including congenital cystic adenomatoid malformation)	4
Exomphalos	4
Confirmed parvovirus infection	4
Twin-to-twin transfusion syndrome	4
Bowel obstruction (including duodenal atresia)	3
Fetomaternal alloimmune thrombocytopenia	3
Monochorionic monoamniotic twins	3
Polyhydramnios	3

Table 1.2 Fetal problems presenting to the Centre for Fetal Diagnosis and Treatment at the Royal Brisbane and Women's Hospital in 2007 (there were 4830 births at this hospital in 2007) continued...	
Problem	Number
Confirmed varicella infection	3
Arthrogryposis, epidermolysis bullosa, hand abnormality, previous congenital anomaly, teratoma	2 each
Amniotic band, carriers of genetic diseases, cataract, caudal regression, intrauterine fetal death of twin, known syndrome, neck mass, pleural effusion, previous neonatal alloimmune thrombocytopenia, previous spherocytosis, small stomach	1 each

The format of the typical antenatal consultation is outlined in Table 1.3. Whether the meeting with parents is a case conference, or involves the neonatologist alone with the parents, the first step is the collection of information. The presenting problem for the fetus and the results of any investigations will be the primary focus. Also important is any relevant information about the mother (including past medical and obstetric history, details of the current pregnancy, any medical problems or medications) or the family (family history, social history). This information should be given to you by the referring obstetrician or maternal fetal medicine specialist. Importantly, they should also let you know what the parents have been told and what their expectations are. Some information may need to be elicited from the parents when you meet them.

The discussion with parents should then include most of the features outlined in Table 1.3. It is important to communicate with the parents in terms that are easily understood. Some parents want a lot of detailed information and others want more general advice. This can be difficult to judge and will have to be done at the time of the interview.

Parents are particularly appreciative of information that helps them to prepare for the baby's delivery—especially details on what will actually happen to baby immediately upon delivery and in the hours thereafter, the expected clinical course and the risk of expected or possible morbidities and mortality rates. Information on particular treatments and procedures that are likely is also useful; e.g., intubation and ventilation, umbilical catheter insertion, prostaglandin infusion. Parents are often reassured by talking to someone who knows how things work in the neonatal nursery.

If specific diagnoses have been made then more reliable estimates of the natural history and prognosis can be given. Examples include delivery at a given gestation or a specific structural anomaly such as transposition of the great arteries or gastroschisis.

If a non-specific abnormality has been discovered then the range of possible diagnoses needs to be discussed. Findings such as polyhydramnios

Table 1.3 The antenatal consult

Collect information	• The referring doctor should have contacted you with details of the case
	• Look at any scans with the obstetrician, maternal fetal medicine specialist or radiologist/ultrasonologist, if possible
	• Determine the degree of diagnostic certainty/uncertainty
	• Determine what the parents have been told and what their expectations are
	• Is an interpreter required?
Talk to parents	• Ask the parents to tell you what they have been told and what their understanding of the problem is
	• Explain the problem
	• Explain what will happen upon delivery
	- likely condition of baby
	- likely and possible resuscitation needed
	- will they get to see/hold the baby?
	• Explain transfer to the neonatal nursery
	- will it be intensive or special care?
	- when will they get to visit?
	• What will happen in the neonatal nursery?
	- likely procedures, laboratory tests, etc
	• Who will be looking after the baby?
	- Medical/nursing/other
	- Who will provide updates on baby's progress?
	• Explain the expected course for the specific problem
	- what is the anticipated length of stay?
	- what are the criteria for discharge?
	• Discuss the possibility of uncertainty regarding prognosis
	• Discuss survival rates
	• Discuss likely and potential short- and long-term morbidities
	- especially the rates of moderate to severe disability
	• Discuss pain management
	• Discuss any impact on the ability to breast feed
Question time	• Allow time for parents' questions
	• Check the parents' understanding of the information provided
Document the plan for baby	• Write in the mother's notes
	- plans for initiation (or not) of life support / comfort care
	- document plan for immediate management post-delivery
Ensure that ancillary information has been arranged	• Other antenatal consults required
	- e.g., genetics, paediatric surgeon, spinal specialists, neurosurgeon, cardiology, nephrology, etc
	• Support groups contact information
	• Availability of social workers
	• Tour the neonatal nursery
	- visitation policy

or echogenic bowel could be due to specific problems or may be found in normal babies. An indication of the worst and best case scenarios can be provided and the spectrum of possibilities in between.

COMMON POINTS FOR DISCUSSION

If required, an interpreter should be available for all discussions with parents.

General discussion should always include an assessment of the degree of certainty or uncertainty of any antenatal diagnosis. It is important to emphasise that one of the important tasks in the early neonatal period will be to confirm any diagnosis made *in utero* with more reliable post-natal investigations. Detail can be provided on what those investigations may include and how long it may take to get results.

For any diagnosis, the impact of any degree of prematurity should be discussed.

Parents frequently want to know when they will be able to hold their baby and the impact of any particular problem on the mother's ability to breast feed. The long-term outlook is particularly important to parents and the rates of long-term survival and disability should be discussed.

Many parents will have made their own searches for information about their baby's problem. When speaking to the parents, it is important to establish their level of knowledge about the problem and address any information which appears unreliable (especially the internet). Parents should be given adequate time to ask questions and to ensure they have understood the information provided.

Depending on the parents' pre-existing knowledge and expectations, the consultation may lead to either reduced or increased anxiety about their baby. In some circumstances it may be appropriate that the latter occurs but follow-up to address such anxiety should be offered. The overriding principle is that the information that is given is reliable, and where uncertainty and doubt exists then the parents should also be told about this. It is important to note that the information that parents can get from people who will actually be looking after their baby cannot usually be provided by anyone else, including obstetric and maternal fetal medicine specialists.

TO DELIVER OR NOT DELIVER?

Many times the opinion of a neonatologist is sought to help determine the best time to deliver a fetus at risk. Often the choice is between delivering a baby early (either as soon as possible or at a later gestation) or delivering at term. Examples include the severely growth restricted fetus who is also extremely premature, fetal hydrops, monochorionic monoamniotic twins and rhesus disease. In these circumstances the fetus may be at risk if they remain *in utero*. The optimal mode of delivery should also be considered.

Clearly when any intervention is contemplated (i.e., early delivery) one must consider not only the potential benefit to mother and fetus, but also any potential harm. Unfortunately many decisions of this type are based solely on mortality rates. This is often the primary focus of the obstetric and maternal fetal specialists that are advising the parents. One of the roles of the neonatologist is to highlight, to both the parents and the obstetric/maternal fetal specialists, the significant morbidities associated with delivery at a much earlier gestation even though delivery of a live baby may be more certain. If the primary goal is to deliver a live baby regardless of the baby's condition or ultimate prognosis, this will tend to lead to delivery at a much earlier gestation when the risks to the preterm infant are much greater.

The question that must be asked is: will intervention at any given gestation give sufficient benefit (greater rates of survival without significant disability) whilst minimising harm (i.e., mortality rates and the incidence of long-term disability). Strategies to reduce antepartum fetal deaths should be replaced with strategies to reduce overall mortality **and** long-term disability.

Ultimately it is best to consider the difference between doing nothing (i.e., continuing the pregnancy) and delivering early, with regard to the ultimate outcome for the baby including not only mortality but also long-term neurodevelopmental outcome, disability and quality of life. **If it is not known that the ultimate outcome will be improved by early delivery (or any intervention) then the fetus should remain *in utero* until it is known.**

Parents need the best data available on mortality and disability rates upon which to base any decision to intervene and deliver a fetus early. Sometimes these data are not available and under these circumstances it is probably best to not intervene. Often the prognosis for a fetus who is delivered early is known but the data for their prognosis if they remain *in utero* is not; early delivery cannot be justified in this instance.

NON-INITIATION OF LIFE SUPPORT

In some situations it is appropriate to not initiate life support upon delivery. This is most often contemplated when a fetus has severe congenital abnormalities or will be born extremely preterm. A plan to not resuscitate should only be instigated after discussion between the obstetric, maternal fetal medicine and paediatric staff responsible for the mother and baby, any allied health staff involved, and the baby's parents. The principles involved have been established at consensus conferences in New South Wales in 1986, 1989 and 1998; and the findings of the latest Australia-wide consensus conference were reported by Lui *et al*[1] in 2006. These principles are broadly consistent with similar consensus statements published in other countries and include:

- consideration must be given to the interests and well being of the infant;
- the initiation or the prolongation of treatment is not necessarily in the best interests of the infant;

▶ the opinion of parents as to the best interests of the infant must be respected and accounted for;
▶ society has the right to intervene when parents' decisions are not clearly in the best interests of the infant;
▶ resources are finite—there may be competing financial claims which are as vital to human life as is neonatal intensive care;
▶ parents must be informed and consulted about all medical treatment or non-treatment regarding their newborn child;
▶ appropriate follow-up is essential, including support for parents of disabled survivors and community services for such infants.

The Australian consensus statement considers it inappropriate to initiate life support in infants born with lethal non-correctable malformations (such as anencephaly and confirmed trisomy 13 or 18), and infants born at a gestational age of less than 23 completed weeks. This must be discussed and planned with the parents antenatally.

There will be many other circumstances when the provision of life support will not be considered. Such circumstances occur when it is likely that, if life support is started, the baby will be dependent on continued medical treatment for survival and is very likely to have a major disability if that treatment were to continue (i.e., very little chance of normal outcome), where death is inevitable and imminent regardless of that treatment, and continued treatment cannot relieve pain and suffering believed to be intolerable.

It cannot be understated that these decisions cannot be made except in close collaboration with the parents who must have the best available information on possible outcomes for the baby including mortality rate and the incidence of long-term disability if baby survives.

REFERENCE

1. Lui K, Bajuk B, Foster K, et al. Perinatal care at the borderlines of viability: a consensus statement based on a NSW and ACT consensus workshop. *Medical Journal of Australia*. 2006;185(9):495–500.

Further Reading

American Academy of Pediatrics, Committee on Fetus and Newborn. Noninitiation or withdrawal of intensive care for high-risk newborns. *Pediatrics*. 2007;119(2):401–403.

Griswold KJ, Fanaroff JM. An evidence-based overview of prenatal consultation with a focus on infants born at the limits of viability. *Pediatrics*. 2010;125:e931–e937.

Halamek LP. The advantages of prenatal consultation by a neonatologist. *J Perinatol*. 2001;21(2):116–120.

Miquel-Verges F, Woods SL, Aucott SW, et al. Prenatal consultation with a neonatologist for congenital anomalies: parental perceptions. *Pediatrics*. 2009;124:e573–e579.

Yee WH, Sauve R. What information do parents want from the antenatal consultation? *Paediatr Child Health*. 2007;12(3):191–196.

CHAPTER 2

Conditions that Require Palliative Care

Lucy Cooke, Anthony Herbert

In some situations it will be appropriate to not initiate life support upon delivery. This is most often contemplated when a fetus has severe congenital abnormalities or will be born extremely preterm. The principles upon which such a decision should be made are discussed in Chapter 1.

CONGENITAL MALFORMATIONS

Congenital malformations are the leading cause of death in the perinatal period. Some fetuses are severely affected or have multiple congenital malformations; many of these conditions are not compatible with long-term survival. Such conditions include:

- major structural abnormalities of the brain (e.g., anencephaly and holoprosencephaly);
- chromosomal abnormalities (e.g., Trisomy 18 and Trisomy 13);
- hypoplastic left heart syndrome and other severe forms of complex congenital heart disease;
- severe neuromuscular conditions;
- severe renal abnormalities (with or without pulmonary hypoplasia); and
- life-threatening skeletal dysplasia.

Life expectancy predictions can be uncertain. Some infants with these conditions do live beyond the first year of life.[1] Health professionals need to be comfortable with this uncertainty and be willing and able to provide support over an extended period of time on occasion.

The use of language in how these diagnoses are explained to parents is very important. "Life limiting diagnosis" is more helpful and sensitive than the phrase "non-viable infant". Any "medical definition" will need to be explained in very compassionate terms to parents who are traumatised by any such diagnosis.

Options Available to Families

The options available to parents in this difficult situation include termination of pregnancy or delivering the baby with a plan for palliative care after birth.

Termination of pregnancy is commonly advised. It may seem intuitive that termination will avoid prolongation of the grieving process however some research suggests that this is not the case.[2] It is important to not pass judgement on parents who make these difficult decisions. A lack of consistent medical information and not being given options can have an impact on the grief that parents will experience.

Parents may prefer to continue the pregnancy and have a palliative care plan after birth. This can be facilitated by an inter-disciplinary team supporting the family. When good pain and symptom management can be provided, this is often a more acceptable option for parents and should be presented as an option. Formulation of a detailed plan for the care of the baby immediately after birth and thereafter (often referred to as a "Birth Plan") is integral to this process.

When a significant abnormality is diagnosed antenatally, at least one study suggested that many factors had an impact on parents' decision making at this time. These included religious beliefs, past experiences and the degree of diagnostic uncertainty. There was consistency among parents with regard to their need to feel supported throughout their decision making process.[3] Early introduction to the palliative care team may be helpful to facilitate this.

Steps in Creating a Birth Plan

If parents elect to continue the pregnancy and for the baby to receive palliative care, a number of important steps must be undertaken in creating a birth plan. This includes an open discussion of all pertinent issues. The discussion needs to be sensitive and non-threatening.

In palliative care, it is important to work out the family's goals or wishes. The family members are encouraged to create a list of what they would like to happen. Not all of their wishes may be possible and it is important to explain why this may be the case. Holding and seeing the baby is often important. Other important considerations include:

▶ Mode of delivery

Spontaneous vaginal delivery is the preferred mode of delivery in the absence of maternal factors which preclude it. Caesarean section may be requested by parents, and should be discussed with the mother's obstetric provider.

▶ Resuscitation

A discussion of resuscitation is important and should be handled sensitively with the family. It is often better to have such discussions ahead of time and allow time for the family to work through any issues or concerns they may have. This may include a discussion of the normal process of resuscitation and how this would fit in terms of appropriateness for the specific case at hand.

▶ Pain and symptom management

Pain relief and feeding tubes are important considerations. Pain relief may be provided through the intravenous, subcutaneous or oral route. There is now a trend to administer medications sublingually and avoid invasive procedures. Nutrition has great meaning to all parents and should be considered (including provision of breast milk) where it is possible and feasible. It is important to discuss the implications of nasogastric tube feeding before birth, so that a clear plan can be documented.

▶ Discharge home
Not all life limiting diagnoses are immediately life threatening, and it is important to distinguish those cases where it may be reasonable to expect that a baby will be able to go home from the hospital and be cared for in the home with appropriate support from a local palliative care or community nursing team. If this is the case, antenatal liaison with these teams as well as the family's GP is imperative, to ensure that the plan can be facilitated in timely fashion after birth. Determining a local hospital and paediatrician who could care for the child if they required admission for symptom management, intercurrent illness or end-of-life care should also be undertaken.

▶ Spiritual needs
This would include consideration of the need for baptism or other important spiritual rituals for the family. It is important to be sensitive to religious and cultural diversity in this context. Different denominations will vary in their approach to whether a dead baby should or can be baptised. It is therefore important to be able to contact the appropriate pastoral carer or chaplain for the individual case at hand.

▶ Memory making
It is very important for the family to find ways to recognise and acknowledge their baby's existence. This may include pictures (including ultrasound and photos at delivery), video, moulds, hair locks, memory boxes, footprints / handprints, memorials and charitable donations. Bathing and dressing the infant should also be considered.

It is also critical that the care plan is communicated to all staff (medical, nursing, allied health and pastoral care) **and documented clearly in the maternal medical record.** This is particularly important as the delivery can occur after hours and on weekends. The whole team needs to support the plan. Attempts should be made to resolve any conflicts or disagreements that may occur within the team or between the team and parents well before the birth.

Bereavement Follow-Up

A family-centred approach is required in providing care to parents, siblings and grandparents prior to and beyond the death of a baby. Attending to the unique needs of siblings, in a developmentally appropriate manner, and involving them in the process of grieving is a cornerstone of both paediatric and perinatal palliative care. The degree of involvement of extended family may vary and health professionals may need to help facilitate this. Reactions from family, friends and health care providers all have a significant impact on the grieving process.

The process of perinatal grief and loss has no predictable course. Within the first year of loss, supportive counselling can decrease anger, depression and anxiety. This may require good listening skills, the ability to remain attentive to the grieving parent and significant time on the part of health professionals. Giving a mother permission to grieve sufficiently will ease her loss and promote her healing. Hope is another important consideration and may relate to the question of further children. Planning for bereavement support prior to the birth of the baby can help with this process.

EXTREME PREMATURITY

Extreme prematurity also carries a high risk of death and a very high risk of long-term disability in survivors. Under these circumstances it may be reasonable and appropriate not to initiate life support. However, death is not usually immediate after delivery and if the decision has been made to not resuscitate and start life support there should be a plan for palliative care after birth. Many of the principles discussed above will also apply in such circumstances. These issues are also discussed in Chapters 3 to 6.

REFERENCES

1. Smith A, Field B, Learoyd BM. Trisomy 18 at Age 21 Years. *Am J Med Gen.* 1989;36:338–339.
2. Salvesen KA, Oyen L, Schmidt N, et al. Comparison of long-term psychological responses of women after pregnancy termination due to fetal anomalies and after perinatal loss. *Ultrasound Obstet Gynecol.* 1997;9(2):80–85.
3. Redlinger-Grosse K, Bernhardt BA, Berg K, et al. The decision to continue: the experiences and needs of parents who receive a prenatal diagnosis of holoprosencephaly. *Am J Med Genet.* 2002 Nov 1;112(4):369–378.

Section 2
Prematurity

CHAPTER 3
Preterm Delivery at 22 Weeks Gestational Age

Mark W Davies, Garry DT Inglis, Charlotte Mooring

Delivery of an infant at 22 completed weeks of gestation occurs infrequently. Less than 0.3% of births occur at this gestation.[1] Out of around 320,000 live births per annum in Australia and New Zealand about four babies (0.13 per 10,000) born at 22 weeks gestational age are admitted to neonatal intensive care units.[2]

The causes for preterm delivery are many and often multifactorial or unknown. They may include infection, rupture of membranes, antepartum haemorrhage, cervical incompetence, trauma, multiple pregnancy, polyhydramnios or idiopathic preterm labour. Maternal problems may require delivery at this gestation. These problems include severe trauma, hypertension, pre-eclampsia and HELLP syndrome, or any medical condition that may endanger the mother if the pregnancy continues.

MANAGEMENT–ANTENATAL

The obstetric management is often supportive and expectant until 23 or 24 weeks is reached unless delivery is indicated for maternal reasons. Less than 2% of obstetricians and less than 5% of paediatricians/neonatologists would encourage active treatment of a baby born at 22 weeks.[3] Therefore, attempts to stop labour or prolong gestation (e.g., with tocolysis), protect the fetal brain (e.g., with magnesium sulphate) and to use steroids is controversial. Any proven infection should be treated and prophylactic antibiotics for group B β haemolytic streptococcus should be considered.

In certain cases, an ultrasound to confirm gestational age, current fetal weight and to check for anomalies may provide useful information to assist counselling.

If delivery threatens at this gestation and there is a likelihood that delivery may not occur until 23–24 weeks gestational age, then it is best that delivery is at a hospital that has an intensive care nursery. Transfer *in utero* is much better than *ex utero*. If delivery at 22 weeks is imminent then *in utero* transfer should not be attempted.

Despite optimal antenatal management, many babies born this preterm will be stillborn. Almost all those born alive will be so sick that they will die soon after birth. At the Royal Brisbane and Women's Hospital from 1996 to 2009 there were five babies born at 22 weeks gestational age who were admitted to the neonatal unit and none survived. There are rare reports of survivors from other hospitals.

IMMEDIATE POSTNATAL MANAGEMENT

In certain circumstances, including delivery at 22 weeks gestational age, it is considered appropriate to not initiate life support. This will always be done with close collaboration between the baby's parents and medical, nursing and allied health staff. It is important to embrace the principles established at consensus conferences in New South Wales in 1986, 1989 and 1998; and the findings of the latest consensus conference held in Australia and reported by Lui et al[4] in 2006. There exists a discretionary zone (grey zone) in neonatal practice. Within this zone, after considered discussion between parents and specialist caregivers, it would be acceptable and reasonable medical practice to either initiate or not initiate life support for that newborn. The location of the grey zone boundaries are at 23^{+0} and 25^{+6} weeks. **Below 23 weeks resuscitation and active treatment is not appropriate.**

The parents should be warned that the duration of the dying process after birth is variable. Whilst most babies will die soon after birth, some will live for many hours. The parents may also benefit from knowing how big the baby will be, what the baby may look like and what signs of life may be present. Parents forewarned of how their baby will appear (e.g., gasping respirations, poor colour) before death may be less distressed during this time.

If the baby is for comfort care only, the parents may want to keep baby with them until it dies. Admission of the baby to the neonatal nursery (with separation from the parents) may not be in the best interest of the family. This situation can be managed in the birth suite.

As for any perinatal death, or any baby requiring prolonged hospital admission, the parents may require psychosocial support and the involvement of a social worker.

HOSPITAL STAY

If baby is born alive and is admitted to an intensive care nursery, survival is rare (see above) and that is despite full support in an intensive care nursery.

All will have breathing problems and require intubation and mechanical ventilation. All will have acute lung disease and develop chronic lung disease if they live long enough. The rare survivors will usually need to go home on oxygen. Feeding problems are universal and many will get some damage to their gut—necrotising enterocolitis (NEC) or gastrointestinal perforation with or without NEC—which usually requires surgery. The risk of acquired infection is very high and this can be very serious for a baby.

More than 33% of babies of 22 weeks gestational age will have a severe intraventricular haemorrhage (IVH). More than 10% of babies of 22 weeks gestational age will develop periventricular leucomalacia (PVL). Most will get severe retinopathy of prematurity (ROP).

The parents should be aware that those babies who receive active treatment and survive the initial period are often severely ill, experience multiple problems and usually die before they get to go home. Under these circumstances, there is concern about the baby's suffering and therefore active resuscitation is rarely considered to be in the best interest of the baby.

LONG-TERM OUTCOME

Rare survivors at 22 weeks gestational age are at very high risk of having long-term problems with their brain development. These problems include delayed development, deafness, blindness, intellectual and cognitive deficits, cerebral palsy, behavioural problems and learning problems. The majority of babies who survive will have at least one of these problems to a moderate or severe degree.

RECURRENCE

This will depend on the cause of the preterm delivery. Some are likely to recur (e.g., cervical incompetence) and others will vary. The parents should be advised to seek advice from an obstetrician, a maternal fetal medicine specialist and/or an obstetric physician before the next pregnancy.

REFERENCES

1. Data from the Queensland Perinatal Data Collection published by Queensland Health in Health Statistics Centre Publications at http://www.health.qld.gov.au/hic/default.asp
2. ANZNN (Australian and New Zealand Neonatal Network). Report of the Australian and New Zealand Neonatal Network 2006. Sydney: ANZNN; 2009.
3. Lavin JP, Kantak A, Ohlinger J, et al. Attitudes of obstetric and pediatric health care providers toward resuscitation of infants who are born at the margins of viability. *Pediatrics*. 2006;118(suppl 2):S169–S176.
4. Lui K, Bajuk B, Foster K, et al. Perinatal care at the borderlines of viability: a consensus statement based on a NSW and ACT consensus workshop. *Medical Journal of Australia*. 2006;185(9):495–500.

CHAPTER 4

Preterm Delivery at 23 Weeks Gestational Age

Mark W Davies, Garry DT Inglis, Ian Jones

Delivery of an infant at 23 completed weeks of gestation occurs infrequently. Less than 0.3% of births are delivered at this gestation.[1] Out of around 320,000 live births per annum in Australia and New Zealand about 40 babies (1.3 per 10,000) born at 23 weeks gestational age are admitted to neonatal intensive care units.[2]

The causes for preterm delivery are many and often multifactorial or unknown. They may include infection, rupture of membranes, antepartum haemorrhage, cervical incompetence, trauma, multiple pregnancy, polyhydramnios or idiopathic preterm labour. Maternal problems may require delivery at this gestation. These problems include severe trauma, hypertension, pre-eclampsia and HELLP syndrome, or any medical condition that may endanger the mother if the pregnancy continues.

MANAGEMENT—ANTENATAL

Tocolysis should be used to stop labour or prolong gestation, unless contraindicated. The mother should be given steroids. Prophylactic antibiotics for group B β haemolytic streptococcus should be considered in established preterm labour. In women at risk of preterm birth, magnesium sulphate should be considered to protect the fetal brain.

If delivery is anticipated at this gestation then **if at all possible** it must happen at a hospital that has an intensive care nursery. Transfer *in utero* is much better than *ex utero* as long-term outcomes are better. At 23 weeks some would consider the risk of birth during *in utero* transfer an acceptable one given the universally bad outcome following birth outside a hospital with a neonatal intensive care unit.

Despite optimal antenatal management, some babies born preterm may be stillborn or will be so sick that they die soon after birth. See Figure 10.1 in Chapter 10.

IMMEDIATE POSTNATAL MANAGEMENT

In certain circumstances, it is considered appropriate to not initiate life support. There exists a discretionary zone or grey zone in neonatal practice which includes newborn infants at 23 weeks gestational age. After careful discussion between parents and specialist caregivers—embracing the principles established at consensus conferences in New South Wales in

1986, 1989 and 1998 and the findings of the latest consensus conference held in Australia and reported by Lui et al[3] in 2006—it would be acceptable and reasonable medical practice to not initiate life support for the newborn born at 23 weeks gestational age. The decision whether to initiate treatment or not at 23 weeks will usually depend on the wishes of the parents and other factors such as the condition of the baby before and at birth, and past obstetric history. Under these circumstances, counselling should always include the option of not starting resuscitation and active treatment and the potential consequences of active intervention (as detailed below).

A consultant neonatologist or paediatrician should be present at the delivery. If the baby is for active treatment, there should also be a second paediatric medical officer present.

The baby will require active resuscitation that will require intubation and mechanical ventilation. Baby will be transferred immediately to the intensive care nursery with continuing respiratory support and insertion of umbilical catheters.

HOSPITAL STAY

Even if baby is born alive and is admitted to an intensive care nursery, more than 50–60% will die. Many who do so may not die for some weeks to months.

Those babies who survive will spend on average about 100 days in intensive care and 144 days in hospital. Some of that time may be spent back at referring hospitals that have a special care nursery.

Respiratory support will be needed as all will have breathing problems which may be due to immaturity or hyaline membrane disease. At 23 weeks gestational age, all will require intubation and mechanical ventilation—the average length of time on a ventilator is about 50 days. All of the ventilated babies will need nasal continuous positive airway pressure (CPAP) once extubated for an average of 45 more days.

Long-term lung problems will also be an issue and 70–100% of babies that survive will develop chronic lung disease (CLD). This will mean more time on a ventilator, more time on oxygen and a longer stay in hospital. Of the babies who survive, 50–60% will need to go home on oxygen.

Feeding problems also need to be considered as babies born this early will not be able to suck and swallow. They will need parenteral nutrition and then enteral tube feeds. Feeds, preferably breast milk, will start as a very small amount and build up slowly over many days to weeks. Often the tube feeds need to stop and start. Breast milk feeds are protective against necrotising enterocolitis (NEC) so women should be encouraged to express breast milk for their infants. A small number (17%) of babies will get some damage to their gut—necrotising enterocolitis or gastrointestinal perforation with or without NEC—and this usually requires a major operation to treat and significant intractable feeding difficulties.

Infection is also a risk as babies born prematurely are at increased risk of infection during their time in the nursery, especially those born earlier than 28 weeks of gestation. This can be very serious for a baby.

All babies will become anaemic and most will require one or more packed red cell transfusions. Iron therapy may be necessary after a few weeks.

Brain injury is also a factor as premature babies have very delicate brains. About one-third of babies of 23 weeks gestational age will have a severe intraventricular haemorrhage (IVH). About 10–15% of babies of 23 weeks gestational age will develop periventricular leucomalacia (PVL).

Eye problems are common at 23 weeks gestational age and 50% of babies who survive will get severe retinopathy of prematurity (ROP). Most, if not all, will require laser surgery for this.

For any perinatal death, or any baby requiring prolonged hospital admission, the parents may require psychosocial support and the involvement of a social worker.

LONG-TERM OUTCOME

Babies born at 23 weeks gestational age are at high risk of having long-term problems with their brain development—delayed development, deafness, blindness, intellectual and cognitive deficits, cerebral palsy, behavioural problems and learning problems. About 55% of babies who survive will have at least one of these problems to a moderate or severe degree. Babies with severe IVH, PVL, severe ROP, severe infection and CLD are at even higher risk of these types of problems.

RECURRENCE

This will depend on the cause of the preterm delivery. Some are likely to recur (e.g., cervical incompetence) and others will vary. The parents should be advised to seek advice from an obstetrician, a maternal fetal medicine specialist and/or an obstetric physician before the next pregnancy.

REFERENCES

1. Data from the Queensland Perinatal Data Collection published by Queensland Health in Health Statistics Centre Publications at http://www.health.qld.gov.au/hic/default.asp
2. ANZNN (Australian and New Zealand Neonatal Network). Report of the Australian and New Zealand Neonatal Network 2006. Sydney: ANZNN; 2009.
3. Lui K, Bajuk B, Foster K, et al. Perinatal care at the borderlines of viability: a consensus statement based on a NSW and ACT consensus workshop. *Medical Journal of Australia.* 2006;185(9):495–500.

CHAPTER 5

Preterm Delivery at 24 Weeks Gestational Age

Mark W Davies, Luke A Jardine

Delivery of an infant at 24 completed weeks of gestation occurs infrequently. Less than 0.3% of births are delivered at this gestation.[1] Out of around 320,000 live births per annum in Australia and New Zealand about 160 babies (0.5 per 1000) born at 24 weeks gestational age are admitted to neonatal intensive care units.[2]

The causes for preterm delivery are many and often multifactorial or unknown. They may include infection, rupture of membranes, antepartum haemorrhage, cervical incompetence, trauma, multiple pregnancy, polyhydramnios or idiopathic preterm labour. Maternal problems may require delivery at this gestation. These problems include severe trauma, hypertension, pre-eclampsia and HELLP syndrome, or any medical condition that may endanger the mother if the pregnancy continues.

MANAGEMENT—ANTENATAL

Tocolysis should be used to stop labour or prolong gestation, unless contraindicated. The mother should be given steroids. Prophylactic antibiotics for group B β haemolytic streptococcus should be considered in established preterm labour. In women at risk of preterm birth, magnesium sulphate should be considered to protect the fetal brain.

If delivery is anticipated at this gestation, then **if at all possible** it must happen at a hospital that has an intensive care nursery. Transfer *in utero* is much better than *ex utero*. At 24 weeks some would consider the risk of birth during *in utero* transfer an acceptable one given the usually poor outcome following birth outside a hospital with a neonatal intensive care unit.

Despite optimal antenatal management, some babies born preterm may be stillborn or will be so sick that they die soon after birth. See Figure 10.1 in Chapter 10.

IMMEDIATE POSTNATAL MANAGEMENT

In certain circumstances, it is considered appropriate to not initiate life support. There exists a discretionary zone or grey zone in neonatal practice which includes newborn infants at 24 weeks gestational age. After careful discussion between parents and specialist caregivers—embracing the principles established at consensus conferences in New South Wales in

1986, 1989 and 1998 and the findings of the latest consensus conference held in Australia and reported by Lui et al[3] in 2006—it would be acceptable and reasonable medical practice to not initiate life support for the newborn born at 24 weeks gestational age. It would also be reasonable to initiate active treatment. The decision whether to initiate treatment or not at 24 weeks will depend on the wishes of the parents and other factors such as the condition of the baby before and at birth and past obstetric history. Under these circumstances, counselling should always include the option of not starting resuscitation and active treatment and the potential consequences of active intervention (as detailed below). In our experience, most parents would opt for planned active treatment if baby is born alive at 24 weeks gestational age. A consultant neonatologist or paediatrician should be present at the delivery. If the baby is for active treatment, there should also be a second paediatric medical officer present.

The baby will require active resuscitation that will usually include intubation and mechanical ventilation; rarely nasal continuous positive airway pressure (CPAP) alone. Baby will be transferred immediately to the intensive care nursery with continuing respiratory support and insertion of umbilical catheters.

HOSPITAL STAY

The statistics provided below are based on the average of all admissions. There are known factors which may slightly improve some outcomes and these include the use of appropriate antenatal steroids, delivery in a hospital with neonatal intensive care facilities, female sex, appropriate weight for gestational age and antenatal administration of magnesium sulphate.

Even if baby is born alive and is admitted to an intensive care nursery, about 40–50% will die. Many who do so may not die for some weeks to months.

Those babies who survive will spend on average about 99 days in intensive care and 142 days in hospital. Some of that time may be spent back at referring hospitals that have a special care nursery.

Respiratory support will be needed as all will have breathing problems which may be due to immaturity or hyaline membrane disease. At 24 weeks gestational age, virtually all will require intubation and mechanical ventilation—the average length of time on a ventilator is about 35–40 days. Almost all (97%) of the ventilated babies will need CPAP once extubated for an average of 44 more days. Most babies at 24 weeks will have apnoea of prematurity. Treatment may include prolonged mechanical ventilation, non-invasive positive pressure ventilation, CPAP and caffeine.

Long-term lung problems will also be an issue and 50–70% of babies will develop chronic lung disease (CLD). This will mean more time on a ventilator, more time on oxygen and a longer stay in hospital. Many babies will require a course of steroids to facilitate their extubation. Of the babies who survive, 35–40% will need to go home on oxygen.

Feeding problems also need to be considered as babies born this early will not be able to suck and swallow. They will need parenteral nutrition and then enteral tube feeds. Feeds, preferably breast milk, will start as a very small amount and build up slowly over many days to weeks. Often the tube feeds need to stop and start. A small number (~8%) of babies will get some damage to their gut—necrotising enterocolitis (NEC) or gastrointestinal perforation with or without NEC—this may require a major operation to treat and significant intractable feeding difficulties.

Jaundice of prematurity will develop in the majority of babies at 24 weeks gestation. High levels of bilirubin have the potential to cross the blood–brain barrier causing acute bilirubin encephalopathy in the short term and kernicterus in the long term. Most babies will be adequately treated with phototherapy and very rarely will require more aggressive forms of treatment.

Cardiac problems are an issue as at 24 weeks gestational age many babies will have problems maintaining their blood pressure and may require inotropic support. A number of babies will have a patent ductus arteriosus (PDA). This may require medication and a major operation to treat.

Infection is also a problem as babies born prematurely are at increased risk of infection during their time in the nursery, especially those born earlier than 28 weeks of gestation. This can be very serious for a baby.

All babies will become anaemic and most will require one or more packed red cell transfusions. Iron therapy may be necessary after a few weeks.

Brain injury is also a factor as premature babies have very delicate brains. Of babies of 24 weeks gestational age, 20–25% will have a severe intraventricular haemorrhage (IVH). About 8% of babies of 24 weeks gestational age will develop periventricular leucomalacia (PVL).

Eye problems are common at 24 weeks gestational age and 30–40 per cent of babies who survive will get severe retinopathy of prematurity (ROP). Most, if not all, will require laser surgery for this. Refractive errors, which may require glasses, are common.

Inguinal hernias are common and will normally be repaired prior to discharge home.

Iatrogenic problems occur as at 24 weeks a number of invasive procedures are required to keep babies alive (e.g., intubation, respiratory support, umbilical catheters, intercostal catheters, central venous access, arterial lines, surgery etc). These procedures have known complications. Some of the more significant iatrogenic problems include vocal cord damage, subglottic stenosis, arterial embolism resulting in loss of digits/limbs, erosion of nasal septum, scarring of the skin and catheter related sepsis.

LONG-TERM OUTCOME

Babies born at 24 weeks gestational age are at high risk of having long term-problems with their brain development—delayed development, deafness, blindness, intellectual and cognitive deficits, cerebral palsy, behavioural problems and learning problems. About 35% of babies who survive will have at least one of these problems to a moderate or severe degree. These figures are very rough estimates. Babies with severe IVH, PVL, severe ROP, severe infection and CLD are at even higher risk of these types of problems.

RECURRENCE

This will depend on the cause of the preterm delivery. Some are likely to recur (e.g., cervical incompetence) and others will vary. The parents should be advised to seek advice from an obstetrician, a maternal fetal medicine specialist and/or an obstetric physician before the next pregnancy.

REFERENCES

1. Data from the Queensland Perinatal Data Collection published by Queensland Health in Health Statistics Centre Publications at http://www.health.qld.gov.au/hic/default.asp.
2. ANZNN (Australian and New Zealand Neonatal Network). Report of the Australian and New Zealand Neonatal Network 2006. Sydney: ANZNN; 2009.
3. Lui K, Bajuk B, Foster K, et al. Perinatal care at the borderlines of viability: a consensus statement based on a NSW and ACT consensus workshop. *Medical Journal of Australia*. 2006;185(9):495–500.

CHAPTER 6

Preterm Delivery at 25 Weeks Gestational Age

Mark W Davies, Luke A Jardine

Delivery of an infant at 25 completed weeks of gestation occurs infrequently. Less than 0.3% of births are delivered at this gestation.[1] Out of around 320,000 live births per annum in Australia and New Zealand, about 205 babies (0.64 in 1000) born at 25 weeks gestational age are admitted to neonatal intensive care units.[2]

The causes for preterm delivery are many and often multifactorial or unknown. They may include infection, rupture of membranes, antepartum haemorrhage, cervical incompetence, trauma, multiple pregnancy, polyhydramnios or idiopathic preterm labour. Maternal problems may require delivery at this gestation. These problems include severe trauma, hypertension, pre-eclampsia and HELLP syndrome, or any medical condition that may endanger the mother if the pregnancy continues.

MANAGEMENT—ANTENATAL

Tocolysis should be used unless contraindicated. The mother should be given steroids. Prophylactic antibiotics for group B β haemolytic streptococcus should be considered in established preterm labour. In women at risk of preterm birth, magnesium sulphate should be considered to protect the fetal brain.

If delivery is anticipated at this gestation, then **if at all possible** it must happen at a hospital that has an intensive care nursery. Transfer *in utero* is much better than *ex utero*.

IMMEDIATE POSTNATAL MANAGEMENT

In certain circumstances it is considered appropriate to not initiate life support. There exists a discretionary zone or grey zone in neonatal practice which includes newborn infants at 25 weeks gestational age. After careful discussion between parent and specialist caregivers—embracing the principles established at consensus conferences in New South Wales in 1986, 1989 and 1998 and the findings of the latest consensus conference held in Australia and reported by Lui et al[3] in 2006—it would be acceptable and reasonable medical practice to not initiate life support for the newborn born at 25 weeks gestational age. However, it is also reasonable, and far more usual, to initiate active treatment. The decision whether to initiate treatment or not at 25 weeks will depend on the wishes of the parents and other factors such as the condition of the baby before and at birth, and past obstetric history. Under these circumstances, counselling should always include the option of not starting resuscitation and active treatment and detail the potential consequences of active intervention (as detailed below). In our experience, most parents would opt for planned active treatment if a baby is born alive at 25 weeks gestational age.

The baby will require active resuscitation that will usually include intubation and mechanical ventilation; rarely nasal continuous positive airway pressure (CPAP) alone. Baby will be transferred immediately to the intensive care nursery with continuing respiratory support and insertion of umbilical catheters.

HOSPITAL STAY

The statistics provided below are based on the average of all admissions. There are known factors which may slightly improve some outcomes and these include the use of appropriate antenatal steroids, delivery in a hospital with neonatal intensive care facilities, female sex, appropriate weight for gestational age and antenatal administration of magnesium sulphate.

Even if baby is born alive and is admitted to an intensive care nursery, about 20–25% will die. Many who do so may not die for some weeks to months.

Those babies who survive will spend on average about 80 days in intensive care and 120 days in hospital. Some of that time may be spent back at referring hospitals that have a special care nursery.

Respiratory support will be needed as all will have breathing problems which may be due to immaturity or hyaline membrane disease. At 25 weeks gestational age, virtually all will require intubation and mechanical ventilation—the average length of time on a ventilator is about 25–30 days. Almost all (98%) of the ventilated babies will need CPAP once extubated for an average of 38 more days. Most babies at 25 weeks will have apnoea of prematurity. Treatment may include prolonged mechanical ventilation, non-invasive positive pressure ventilation, CPAP and caffeine.

Long-term lung problems will also be an issue and 50–65% of babies will develop chronic lung disease (CLD). This will mean more time on a ventilator, more time in oxygen and a longer stay in hospital. Many babies will require a course of steroids to facilitate their extubation. Of the babies who survive, 15–20% will need to go home on oxygen.

Feeding problems also need to be considered as babies born this early will not be able to suck and swallow. They will need parenteral nutrition and then enteral tube feeds. Feeds, preferably breast milk, will start as a very small amount and build up slowly over many days to weeks. Often the tube feeds need to stop and start. A small number (~7%) of babies will get some damage to their gut—necrotising enterocolitis (NEC) or gastrointestinal perforation with or without NEC—this may require a major operation to treat and significant intractable feeding difficulties.

Jaundice of prematurity will develop in the majority of babies at 25 weeks gestation. High levels of bilirubin have the potential to cross the blood–brain barrier causing acute bilirubin encephalopathy in the short term and kernicterus in the long term. Most babies will be adequately treated with phototherapy and very rarely will require more aggressive forms of treatment.

Cardiac problems are an issue as at 25 weeks gestational age many babies will have problems maintaining their blood pressure and may require inotropic support. A number of babies will have a patent ductus arteriosus (PDA). This may require medication and a major operation to treat.

Infection is also a problem as babies born prematurely are at increased risk of infection during their time in the nursery, especially those born earlier than 28 weeks of gestation. This can be very serious for a baby.

All babies will become anaemic and most will require one or more packed red cell transfusions. Iron therapy may be necessary after a few weeks.

Brain injury is also a factor as premature babies have very delicate brains. Of babies of 25 weeks gestational age, 10–15% will have a severe intraventricular haemorrhage (IVH). About 5% of babies of 25 weeks gestational age will develop periventricular leucomalacia (PVL).

Eye problems are common at 25 weeks gestational age and 20–25% of babies who survive will get severe retinopathy of prematurity (ROP). Most, if not all, will require LASER surgery for this. Refractive errors, which may require glasses, are common.

Inguinal hernias are common and will normally be repaired prior to discharge home.

Iatrogenic problems occur as at 25 weeks a number of invasive procedures are required to keep babies alive (e.g., intubation, respiratory support, umbilical catheters, intercostal catheters, central venous access, arterial lines, surgery, etc.). These procedures have known complications. Some of the more significant iatrogenic problems include vocal cord damage, subglottic stenosis, arterial embolism resulting in loss of digits/limbs, erosion of nasal septum, scarring of the skin and catheter related sepsis.

LONG-TERM OUTCOME

Babies born at 25 weeks gestational age are at high risk of having long-term problems with their brain development—delayed development, deafness, blindness, intellectual and cognitive deficits, cerebral palsy, behavioural problems and learning problems. About 30% of babies who survive will have at least one of these problems to a moderate or severe degree. These figures are very rough estimates. Babies with severe IVH, PVL, severe ROP, severe infection and CLD are at even higher risk of these types of problems.

RECURRENCE

This will depend on the cause of the preterm delivery. Some are likely to recur (e.g., cervical incompetence) and others will vary. The parents should be advised to seek advice from an obstetrician, a maternal fetal medicine specialist and/or an obstetric physician before the next pregnancy.

REFERENCES

1. Data from the Queensland Perinatal Data Collection published by Queensland Health in Health Statistics Centre Publications at http://www.health.qld.gov.au/hic/default.asp.
2. ANZNN (Australian and New Zealand Neonatal Network). Report of the Australian and New Zealand Neonatal Network 2006. Sydney: ANZNN; 2009.
3. Lui K, Bajuk B, Foster K, et al. Perinatal care at the borderlines of viability: a consensus statement based on a NSW and ACT consensus workshop. *Medical Journal of Australia.* 2006;185(9):495–500.

CHAPTER 7

Preterm Delivery at 26 Weeks Gestational Age

Mark W Davies, Luke A Jardine

Delivery of an infant at 26 completed weeks of gestation occurs infrequently. Less than 0.3% of births are delivered at this gestation.[1] Out of around 320,000 live births per annum in Australia and New Zealand about 280 babies (0.88 in 1000) born at 26 weeks gestational age are admitted to neonatal intensive care units.[2]

The causes for preterm delivery are many and often multifactorial or unknown. They may include infection, rupture of membranes, antepartum haemorrhage, cervical incompetence, trauma, multiple pregnancy, polyhydramnios or idiopathic preterm labour. Maternal problems may require delivery at this gestation. These problems include severe trauma, hypertension, pre-eclampsia and HELLP syndrome, or any medical condition that may endanger the mother if the pregnancy continues.

MANAGEMENT—ANTENATAL

Tocolysis should be used unless contraindicated. The mother should be given steroids. Prophylactic antibiotics for group B β haemolytic streptococcus should be considered in established preterm labour. In women at risk of preterm birth, magnesium sulphate should be considered to protect the fetal brain.

If delivery is anticipated at this gestation, then **if at all possible** it must happen at a hospital that has an intensive care nursery. Transfer *in utero* is much better than *ex utero*.

IMMEDIATE POSTNATAL MANAGEMENT

In certain circumstances it is considered appropriate to not initiate life support. However, at 26 weeks there is indication to treat unless there are exceptional circumstances. This is consistent with the principles established at consensus conferences in New South Wales in 1986, 1989 and 1998; and the findings of the latest consensus conference held in Australia and reported by Lui et al[3] in 2006.

The baby will usually require active resuscitation including intubation and mechanical ventilation. All babies will need respiratory support started in the delivery room and some babies may only need nasal continuous positive airway pressure (CPAP). The baby will be transferred immediately to the intensive care nursery with continuing respiratory support and insertion of umbilical catheters.

HOSPITAL STAY

The statistics provided below are based on the average of all admissions. There are known factors which may slightly improve some outcomes and these include the use of appropriate antenatal steroids, delivery in a hospital with neonatal intensive care facilities, female sex, appropriate weight for gestational age and antenatal administration of magnesium sulphate.

Even if baby is born alive and is admitted to an intensive care nursery, about 10–15% will die. Many who do so may not die for some weeks to months.

Those babies who survive will spend on average about 60 days in intensive care and 100 days in hospital. Some of that time may be spent back at referring hospitals that have a special care nursery.

Respiratory support will be needed as all will have breathing problems which may be due to immaturity or hyaline membrane disease. At 26 weeks gestational age almost all will require intubation and mechanical ventilation—the average length of time on a ventilator is about 15–20 days. Almost all (99%) of the ventilated babies will need CPAP once extubated for an average of 33 more days. Most babies at 26 weeks will have apnoea of prematurity. Treatment may include prolonged mechanical ventilation, non-invasive positive pressure ventilation, CPAP and caffeine.

Long-term lung problems will also be an issue and 40% of babies will develop chronic lung disease (CLD). This will mean more time on a ventilator, more time in oxygen and a longer stay in hospital. Many babies will require a course of steroids to facilitate their extubation. Of the babies who survive, 5–10% will need to go home on oxygen.

Feeding problems also need to be considered as babies born this early will not be able to suck and swallow. They will need parenteral nutrition and then enteral tube feeds. Feeds, preferably breast milk, will start as a very small amount and build up slowly over many days to weeks. Often the tube feeds need to stop and start. A small number (~3%) of babies will get some damage to their gut—necrotising enterocolitis (NEC) or gastrointestinal perforation with or without NEC—this may require a major operation to treat and significant intractable feeding difficulties.

Jaundice of prematurity will develop in the majority of babies at 26 weeks gestation. High levels of bilirubin have the potential to cross the blood–brain barrier causing acute bilirubin encephalopathy in the short term and kernicterus in the long term. Most babies will be adequately treated with phototherapy and very rarely will require more aggressive forms of treatment.

Cardiac problems are an issue as at 26 weeks gestational age many babies will have problems maintaining their blood pressure and may require inotropic support. A number of babies will have a patent ductus arteriosus (PDA). This may require medication and a major operation to treat.

Infection is also a problem as babies born prematurely are at increased risk of infection during their time in the nursery, especially those born earlier than 28 weeks of gestation. This can be very serious for a baby.

All babies will become anaemic and most will require one or more packed red cell transfusions. Iron therapy may be necessary after a few weeks.

Brain injury is also a factor as premature babies have very delicate brains. Of babies of 26 weeks gestational age, 8–12% will have a severe intraventricular haemorrhage (IVH). About 5% of babies of 26 weeks gestational age will develop periventricular leucomalacia (PVL).

Eye problems can also occur at 26 weeks gestational age and 15–20% of babies who survive will get severe retinopathy of prematurity (ROP). Most, if not all, will require laser surgery for this. Refractive errors, which may require glasses, are common.

Inguinal hernias are common and will normally be repaired prior to discharge home.

Iatrogenic problems occur as at 26 weeks a number of invasive procedures are required to keep babies alive (e.g., intubation, respiratory support, umbilical catheters, intercostal catheters, central venous access, arterial lines, surgery, etc). These procedures have known complications. Some of the more significant iatrogenic problems include vocal cord damage, subglottic stenosis, arterial embolism resulting in loss of digits/limbs, erosion of nasal septum, scarring of the skin and catheter related sepsis.

LONG-TERM OUTCOME

Babies born at 26 weeks gestational age are at high risk of having long-term problems with their brain development—delayed development, deafness, blindness, intellectual and cognitive deficits, cerebral palsy, behavioural problems and learning problems. About 25% of babies who survive will have at least one of these problems to a moderate or severe degree. These figures are very rough estimates. Babies with severe IVH, PVL, severe ROP, severe infection and CLD are at even higher risk of these types of problems.

RECURRENCE

This will depend on the cause of the preterm delivery. Some are likely to recur (e.g., cervical incompetence) and others will vary. The parents should be advised to seek advice from an obstetrician, a maternal fetal medicine specialist and/or an obstetric physician before the next pregnancy.

REFERENCES

1. Data from the Queensland Perinatal Data Collection published by Queensland Health in Health Statistics Centre Publications at http://www.health.qld.gov.au/hic/default.asp.
2. ANZNN (Australian and New Zealand Neonatal Network). Report of the Australian and New Zealand Neonatal Network 2006. Sydney: ANZNN; 2009.
3. Lui K, Bajuk B, Foster K, et al. Perinatal care at the borderlines of viability: a consensus statement based on a NSW and ACT consensus workshop. *Medical Journal of Australia.* 2006;185(9):495–500.

CHAPTER 8

Preterm Delivery at 27 Weeks Gestational Age

Mark W Davies, Luke A Jardine

Delivery of an infant at 27 completed weeks of gestation occurs infrequently. Less than 0.3% of births are delivered at this gestation.[1] Out of around 320,000 live births per annum in Australia and New Zealand about 333 babies (1.0 in 1000) born at 27 weeks gestational age are admitted to neonatal intensive care units.[2]

The causes for preterm delivery are many and often multifactorial or unknown. They may include infection, rupture of membranes, antepartum haemorrhage, cervical incompetence, trauma, multiple pregnancy, polyhydramnios or idiopathic preterm labour. Maternal problems may require delivery at this gestation. These problems include severe trauma, hypertension, pre-eclampsia and HELLP syndrome, or any medical condition that may endanger the mother if the pregnancy continues.

MANAGEMENT—ANTENATAL
Tocolysis should be used unless contraindicated. The mother should be given steroids. Prophylactic antibiotics for group B β haemolytic streptococcus should be considered in established preterm labour. In women at risk of preterm birth, magnesium sulphate should be considered to protect the fetal brain.

If delivery is anticipated at this gestation, then **if at all possible** it must happen at a hospital that has an intensive care nursery. Transfer *in utero* is much better than *ex utero*.

IMMEDIATE POSTNATAL MANAGEMENT
At 27 weeks there is indication to treat unless there are exceptional circumstances. This is consistent with the principles established at consensus conferences in New South Wales in 1986, 1989 and 1998; and the findings of the latest consensus conference held in Australia and reported by Lui et al[3] in 2006.

Most babies will require active resuscitation including intubation and mechanical ventilation. Virtually all babies will need respiratory support started in the delivery room and some babies may only need nasal continuous positive airway pressure (CPAP). The baby will be transferred immediately to the intensive care nursery with continuing respiratory support and insertion of umbilical catheters.

HOSPITAL STAY

The statistics provided below are based on the average of all admissions. There are known factors which may slightly improve some outcomes and these include the use of appropriate antenatal steroids, delivery in a hospital with neonatal intensive care facilities, female sex, appropriate weight for gestational age and antenatal administration of magnesium sulphate.

Even if baby is born alive and is admitted to an intensive care nursery, about 10–12% will die. Many who do so may not die for some weeks to months.

Those babies who survive will spend on average about 43 days in intensive care and 85 days in hospital. Some of that time may be spent back at referring hospitals that have a special care nursery.

Respiratory support will be needed as almost all will have breathing problems which may be due to immaturity or hyaline membrane disease. At 27 weeks gestational age, 80–85% will require intubation and mechanical ventilation—the average length of time on a ventilator is about 15 days. Almost all (98%) of the ventilated babies will need CPAP once extubated for an average of 29 more days. About 15% of babies will only ever need CPAP for an average of 14 days. Most babies at 27 weeks will have apnoea of prematurity. Treatment may include prolonged mechanical ventilation, non-invasive positive pressure ventilation, CPAP and caffeine.

Long-term lung problems will also be an issue and 35–40% of babies will develop chronic lung disease (CLD). This will mean more time on a ventilator, more time in oxygen and a longer stay in hospital. Many babies will require a course of steroids to facilitate their extubation. Of the babies who survive, 5–10% will need to go home on oxygen.

Feeding problems also need to be considered as babies born this early will not be able to suck and swallow. They will need parenteral nutrition and then enteral tube feeds. Feeds, preferably breast milk, will start as a very small amount and build up slowly over many days to weeks. Often the tube feeds need to stop and start. A small number (~3%) of babies will get some damage to their gut—necrotising enterocolitis (NEC) or gastrointestinal perforation with or without NEC—this may require a major operation to treat and significant intractable feeding difficulties.

Jaundice of prematurity will develop in the majority of babies at 27 weeks gestation. High levels of bilirubin have the potential to cross the blood–brain barrier causing acute bilirubin encephalopathy in the short term and kernicterus in the long term. Most babies will be adequately treated with phototherapy and very rarely will require more aggressive forms of treatment.

Cardiac problems are an issue as at 27 weeks gestational age many babies will have problems maintaining their blood pressure and may require inotropic support. A number of babies will have a patent ductus arteriosus (PDA). This may require medication and a major operation to treat.

Infection is also a problem as babies born prematurely are at increased risk of infection during their time in the nursery, especially those born earlier than 28 weeks of gestation. This can be very serious for a baby.

All babies will become anaemic and many will require one or more packed red cell transfusions. Iron therapy may be necessary after a few weeks.

Brain injury is also a factor as premature babies have very delicate brains. Of babies of 27 weeks gestational age, 5–10% will have a severe intraventricular haemorrhage (IVH). About 4% of babies of 27 weeks gestational age will develop periventricular leucomalacia (PVL).

Eye problems can also occur at 27 weeks gestational age and 3% of babies who survive will get severe retinopathy of prematurity (ROP). Most, if not all, will require laser surgery for this. Refractive errors, which may require glasses, are common.

Inguinal hernias are common and will normally be repaired prior to discharge home.

Iatrogenic problems occur as at 27 weeks a number of invasive procedures are required to keep babies alive (e.g., intubation, respiratory support, umbilical catheters, intercostal catheters, central venous access, arterial lines, surgery, etc). These procedures have known complications. Some of the more significant iatrogenic problems include vocal cord damage, subglottic stenosis, arterial embolism resulting in loss of digits/limbs, erosion of nasal septum, scarring of the skin and catheter related sepsis.

LONG-TERM OUTCOME

Babies born at 27 weeks gestational age are at high risk of having long-term problems with their brain development—delayed development, deafness, blindness, intellectual and cognitive deficits, cerebral palsy, behavioural problems and learning problems. About 20% of babies who survive will have at least one of these problems to a moderate or severe degree. These figures are very rough estimates. Babies with severe IVH, PVL, severe ROP, severe infection and CLD are at even higher risk of these types of problems.

RECURRENCE

This will depend on the cause of the preterm delivery. Some are likely to recur (e.g., cervical incompetence) and others will vary. The parents should be advised to seek advice from an obstetrician, a maternal fetal medicine specialist and/or an obstetric physician before the next pregnancy.

REFERENCES

1. Data from the Queensland Perinatal Data Collection published by Queensland Health in Health Statistics Centre Publications at http://www.health.qld.gov.au/hic/default.asp
2. ANZNN (Australian and New Zealand Neonatal Network). Report of the Australian and New Zealand Neonatal Network 2006. Sydney: ANZNN; 2009.
3. Lui K, Bajuk B, Foster K, et al. Perinatal care at the borderlines of viability: a consensus statement based on a NSW and ACT consensus workshop. *Medical Journal of Australia*. 2006;185(9):495–500.

CHAPTER 9

Preterm Delivery at 28–32 Weeks Gestational Age

Ulrike Brandenburg, David Millar, Luke A Jardine

Delivery of an infant between 28 and 32 weeks gestational age is uncommon. Less than 1% of births are delivered at this gestation.[1] Out of approximately 295,000 live births per annum in Australia, 2200 babies (7.5 in 1000) are born between 28 and 32 weeks gestation and most of them are admitted to a neonatal intensive care nursery.

The causes of delivery at this gestation are many and often multifactorial or unknown.[2] They may include spontaneous preterm labour. Common causes of preterm labour include: infection (e.g., chorioamnionitis, urinary tract infection), premature pre-labour rupture of membranes (PPROM), cervical incompetence, polyhydramnios and antepartum haemorrhage. At higher risk for preterm delivery are women with close temporal proximity (<6 months) to a previous delivery, a history of previous preterm delivery and multiple gestation. In Australia, Indigenous ethnicity and low socioeconomic state remain risk factors for preterm births. Maternal problems that may require delivery at this gestation include trauma, preeclampsia and HELLP syndrome, or any other medical condition that may endanger the mother if the pregnancy continues. A number of conditions in the fetus may indicate early delivery; many of these are discussed elsewhere in this book.

MANAGEMENT—ANTENATAL

Tocolysis should be used unless contraindicated. Tocolysis does not reduce the rate of preterm birth but can delay delivery by about 48 hours to allow transfer to a perinatal centre and administration of steroids.

The mother should be given steroids (12 mg betamethasone intramuscular repeated once after 24 hours) to reduce neonatal morbidity and mortality from respiratory distress syndrome, intraventricular haemorrhage, necrotising enterocolitis and a patent ductus arteriosus.

Antibiotic treatment (generally erythromycin) in the presence of preterm rupture of membranes decreases the risk of neonatal infection and corresponding morbidity and can prolong pregnancy by reducing chorioamnionitis. Preparations with clavulanic acid (augmentin) should be avoided as it may increase the risk of necrotising enterocolitis. Where indicated, magnesium sulphate should be considered in women at risk of preterm birth to protect the fetal brain (generally <30 weeks).

Ideally, delivery should happen at a hospital where there are facilities to manage preterm babies. Every attempt should be made to transfer the baby *in utero* to a suitable hospital if it is safe to do so. At the gestation of 28–32 weeks, *in utero* transfer significantly decreases mortality and morbidity compared to *ex utero* transport.[3]

Cervical length measurement can help to discriminate between high and low risk of early delivery (<20 mm *versus* >30 mm). Fetal fibronectin (FFN test) in cervicovaginal secretions has a high negative predictive value (only 1% of women with negative test result deliver within one week) and may provide useful information about the need to transfer. Unfortunately, it has poor positive predictive value in the presence of PPROM or vaginal bleeding.[3]

Parental counselling should include neonatal mortality and morbidity risks as outlined below (and detailed in Chapter 10) and the requirement of transfer of the infant to a tertiary perinatal centre. If time permits, a parental tour of the neonatal nursery is recommended.

IMMEDIATE POSTNATAL MANAGEMENT

All infants between 28 and 32 weeks gestation should have life support, if required, except those with definite lethal congenital malformations. Resuscitation and stabilisation should proceed according to local guidelines. Respiratory support with either continuous positive airway pressure (CPAP) or mechanical ventilation is commonly required. Intratracheal surfactant administration may be needed for respiratory distress syndrome.

Infants of these gestations will have a low birth weight (LBW) and are at increased risk of hypothermia and hypoglycaemia.[4] A heat source and glucose/dextrose 10% infusion should be available. Vascular access will be required (either umbilical vessel catheters or a peripheral cannula depending on the baby's condition). In most cases a blood culture will need to be collected and the baby commenced on intravenous antibiotics.

Increased morbidity and mortality associated with *ex utero* transport can be minimised by keeping vital parameters (temperature, blood glucose level, blood pressure, pH, oxygenation and arterial carbon dioxide) within normal limits before and during transport.[2,3,4]

SURVIVAL AND HOSPITAL STAY

The statistics provided below are based on the average of all admissions. See also Chapter 10. There are known factors which may slightly improve some outcomes and these include the use of appropriate antenatal steroids, delivery in a hospital with neonatal intensive care facilities, female sex, appropriate weight for gestational age and antenatal administration of magnesium sulphate.

Most infants born between 28 and 32 weeks gestation will survive with mortality being <10% in the 28 week group and decreasing further with increasing gestational age.

All will require admission to a neonatal nursery, most of them to the intensive care nursery, for a variety of potential problems. Many of the issues are similar to those of earlier gestation; however, mortality and morbidity are inversely related to gestational age.

Respiratory support may be needed with more than half of these infants having breathing problems. However, many of the infants >30 weeks gestation will be managed with CPAP alone. The proportion of babies that require intubation and mechanical ventilation will vary from around 18–72% depending on the gestation (see Figure 10.3 in Chapter 10). The average length of time spent on the ventilator is less than 4 days. Long-term lung problems are infrequent with <15% developing chronic lung disease. Treatment with home oxygen therapy is rare.

Feeding problems also need to be considered as infants born at this stage are unable to coordinate suck and swallowing. Most will require enteral tube feeds, preferably with expressed breast milk. Enteral feeds are usually gradually increased and partial parenteral nutrition may be required until full feeds are tolerated. Infants born between 28 and 32 weeks gestation rarely develop necrotising enterocolitis (<2%). However, necrotising enterocolitis remains a very serious condition with an associated mortality and morbidity.

Jaundice will be a factor as most infants born at this gestation will develop jaundice in the first week of life. Most cases are due to immaturity of the liver's ability to excrete bilirubin. Preterm infants are more at risk of bilirubin encephalopathy than more mature infants. Most are adequately treated with phototherapy and very rarely will require more aggressive forms of treatment.

Apnoea of prematurity is a common problem in infants born between 28 and 32 weeks gestation. Treatment is with a combination of caffeine or respiratory support (CPAP).

Anaemia can be a problem as haemoglobin levels fall after birth in all newborn infants. Blood sampling amplifies this physiological process. Packed red cell transfusions may be necessary as may iron therapy after a few weeks.

Infection is also a problem as these infants' immune systems are underdeveloped. Serious infections, with bacteria, fungi or viruses, may affect the blood, central nervous system or lungs, although less frequently than those more prematurely. Infections are treated with antibiotics, antifungals or antivirals.

Ductus arteriosus, the delayed physiological closure of the ductus arteriosus, in preterm infants is common, especially in those with respiratory distress syndrome. Treatment options include observation, medical closure (indometacin or ibuprofen) or rarely, at this gestation, surgical duct ligation.

Brain injury is a factor, although less common than in more preterm infants. These infants are still at risk of developing intraventricular and intraparenchymal haemorrhage (<14% infants). Less than 2% of infants at this gestation will develop periventricular leukomalacia. Routine cranial ultrasound scanning is often performed to look for these complications.

Retinopathy of prematurity is uncommon in this gestation with <3% having severe ROP. Treatment with laser to the retina may be necessary to prevent blindness but is rarely required in this gestation group.

Iatrogenic problems are less common at these gestations, but a number of invasive procedures are still required to keep these babies alive (e.g., intubation, respiratory support, umbilical catheters, intercostal catheters, central venous access, arterial lines, surgery, etc). These procedures have known complications. Some of the more significant iatrogenic problems include vocal cord damage, subglottic stenosis, arterial embolism resulting in loss of digits/limbs, erosion of the nasal septum, scarring of the skin and catheter related sepsis.

LONG-TERM OUTCOME

The majority (65%) of babies born between 28 and 32 weeks gestation will have a completely normal outcome. The incidence of long-term problems is inversely proportional to gestational age. Long-term problems include delayed development, deafness, blindness, intellectual and cognitive deficits, cerebral palsy, behavioural problems and learning problems. Less than 5% of survivors from this gestational age group will develop these problems to a severe degree. There is also a higher risk of developmental co-ordination disorder and attention deficit hyperactivity disorder in later childhood compared to term infants. Long-term follow-up with a general paediatrician or the family doctor would be advised.

RECURRENCE

Recurrence will depend on the cause of the preterm delivery. Some are likely to recur (e.g., cervical incompetence) and others will vary. The parents should be advised to seek advice from an obstetrician, a maternal fetal medicine specialist and/or an obstetric physician before the next pregnancy.

REFERENCES

1. The National Perinatal Statistics Unit (NPSU) of the Australian Institute of Health and Welfare (AIHW): Australia's mothers and babies 2008 Perinatal statistics series no 24 (Nov 2010).
2. Goldenberg RL, Culhane JF, Iams JD, et al. Epidemiology and causes of preterm birth. *Lancet.* 2008 Jan 5;371(9606):75–84.
3. Shlossman P, Manley J, Sciscione A, et al. An analysis of neonatal morbidity and mortality in maternal (in-utero) and neonatal transport at 24–34 weeks gestation. *Am J Perinatol.* 1997;14(8):449–456.
4. McCall EM, Alderdice F, Halliday HL, et al. Interventions to prevent hypothermia at birth in preterm and/or low birthweight infants. *Cochrane Database Syst Rev.* 2010 Mar 17;(3):CD004210.

CHAPTER 10

Morbidity and Mortality Statistics for Births at Less Than 32 Weeks Gestational Age

Mark W Davies

The preceding chapters have detailed various outcomes for preterm infants, week by week, up to 32 weeks gestational age. It is sometimes useful to compare various outcomes by gestational age, especially when there is some choice in the timing of delivery. The figures in this chapter will help in comparing outcomes by gestational age.

The following statistics for survival and morbidity relate to outcomes of interest at the time of hospital discharge. The outcomes shown are for babies born at the Royal Brisbane and Women's Hospital (RBWH), Brisbane from 2005–2009 inclusive, with some smoothing of the data. The data are also broadly consistent with other data sources in Australia and New Zealand and internationally. These data, while specific for the RBWH, will give broadly applicable numbers which will be of some use when counselling parents.

SURVIVAL

Figure 10.1 details survival to hospital discharge for three groups. The first population consists of those fetuses alive at the start of labour. For those at the limits of viability the mortality is high and the overall survival is much lower than those babies that are born alive and those that get admitted to the neonatal unit. There is considerable risk of the fetus dying in labour at 23 weeks gestational age and some that are born alive do not survive long enough to be admitted to the neonatal unit.

For the extremely preterm there are significant improvements in survival for each completed week of gestation. There is usually no significant improvement in survival beyond 28 weeks gestational age.

MORBIDITY

Most of the major morbidities and their consequences are detailed in Figures 10.2 to 10.13. Most of these decrease considerably with each completed week of gestation from 23 to 33 weeks gestational age. While there are few gains to be made with regard to survival beyond 28 weeks gestational age, there are significant gains to be made with regard to morbidity. Overall length of stay in hospital, the likelihood of needing respiratory support and long-term neurodevelopmental outcome all improve

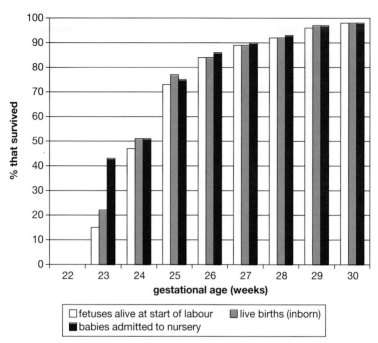

Figure 10.1 Survival statistics.

with increasing gestational age even beyond 28 weeks. These considerations are important when the timing of delivery of a fetus at risk is being considered.

Many preterm infants have multiple problems during their stay in the neonatal nursery. Figures 10.11 and 10.12 are therefore useful in that they provide data on those babies that have one or more problems, or more importantly reveal the proportion of infants that survive to hospital discharge without any major morbidity or without any major neurosensory morbidity by the time of discharge from hospital.

For the purposes of the data in Figure 10.11, Major Neonatal Morbidity is defined as those babies that have one or more of the following: oxygen/CPAP at 36 weeks, definite necrotising enterocolitis (NEC), stage 3 or 4 retinopathy of prematurity (ROP), grade 3 or 4 intraventricular haemorrhage (IVH), periventricular leukomalacia (PVL), porencephalic cyst, or hydrocephalus.

For the purposes of the data in Figure 10.12, Major Neonatal Neurosensory Morbidity is defined as those babies that have one or more of

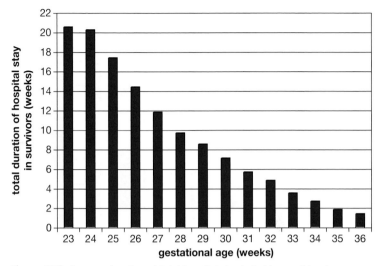

Figure 10.2 Average duration of total hospital stay in babies surviving to discharge.

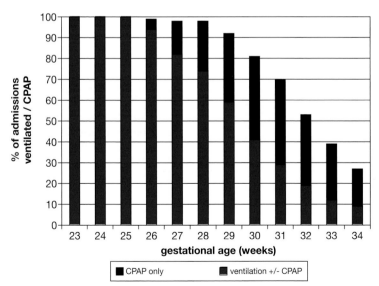

Figure 10.3 Proportion of babies admitted who had respiratory support.

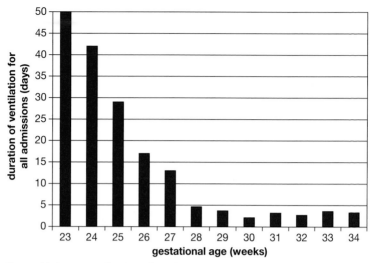

Figure 10.4 Average duration of mechanical ventilation for all admissions.

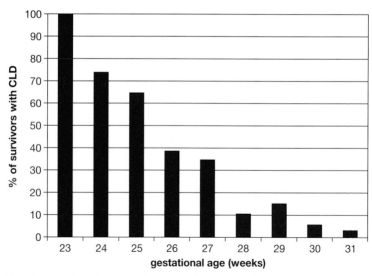

Figure 10.5 Proportion of survivors with chronic lung disease.

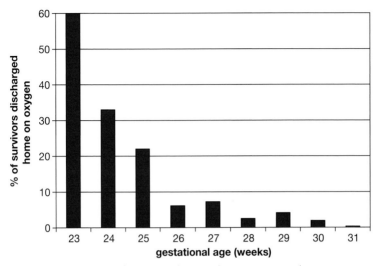

Figure 10.6 Proportion of survivors who went home on oxygen therapy.

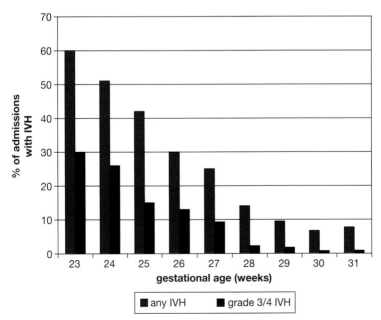

Figure 10.7 Proportion of all admissions who had intraventricular haemorrhage (IVH).

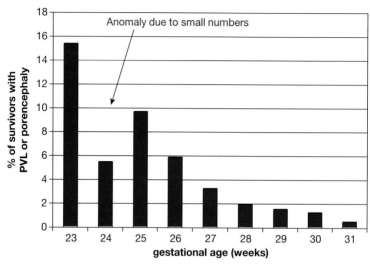

Figure 10.8 Proportion of all survivors who had periventricular leucomalacia (PVL) or porencephaly.

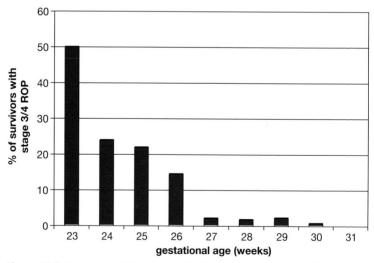

Figure 10.9 Proportion of all survivors who had severe retinopathy of prematurity (ROP).

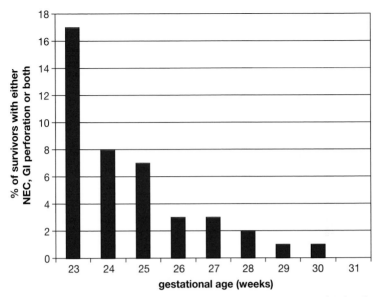

Figure 10.10 Proportion of babies who had either necrotising enterocolitis (NEC), gastrointestinal perforation or both.

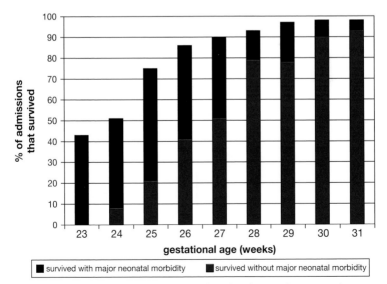

Figure 10.11 Proportion of all survivors with and without Major Neonatal Morbidity.

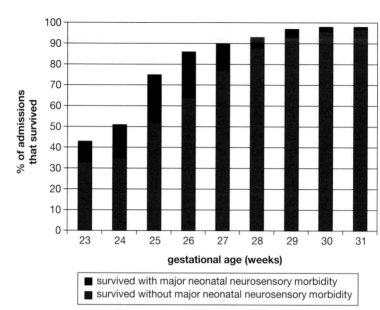

Figure 10.12 Proportion of all survivors with and without Major Neonatal Neurosensory Morbidity.

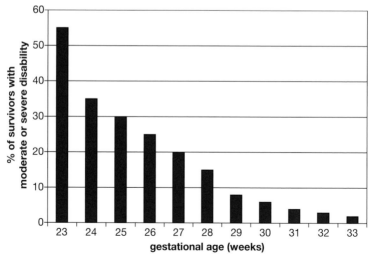

Figure 10.13 Proportion of all survivors with long-term moderate or severe disability.

the following: stage 3 or 4 ROP, grade 3 or 4 IVH, PVL, porencephalic cyst, or hydrocephalus.

LONG-TERM OUTCOME

Preterm infants are at risk for adverse neurodevelopmental outcome. This may include non-specific developmental delay, cerebral palsy (CP), intellectual deficit, deafness and blindness.

The following data are derived from combining the data from a few recent studies and follow-up data from RBWH. They are a rough guide only; the confidence intervals around them are wide. The following definitions for the level of disability are an example of those used.

Moderate disability—Developmental Quotient between 2 and 3 standard deviations below the mean, deaf, moderate CP (walk with aids).

Severe disability—Developmental Quotient more than 3 standard deviations below the mean, blind, severe CP (unable to walk).

Section 3
Non-Specific Antenatal Findings

CHAPTER 11
Reduced Liquor Volumes

Scott G Petersen, Colm PF O'Donnell

Reduced volumes of liquor, or amniotic fluid, can be described as either oligohydramnios or anhydramnios. Oligohydramnios describes the condition of too little, or less than expected, amniotic fluid surrounding the fetus. Anhydramnios implies there is no measureable fluid around the baby.

DEFINITION

Oligohydramnios is suspected either:
▶ clinically, when the fundal height is less than expected and the fetus is easily palpated; or
▶ on an ultrasound scan, if there is either a maximum vertical pocket (MVP) of amniotic fluid of ≤2 cm, or an amniotic fluid index (AFI) of <5 cm.

In pregnancies with oligohydramnios the amniotic fluid volume at term is usually <500 mL. The assessment of amniotic fluid volume is discussed in Box 11.1.

The physiology and regulation of amniotic fluid are discussed in Box 11.2.

INCIDENCE

The incidence of oligohydramnios varies with the population screened, the timing of assessment and the method of measurement. The overall incidence in normal singleton pregnancies is 1%.[1] The incidence after 34 weeks gestation is 2%[2] and after 40 weeks is 11%.[3]

CAUSES

Oligohydramnios is a consequence of either an increased loss of amniotic fluid, reduced production of amniotic fluid or a combination of both. The aetiology influences the severity and the gestational age at which it is diagnosed. The cause for any oligohydramnios is determined by assessing maternal condition, looking for any specific antenatal complications, and obstetric ultrasound. Often no cause is identified, particularly in cases where measurements are just below the clinical cut-off values.

Maternal Causes

Maternal causes include:

▶ vascular disease leading to uteroplacental insufficiency (e.g., chronic hypertension, vascular disease, nephropathy, thrombophilia, diabetes);
▶ drug use (e.g., angiotensin converting enzyme inhibitors, prostaglandin synthetase inhibitors, trastuzumab); and
▶ dehydration.

Obstetric Complications

Obstetric complications that can cause oligohydramnios include:

▶ preterm pre-labour rupture of membranes (PPROM);
▶ placental pathology with utero-placental insufficiency (e.g., preeclampsia, fetal growth restriction, abruption); and
▶ multiple pregnancies with placental complications (see Chapters 23 and 24).

Fetal Anomalies

Fetal causes of oligohydramnios include:

▶ structural abnormalities—from a study of 145 pregnancies with oligohydramnios[4] the following causes were found:
  • renal pathology (renal abnormalities; urogenital tract obstruction) 65%,
  • multiple abnormalities 12%,
  • central nervous system abnormalities 5%,
  • skeletal system abnormalities 4%,
  • cardiovascular system abnormalities 3%,
  • other 4%; and
▶ chromosomal abnormalities.

Idiopathic

Idiopathic cases are usually seen in pregnancies beyond 40 weeks gestation. These are managed based on routine obstetric indicators.

Timing of Onset

The time of onset is useful in helping to determine the cause and also helps determine the prognosis.

1. With onset in the first trimester:
  • the aetiology is usually unclear but it is considered to be related to the implantation process as fluid flow is related to membranous pathways (as opposed to fetal fluid production (i.e., urine) that occurs later in pregnancy) and
  • the prognosis is poor unless the oligohydramnios is correctable by management of maternal hydration status.

2. With onset in the second trimester:
- fetal causes are common given the increased urine component in amniotic fluid; and
- a case series of 128 fetuses with oligohydramnios between 13 and 24 weeks of gestation reported the following causes:[5]
  - fetal abnormality 51% (9% with aneuploidy),
  - preterm premature rupture of membranes 34%,
  - placental abruption 7%,
  - fetal growth restriction 5%,
  - unknown 4%.

3. With onset in the third trimester the most common aetiologies include:
  - preterm pre-labour rupture of membranes,
  - utero-placental insufficiency,
  - fetal abnormality,
  - idiopathic,
  - post-term pregnancy beyond 40 weeks.

CONSEQUENCES

The prognosis for the fetus is principally determined by the cause of the oligohydramnios. The cause also determines management. It is vital therefore that, where possible, the cause of oligohydramnios is identified.

The complications associated with oligohydramnios also vary according to the gestation at onset. Generally the earlier that it occurs the more significant the consequences.

Adverse consequences include:
- miscarriage;
- preterm birth;
- perinatal mortality and morbidity:
  - congenital abnormality,
  - growth restriction,
  - infection;
- maternal morbidity:
  - need for operative delivery,
  - infection;
- fetal developmental consequences:
  - pulmonary hypoplasia and subsequent bronchopulmonary dysplasia—these are almost universal in cases of bilateral renal agenesis, and there is no reliable direct prenatal technique to diagnosis pulmonary hypoplasia,
  - talipes is associated with oligohydramnios and increases the likelihood of pulmonary hypoplasia;
  - musculoskeletal abnormalities (arthrogryposis sequence); and
- fetal malpresentation, especially breech presentation.

The adverse consequences are considered to be more significant if there is:

- anhydramnios;
- no fluid demonstrable in the fetal stomach or bladder;
- onset before week 24;
- fetal abnormality;
- fetal growth restriction;
- abnormal Doppler studies; and
- maternal disease (e.g., pre-eclampsia).

In unselected populations, not controlling for cause, oligohydramnios has been associated with the following poor outcomes:

- an increased risk of caesarean section for fetal distress with a relative risk of 2.2;[6]
- Apgar scores <7 at 5 minutes with a relative risk of 5.2;[6]
- increased perinatal mortality with the risk increased 13-fold overall, 47-fold if severe.[7]

In a study of pregnancies with oligohydramnios where *preterm pre-labour rupture of membranes* and congenital anomalies were excluded as causes, perinatal morbidity was reported in 11% of cases with normal Doppler studies compared to 80% with abnormal Doppler studies.[8]

TIMING OF ONSET

Oligohydramnios diagnosed in the second trimester carries a higher perinatal mortality rate than a diagnosis in the third trimester[5]—only 11% of 128 fetuses with oligohydramnios diagnosed between 13 and 24 weeks survived the perinatal period. Many of these pregnancies were terminated (predominantly for fetal abnormalities and following *preterm pre-labour rupture of membranes*). By contrast, only 15% of the 122 diagnosed in the third trimester did not survive the perinatal period (and most of these had congenital anomalies).

MANAGEMENT—ANTENATAL

The finding of oligohydramnios should prompt further investigation to determine the cause. A detailed ultrasound scan should be done to identify signs of fetal compromise or other complications. The possibility of intervention should be considered.

Investigation should be directed towards the likely cause (see below) and may include:

- amniotic fluid protein detection test (e.g., AmniSure, Actim PROM) for *preterm pre-labour rupture of membranes*;
- amniocentesis, if possible, or chorionic villous sampling to look for chromosomal anomalies; and
- fetal magnetic resonance imaging (MRI) to determine the extent of any structural anomalies suggested by ultrasound.

The need for intervention is determined by maternal well being, the cause of the oligohydramnios and fetal well being. Prompt delivery may be required for maternal or fetal indications.

Amnioinfusion (the instillation of 0.9% saline into the amniotic cavity) is a temporary measure used to either facilitate ultrasound assessment of the fetus for structural abnormalities or to reduce cord compression during labour.

The most common causes of oligohydramnios and the management of each are detailed below.

Pre-Labour Rupture of Membranes

Three per cent of pregnancies are complicated by *preterm pre-labour rupture of membranes*. The diagnosis is largely made on clinical grounds. An amniotic fluid protein detection test (e.g., Amnisure) may help.

Management is determined by gestation and whether there is any evidence of chorioamnionitis or abruption. Treatment should include:

▶ maternal administration of antenatal steroids for fetal lung maturation, magnesium sulphate infusion for fetal neuroprotection and antibiotics for prolongation of the pregnancy and the prevention or treatment of infection;

▶ *in utero* transfer to a maternity hospital with an intensive care nursery if <32 weeks gestation;

▶ observe for signs of chorioamnionitis, abruption or labour; and

▶ counsel the parents about the implications for pulmonary and musculoskeletal development if preterm pre-labour rupture of membranes has occurred <24 weeks gestation:[9]

- pulmonary hypoplasia—the average prevalence is 9% (related to gestation at onset and severity), but is only reported in <1.4% of cases after 26 weeks,
- musculoskeletal abnormality—the average prevalence is 7% (related to duration of oligohydramnios); it is usually correctable with postnatal growth and development, physiotherapy and/or surgery.

Fetal Anomaly

Fetal anomalies may be identified with ultrasound in the context of oligohydramnios. These anomalies may be the cause of the oligohydramnios (e.g., renal agenesis), be associated with and suggest the cause of the oligoydramnios (e.g., talipes and hand abnormalities indicating Edwards syndrome) or be a consequence of the oligohydramnios (e.g., talipes).

Again, the cause of oligohydramnios determines prognosis and treatment. For example, a diagnosis of trisomy 13 confers dismal prognosis (see Chapter 29). Similarly, if fetal kidneys cannot be identified, lethal pulmonary hypoplasia is likely and lethal renal failure without renal replacement therapy almost certain (see Chapter 43). In contrast, the prognosis for fetuses with talipes caused by oligohydramnios due to *preterm pre-labour rupture of membranes* is less grim.

The woman should be referred to a maternal fetal medicine specialist for consideration of fetal therapy for urinary tract obstruction (see Chapter 43).

The parents should be counselled about the implications for pulmonary and musculoskeletal development if the oligohydramnios occurred before 24 weeks gestation. The possibility of aneuploidy (and its implications) which may not be excluded prenatally should be discussed.

Uteroplacental Insufficiency

The indications for delivery are based on either the maternal or fetal condition.

Monitoring of the maternal condition is based on clinical observations and the results of laboratory investigations (e.g., full blood count and film examination, urea and electrolytes, liver function, urinalysis).

Monitoring of the fetal condition is based on cardiotocography and ultrasound assessment of fetal growth and well being by Doppler velocimetry (see Chapter 25).

Maternal Dehydration

Normal hydration should be restored by replacement with water or intravenous hypotonic solution. The use of hypotonic solutions causes a reduction in maternal osmolality and creates a gradient for the transfer of water from the mother to the fetus (and amniotic fluid via the fetus). Isotonic volume replacement to the mother will not have the same effect.[10]

Idiopathic Isolated Oligohydramnios

Any association between increased perinatal morbidity and mortality is lost after correction for any fetal abnormality and maternal condition.[8,11,12]

Indications for delivery are based on either maternal or fetal condition:

- monitoring of the maternal condition is clinically based;
- monitoring of the fetal condition is based on cardiotocography and ultrasound assessment of fetal growth and well being (including Doppler studies of the middle cerebral artery); and
- obstetric intervention for oligohydramnios may be associated with a higher rate of caesarean delivery for non-reassuring fetal status.[11,12]

Post-Term Pregnancy Beyond 40 Weeks

The Royal College of Obstetrics & Gynaecology (RCOG) recommends women with uncomplicated pregnancies be offered induction of labour from 41 weeks of pregnancy (based on certain dating) to prevent fetal death.[13]

POSTNATAL MANAGEMENT

The postnatal management is principally determined by the cause and severity of oligohydramnios and the gestational age at birth.

As discussed above, there is a high likelihood that the baby will be delivered preterm. The implications of prematurity are discussed in Chapters 4 to 9.

The condition of the baby at birth may be worsened by antenatal utero-placental insufficiency and intrapartum events (umbilical cord compression, acute on chronic hypoxia).

Pulmonary hypoplasia is associated with very high rates of mortality. It is, however, very difficult to predict the presence or severity of pulmonary hypoplasia antenatally.[14] Pulmonary hypoplasia is diagnosed postnatally by the degree of respiratory support needed and the appearance on chest X-ray (or on post-mortem examination). If there is any pulmonary hypoplasia (in addition to any prematurity) the baby will need intubation and mechanical ventilation from birth. Baby will be transferred as soon as possible to the intensive care nursery with continuing respiratory support and insertion of umbilical catheters.

The possibility of infection should be covered with antibiotics, started as soon as possible after birth.

Any musculoskeletal problems are usually correctable with postnatal growth and development, physiotherapy and/or surgery.

ETHICS

Decisions regarding palliative care and active management with full neonatal resuscitation are complex and require multidisciplinary counselling of the parents (by the obstetrician, a maternal fetal medicine specialist and neonatologist) before delivery. The anticipated postnatal course and plans for active treatment or comfort care only should be detailed and communicated to the neonatal staff.

Box 11.1   ASSESSMENT OF AMNIOTIC FLUID VOLUME

Measuring amniotic fluid

In clinical practice, amniotic fluid volume is estimated with ultrasound using the following methods:

Single deepest pocket (SDP) or maximal vertical pocket (MVP) technique

This was the first technique developed to estimate amniotic fluid volume by measuring the maximal vertical (anteroposterior) depth of the single largest pocket of fluid without fetal parts or umbilical cord:[1]

- oligohydramnios—≤2 cm;
- normal—2.1 to 8 cm; and
- polyhydramnios—>8 cm.

   The maximal vertical pocket varies significantly with gestational age, ranging from 5.7 cm at week 28 to 4.8 cm at term, with a peak value of 5.8 cm at week 32.[2]

   This is considered the best technique to estimate the amniotic fluid volume in the sacs of multiple pregnancies.

Amniotic fluid index (AFI)

This is the most widely used ultrasound method to estimate amniotic fluid volume and the best method for identifying abnormal amniotic fluid volumes in singleton pregnancies.[3]

The gravid uterus is divided into quadrants by dividing the uterus vertically using the linea nigra, and horizontally using a line drawn at right angles to the linea nigra through the umbilicus. The amniotic fluid index is calculated by adding the measured maximal vertical (anteroposterior) depths of the largest pockets of fluid without fetal parts or umbilical cord from the four quadrants of the uterus (see Figure 11.1). One centimetre (cm) of amniotic fluid index is considered equivalent to a volume of 30 cm^3:

- oligohydramnios—0 to <5 cm;
- normal—5 to 25 cm; and
- polyhydramnios—>25 cm.

The amniotic fluid index varies significantly with gestational age[4] and mimics the normogram determined by Brace and Wolf based on dye-dilutional technique.[5] The median amniotic fluid index is 15 cm at week 32 and 11 cm at week 42 with the 5th–95th percentile in normal singleton pregnancies ranging between 7 and 21 cm.[5] Adverse pregnancy outcomes (fetal complications, poor tolerance of labour and perinatal death) are associated with amniotic fluid index values <5 cm and >25 cm.[6]

Two-diameter pocket

This method multiplies the vertical depth of the maximal vertical pocket in the uterus by its largest horizontal diameter:

- oligohydramnios—0–15 cm^2;
- normal—15.1–50 cm^2; and
- polyhydramnios—>50 cm^2.

All the ultrasound methods of estimating amniotic fluid volume appear to identify pregnancies with normal amniotic fluid volumes more reliably than pregnancies with abnormal amniotic fluid volumes. Each method has poor sensitivity (<30%) for detecting abnormal amniotic fluid volume based on dye-dilution measurement.[3,7] This may be affected by operator experience, pressure created by application of the ultrasound transducer, scanning conditions and fetal position and fetal movements.

In clinical practice, ultrasound estimation of amniotic fluid volume is just one component of antenatal fetal well being surveillance that is used in conjunction with other ultrasound assessments (fetal anatomy, fetal biometry, Doppler studies and biophysical profile) and cardiotocography. An isolated finding of abnormal amniotic fluid volume must be interpreted with caution given the potential for maternal and neonatal morbidity related to obstetric intervention.

References

1. Chamberlain MB, Manning FA, Morrison I, et al. Ultrasound evaluation of amniotic fluid I. The relationship of marginal and decreased amniotic fluid volume to perinatal outcome. *Am J Obstet Gynecol.* 1984;150:245–249.
2. Bottoms SF, Welch RA, Zador IE, et al. Limitations of using maximum vertical pocket and other sonographic evaluations of amniotic fluid volume to predict fetal growth: technical or physiologic. *Am J Obstet Gynecol.* 1986;155:154–158.

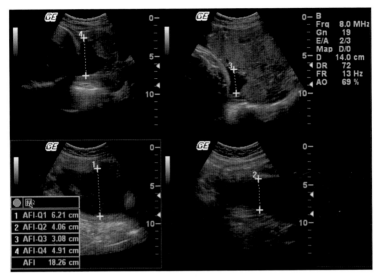

Figure 11.1 Measurement of the amniotic fluid index.

3. Schrimmer DB, Moore TR. Sonographic evaluation of amniotic fluid volume. *Clinical Obstetrics & Gynecology*. 2002;45(4):1026–1038.
4. Moore TR, Cayle JE. The amniotic fluid index in normal human pregnancy. *Am J Obstet Gynecol*. 1990;162(5):1168–1173.
5. Brace RA, Wolf EJ. Normal amniotic fluid volume changes throughout pregnancy. *Am J Obstet Gynecol*. 1989;161:382–388.
6. Phelan JP, Ahn MO, Smith CV, et al. Amniotic fluid index measurements during pregnancy. *J Reprod Med*. 1987;32:601–604.
7. Magann EF, Doherty DA, Chauhan SP, et al. How well do the amniotic fluid index and single deepest pocket indices (below the 3rd and 5th and above the 95th and 97th percentiles) predict oligohydramnios and hydramnios? *Am J Obstet Gynecol*. 2004;190:164.

Box 11.2   PHYSIOLOGY OF AMNIOTIC FLUID

Amniotic fluid is the clear fluid that surrounds the fetus in the amniotic sac; its volume and composition varies throughout gestation. Amniotic fluid should not be confused with coelomic fluid which is similar to maternal plasma and is found in the extra-embryonic coelomic cavity between the amnion and chorion before this space is obliterated by week 14.[1]

Compared to fetal or maternal blood, amniotic fluid has low sodium and chloride concentrations, and a lower osmolality that decreases as the pregnancy progresses (260 mOsm/kg at term compared to a blood osmolality of 280 mOsm/kg).

Role of amniotic fluid

Amniotic fluid has many functions that are important for normal fetal growth and development.[2] These include:

- provides space for growth and movement, and cushions the umbilical cord from compression;
- protects against external factors, such as trauma and infection;
- maintains a constant temperature;
- provides fluid, nutrients, hormones, growth factors and antibacterial agents including antibodies; and
- provides the optimal sterile environment for normal development of the respiratory, musculoskeletal and gastrointestinal systems.

Amniotic fluid also contains biochemical markers that may be measured to provide clinically useful information (e.g., lecithin:sphingomyelin ratio indicating surfactant production and fetal lung maturity; alpha-fetoprotein and acetyl-cholinesterase indicating the presence of an open neural tube defect).

Regulation of amniotic fluid

Regulation of the amniotic fluid volume by the fetus commences in mid-gestation (second trimester) when the fetus begins to produce urine and swallow increasing volumes.[2] Amniotic fluid is continuously produced and cleared and its volume is regulated by the balance between the two processes. While the total volume of amniotic fluid is turned over daily, the volume of amniotic fluid present at any time does not usually vary greatly from day to day.

Amniotic fluid volume is regulated via six pathways. Amniotic fluid is produced by 1) fetal urine production and 2) fetal lung fluid secretion; it is cleared by 3) fetal swallowing; and it may be produced or cleared by 4) intramembranous transfer within the fetal compartment (exchange into fetal blood across membranes), 5) transmembranous transfer within the maternal and placental compartments and 6) transmucosal secretions from the fetal compartment (e.g., skin before keratinisation and oral-nasal cavities).[4]

Ultimately all amniotic fluid is derived from the mother via the placenta and changes in maternal hydration are recognised to affect amniotic fluid volumes via transplacental osmotic gradients.[3] The transmembranous and intramembranous pathways permit bidirectional flow of water across osmotic gradients, and solutes by diffusion. Regulation of solutes (e.g., sodium and chloride) within the amniotic fluid occurs primarily via the intramembranous pathway. The relative importance of each of these pathways changes with advancing gestation.[5] Production in the first trimester is mainly from transmembranous transfer and transmucosal secretions. In the second and third trimester production is primarily from fetal urine and lung fluid (transmucosal and membranous pathways remain as minor sources). By week 20 amniotic fluid is composed mostly of fetal urine. Clearance of amniotic fluid in the first and second trimester is primarily by fetal swallowing and the intramembranous pathway. Clearance also occurs across membranes into the maternal blood (transmembranous pathway). In the third trimester (from week 28) fetal swallowing is the major pathway to clear amniotic fluid.

1. Fetal urine production

Fetal urine production[4] commences when the cloacal membrane degenerates around week 8 and the rate of production increases with advancing gestation. The amniotic fluid volumes are 2–5 mL at 22 weeks of gestation and 800–1200 mL (0.2 mL/minute/ kg) at term.

Fetal renal function near-term responds to hormonal signals (e.g., vasopressin) and maternal medication use (e.g., prostaglandin synthetise inhibitors) with alteration in urinary volume and osmolality.

Fetal urinary flow rates decrease with conditions associated with poor fetal condition (e.g., placental insufficiency) and increase with conditions associated with a hyperdynamic circulation (e.g., fetal anaemia, chorioangioma, supraventricular tachycardia, twin-to-twin transfusion syndrome). Acute hypoxia decreases fetal urine production.

2. Fetal lung fluid secretion

Fetal lung fluid is produced at a rate of 170 mL/day at term, half of which is swallowed.[4] The presence of fetal lung fluid in amniotic fluid provides the rationale for fetal lung maturity testing. Fetal lung fluid production decreases with asphyxia and ceases during labour when the fluid is absorbed into the pulmonary lymphatics.[6]

3. Fetal swallowing

Fetal swallowing commences by week 8 and increases throughout gestation with progressively increasing volumes and coordination.[7] The volume swallowed is 500–1000 mL/day (155 mL/kg/day) at term, with the increase in the volume swallowed considered to contribute to the reduction of amniotic fluid volume towards term and post-term.[4,8]

Fetal swallowing activity is linked to fetal neuro-behaviour and influenced by central and systemic dipsogenic mechanisms, hypoxia, hypotension and plasma osmolality changes. Acute hypoxia is associated with a decrease in fetal swallowing activity. Reduced fetal swallowing is associated with fetal anomalies (e.g., anencephaly).

4. Intramembranous flow

Intramembranous flow accounts for 200–400 mL/day at term.[4] Intramembranous flow is driven by the osmotic gradient between fetal plasma and amniotic fluid and may be regulated by prostaglandins and angiogenic factors (e.g., vascular endothelial growth factor) via aquaporin water channels.[3,4] Intramembranous flow may be up-regulated as part of adaptive fetal responses in cases of gastrointestinal obstruction or reduced fetal swallowing.[9]

5. Transmucosal oral-nasal secretions

Transmucosal oral-nasal secretions accounts for 25 mL/day at term.[4]

6. Transmembranous flow

Transmembranous flow accounts for 10 mL/day at term.[4]

Volume of amniotic fluid

The amniotic fluid volume increases significantly from week 8 when the embryonic period of development ends (10–20 mL at week 10). The volume peaks around week 34 (800–1000 mL) and declines towards term (about 700 mL, range 250–1400 mL).[10,11] The largest variability in volume occurs in the third trimester, probably due to greater variation in fetal urine production and swallowing.

Abnormal amniotic fluid volume is associated with adverse perinatal outcomes and hence it is measured during antenatal fetal well being surveillance. Assessment of amniotic fluid volume is recommended at each antenatal visit as part of standard prenatal care with determination of amniotic fluid volume at every ultrasound performed from the second trimester. Abnormal amniotic fluid volume may suggest the diagnosis of pre-labour rupture of membranes, fetal anomalies (both structural and chromosomal) and poor fetal condition.

Factors established as affecting amniotic fluid volume include postmaturity (>42 weeks), maternal hydration, maternal vascular disease (associated with utero-placental insufficiency), diabetes in pregnancy, maternal medications (e.g., prostaglandin synthetase inhibitors), altitude, fetal anomalies and fetal growth (e.g., macrosomia and growth restriction). Maternal smoking has not been shown to affect amniotic fluid volume.

References

1. Campbell J, Wathen N, Macintosh M, et al. Biochemical composition of amniotic fluid and extraembryonic coelomic fluid in the first trimester of pregnancy. *Br J Obstet Gynaecol*. 1992;99:563.
2. Brace RA. Physiology of amniotic fluid volume regulation. *Clin Obstet Gynecol*. 1997;40:280–289.
3. Moore TR. Amniotic fluid dynamics reflect fetal and maternal health and disease. *Obstet Gynecol*. 2010;116:759.
4. Brace, RA, Ross, MG. Amniotic fluid volume regulation. In: Brace RA, Hanson MA, Rodeck CH, eds. *Fetus and Neonate—Volume 4: Body fluids and kidney function*. Cambridge University Press; 1998:88.
5. Brace RA. Progress toward understanding the regulation of amniotic fluid volume: water and solute fluxes in and through the fetal membranes. *Placenta*. 1995;16:1.
6. Harding, R. Development of the respiratory system. In: Thorburn GD, Harding R, eds. *Textbook of Fetal Physiology*. Oxford Medical Publications; 1994:140.
7. Grassi R, Farina R, Floriani I, et al. Assessment of fetal swallowing with gray-scale and color Doppler sonography. *AJR Am J Roentgenol*. 2005;185:1322.
8. Ross MG, Nijland MJM. Fetal Swallowing: Relation to Amniotic Fluid Regulation. *Clinical Obstetrics and Gynecology*. Volume 1997;40(2):352–365.
9. Jang PR, Brace RA. Amniotic fluid composition changes during urine drainage and tracheoesophageal occlusion in fetal sheep. *Am J Obstet Gynecol*. 1992;167:1732–1741.
10. Brace RA, Wolf EJ. Normal amniotic fluid volume changes throughout pregnancy. *Am J Obstet Gynecol*. 1989;161:382–388.
11. Magann EF, Bass JD, Chauhan SP, et al. Amniotic fluid volume in normal singleton pregnancies. *Obstet Gynecol*. 1997;90:524.

REFERENCES

1. Magann EF, Bass JD, Chauhan SP, et al. Amniotic fluid volume in normal singleton pregnancies. *Obstet Gynecol*. 1997;90:524.
2. Casey BM, McIntire DD, Bloom SL, et al. Pregnancy outcomes after antepartum diagnosis of oligohydramnios at or beyond 34 weeks' gestation. *Am J Obstet Gynecol*. 2000;182(4):909–912.

3. Locatelli A, Zagarella A, Toso L, et al. Serial assessment of amniotic fluid index in uncomplicated term pregnancies: prognostic value of amniotic fluid reduction. *J Matern Fetal Neonatal Med.* 2004;15(4):233.

4. Hill LM. Oligohydramnios: sonographic diagnosis and clinical implications. *Clin Obstet Gynecol.* 1997;40:314–327.

5. Shipp TD, Bromley B, Pauker S, et al. Outcome of singleton pregnancies with severe oligohydramnios in the second and third trimesters. *Ultrasound Obstet Gynecol.* 1996;7:108–113.

6. Chauhan S, Sanderson M, Hendrix N, et al. Perinatal outcome and amniotic fluid index in the antepartum and intrapartum periods: A meta-analysis. *Am J Obstet Gynecol.* 1999;181:1473–1478.

7. Chamberlain MB, Manning FA, Morrison I, et al. Ultrasound evaluation of amniotic fluid I. The relationship of marginal and decreased amniotic fluid volume to perinatal outcome. *Am J Obstet Gynecol.* 1984;150:245–249.

8. Carroll BC, Bruner JP. Umbilical artery Doppler velocimetry in pregnancies complicated by oligohydramnios. *J Reprod Med.* 2000;45:562–566.

9. McElrath T. Midtrimester premature rupture of membranes. Up-To-Date, 2009.

10. Moore TR. Amniotic fluid dynamics reflect fetal and maternal health and disease. *Obstet Gynecol.* 2010;116:759.

11. Kreiser D, El-Sayed Y, Sorem KA, et al. Decreased amniotic fluid index in lowrisk pregnancy. *J Reprod Med.* 2001;46:743–746.

12. Conway DL, Adkins WB, Schroeder B, et al. Isolated oligohydramnios in the term pregnancy: is it a clinical entity? *J Matern Fetal Med.* 1998;7:197–200.

13. RCOG. Induction of Labour: Evidence-based Clinical Guideline Number 9. RCOG Clinical Effectiveness Support Unit, 2001.

14. Everest NJ, Jacobs SE, Davis PG, et al. Outcomes following prolonged preterm premature rupture of the membranes. *Arch Dis Child Fetal Neonatal Eed.* 2008;93:F207–F211.

Further Reading

Conway DL, Groth S, Adkins WB, et al. Management of isolated oligohydramnios in the term pregnancy: a randomized clinical trial. *Am J Obstet Gynecol.* 2000;182:S21.

Ek S, Andersson A, Johansson A, et al. Oligohydramnios in uncomplicated pregnancies beyond 40 completed weeks. A prospective, randomised, pilot study on maternal and neonatal outcomes. *Fetal Diagn Ther.* 2005;20:182.

Nabhan AF, Abdelmoula YA. Amniotic fluid index versus single deepest vertical pocket as a screening test for preventing adverse pregnancy outcome. *Cochrane Database Syst Rev.* 2008;CD006593.

Sherer DM. Amniotic fluid dynamics and isolated oligohydramnios. *American Journal of Perinatology.* 2002;19(5):253–266.

Magann EF, Chauhan SP, Doherty DA, et al. AFI versus SDP in amniotic fluid volume estimation. *Am J Perinatol.* 2007;24:549–556.

CHAPTER 12

Polyhydramnios

Scott G Petersen, Colm PF O'Donnell

Polyhydramnios describes the condition of too much, or more than expected, amniotic fluid (liquor) surrounding the fetus. Polyhydramnios is suspected either clinically (i.e., a fundal height greater than expected and fetus not readily palpable) or on ultrasound assessment (maximum vertical pocket >8 cm; amniotic fluid index >25 cm). The fluid volume in a pregnancy with polyhydramnios at term would be greater than 2500 mL. Cause is not implied in the definition. The assessment of amniotic fluid volume is discussed in Box 11.1. The physiology and regulation of amniotic fluid are discussed in Box 11.2.

The measurement cut-offs defining polyhydramnios have been based around clinical outcomes but not normograms. The identification of polyhydramnios should prompt further assessment of fetal and maternal condition, and consideration of obstetric intervention as indicated.

Polyhydramnios is categorised based on amniotic fluid index (see Box 11.1):[1,2]
- mild, 25.1–30 cm, 66% of cases;
- moderate, 30.1–35 cm, 22% of cases; and
- severe, >35 cm, 12% of cases.

INCIDENCE

The incidence varies with the population screened and the method of measurement.[1] Polyhydramnios affects 0.2–1.6% of singleton pregnancies and most commonly occurs in the second half of pregnancy (the vast majority of cases are diagnosed in the third trimester). Some 6–15% of singleton pregnancies have an amniotic fluid index above the 95th percentile (21 cm).

CAUSES

Polyhydramnios occurs as a consequence of either:
- conditions resulting in a reduction in amniotic fluid clearance (primarily reduced fetal swallowing); or
- an increase in urine production.

The aetiology influences the severity and the gestational age at diagnosis. The aetiology of polyhydramnios is determined by assessment of maternal condition and obstetric ultrasound assessment of fetal growth, well being and anatomy. A cause may not be identifiable with measurements just above the clinical cut-off values.

Idiopathic
Idiopathic causes (i.e., not associated with any pathological cause) account for 50–60% of all cases. About 94% of cases are mild; and the amniotic fluid index reduces in at least 75% of these with time. In the absence of specific maternal or fetal conditions, mild polyhydramnios is usually associated with a large for gestational age fetus.

Maternal
Maternal conditions with polyhydramnios include:
◗ diabetes mellitus with hyperglycaemia; and
◗ infection with transplacental transmission:
  • parvovirus B19,
  • cytomegalovirus,
  • syphilis,
  • toxoplasmosis.

Obstetric Complications
Obstetric complications that have a greater incidence of polyhydramnios include multiple pregnancies with chorionicity-related transfusional complications (e.g., twin-to-twin transfusion syndrome, twin reversed arterial perfusion sequence).

Placental Pathology
Conditions with a hyperdynamic circulation (e.g., chorioangioma).

Fetal Growth
Polyhydramnios can complicate pregnancies with a large for gestational age fetus.

Fetal Anomalies
Many fetal abnormalities are associated with polyhydramnios. These include:
◗ structural abnormalities:
  • upper gastrointestinal tract obstruction, classically oesophageal atresia,
  • central nervous system abnormalities (especially those that lead to decreased swallowing),
  • oropharyngeal abnormalities,
  • micrognathia;
◗ chromosomal abnormalities:
  • Down syndrome,
  • Edwards syndrome and triploidy (usually have growth restriction),
  • 22q deletion (DiGeorge syndrome);
◗ mass lesions or tumours associated with sequestration and a hyperdynamic circulation:
  • sacrococcygeal teratoma,
  • mass lesions in the oropharynx.

Fetal Medical Conditions

Fetal medical conditions with polyhydramnios include:
▶ hydrops:
  • immune,
  • non-immune, including fetal anaemia from fetomaternal haemorrhage, α-thalassaemia or glucose-6-phosphatase deficiency;
▶ cardiac dysfunction:
  • arrhythmia,
  • hyperdynamic circulation;
▶ renal function abnormalities (e.g., Bartter syndrome); and
▶ neuromuscular conditions.

Timing of Onset

Onset in the first trimester is rare. Polyhydramnios in the second trimester usually occurs in the context of multiple pregnancies with chorionicity-related transfusional complications and with medical conditions of either the mother or the fetus.

In the third trimester the causes include maternal, placental and fetal conditions or abnormalities. The most common aetiologies include:[3]
▶ fetal abnormalities in 20% (range 8–45%);
▶ maternal diabetes mellitus in 5–26%;
▶ multiple pregnancy complications in 8–10%;
▶ fetal anaemia in 1–11%;
▶ infection; and
▶ idiopathic.

An identifiable cause was reported in 17% of cases with mild polyhydramnios compared with 91% with severe polyhydramnios.[4] Dashe et al[2] reported that fetal abnormalities were identified antenatally in 80% of cases of pregnancies with polyhydramnios, with the abnormality being the specific cause of the polyhydramnios in 8%, 12% and 31% of mild, moderate and severe cases respectively. Fetal anomalies that were missed included tracheo-oesophageal fistula, cardiac septal defects and cleft palate. About 10% of fetuses with abnormalities had aneuploidy; in absence of fetal anomaly, the rate of aneuploidy was 1%.

Only 50% of fetuses with oesophageal atresia and 66% of fetuses with duodenal or proximal jejunal atresia develop polyhydramnios, which reflects functional partial obstruction related to tracheo-oesophageal fistula or adaptative increase in intramembranous pathway clearance.[5]

COMPLICATIONS

The perinatal complications associated with polyhydramnios vary according to cause and gestation at onset. Polyhydramnios is associated with specific obstetric complications.[1,6]

Perinatal mortality and morbidity associated with polyhydramnios includes:

- congenital abnormalities;
- prematurity;
- infection;
- birth trauma with shoulder dystocia associated with a large for gestational age fetus (19–37% cases are LGA);
- cord prolapse; and
- haemodynamic instability and neurological injury in multiple pregnancies with chorionicity-related transfusional complications (see Chapter 23).

Maternal morbidity with polyhydramnios includes:

- discomfort and respiratory difficulties;
- operative delivery;
- birth trauma;
- infection;
- postpartum haemorrhage; and
- amniotic fluid embolism.

There is an increased risk of preterm birth and the risk depends on the cause, especially pre-gestational diabetes[7] and fetal abnormalities. Preterm delivery is not associated with idiopathic causes.

Pre-labour rupture of membranes can lead to cord prolapse or placental abruption.

Fetal malpresentation is more common with polyhydramnios. About 5% will have an unstable lie with transverse lie and shoulder presentation. Cord presentation and breech presentation are also more likely.

The adverse consequences of polyhydramnios are considered more significant if associated with:

- fetal abnormality;
- fetal growth restriction;
- maternal disease;
- fetal infection; and
- birth trauma and emergencies.

In unselected populations not controlling for cause, polyhydramnios has been correlated with poor pregnancy outcome with a 2–5-fold increase in perinatal mortality, even if idiopathic.[1,6] The risk of complications correlates with the severity and underlying cause; complications are less likely if the volume of fluid does not increase and reduces over time.[8]

ANTENATAL MANAGEMENT

The identification of polyhydramnios should prompt further assessment to determine a cause, and to identify any signs of fetal abnormality or compromise. Intervention may involve fetal therapy or early delivery.

Fetal therapy has been validated in the management of twin-to-twin transfusion syndrome (see Chapter 24)[9] and fetal anaemia (i.e., fetal red blood cell transfusion).[10]

Amniodrainage to reduce the amniotic fluid volume is a non-validated clinical tool that aims to reduce maternal morbidity and may prolong the pregnancy, reduce the pressure associated with decreased umbilical cord pH and oxygen. It can also provide amniotic fluid for prenatal diagnosis (biochemical analysis of amniotic fluid and exclusion of aneuploidy and fetal infection).

The maternal administration of prostaglandin synthetase inhibitors (e.g., indomethacin or sulindac) before 34 weeks has been used clinically to reduce fetal urine output.[11]

The pregnancy should be monitored closely for signs of preterm labour and membrane rupture. Labour has to be managed cautiously given the risk of malpresentation and cord prolapse which are obstetric emergencies requiring caesarean delivery in the majority of cases. There is also an increased risk of birth trauma from a large for gestational age fetus.

If there is a fetal abnormality then the outcomes, and therefore the counselling required, will be related to the specific anomalies and/or any aneuploidy. The parents should be counselled about the implications of aneuploidy which may not be excluded prenatally.

Specific fetal therapy is offered in cases of twin-to-twin transfusion syndrome and other potentially treatable fetal conditions, including:

▶ fetal arrhythmia;
▶ mass lesions;
▶ pleural effusions; and
▶ anaemia—the management of fetal anaemia depends on the cause and the fetal condition; *in utero* transfusion is considered if there is fetal compromise or a persistent pathophysiological mechanism.

Monitoring of the fetal condition is based on cardiotocography and obstetric ultrasound assessment of fetal growth and well being by Doppler velocimetry. The parents should be counselled about the implications for neonatal management.

Placental masses are managed by monitoring of the fetal condition with cardiotocography and obstetric ultrasound assessment of fetal growth and well being.

If there is pre-labour rupture of membranes, then exclude malpresentation and cord prolapse. The management depends on the gestation and whether there are any clinical signs of chorioamnionitis or abruption. If there is any malpresentation then consider external cephalic version with stabilising induction of labour to aim for a vaginal birth. If the fetus is a large for gestational age fetus then routine intrapartum management is indicated; shoulder dystocia is common and should be expected.

The management of maternal diabetes is discussed in Chapter 14.

Cases of idiopathic isolated polyhydramnios should have a detailed obstetric ultrasound scan to assess for any fetal abnormality, including assessment of structures associated with tracheo-oesophageal fistula (e.g., the VATER/VACTERL association). There is an increased risk of perinatal morbidity and mortality.[1,12] Delivery is considered from 37 weeks gestation if there is any maternal compromise or a favourable cervix; consider a stabilising induction of labour to aim for a vaginal birth.

NEONATAL MANAGEMENT

The management of the baby is largely determined by the cause and severity of the polyhydramnios and the gestational age at birth. There is a high likelihood that the baby will be delivered preterm; the implications of prematurity are discussed in Chapters 4 to 9.

Neonatal condition at birth may be related to antenatal utero-placental insufficiency, intrapartum events (e.g., cord prolapse, malpresentation with umbilical cord compression and traumatic birth, acute or chronic hypoxia, shoulder dystocia).

Given the difficulty in prenatal diagnosis of oropharyngeal abnormalities and tracheo-oesophageal fistula (90% of which are associated with oesophageal atresia, see Chapter 40), neonatal assessment should aim to exclude these conditions at birth and before feeding.

The baby should be examined in detail soon after birth looking for causes of reduced fetal swallowing, increased urine output or other abnormalities, including:

- upper gastrointestinal obstruction (especially oesophageal or duodenal atresia)—a feeding tube should be passed into the stomach to exclude oesophageal atresia;
- central nervous system defects (e.g., anencephaly, neuromuscular disorders affecting swallowing);
- abdominal wall defects;
- severe skeletal dysplasias;
- evidence of chromosomal abnormalities—this should prompt chromosomal studies;
- respiratory tract abnormalities (e.g., congenital cyst-adenomatoid malformation);
- congenital diaphragmatic hernia; and
- cardiac anomalies.

Polyhydramnios may be associated with hydrops fetalis. In multiple gestations, consider twin-twin transfusion syndrome.

Monitor the baby's urine output to check for polyuric renal disorders.

Infants who are large for gestational age should be examined for signs of macrosomia and monitored for hypoglycaemia. The blood glucose level should be checked shortly after birth and regularly thereafter until normal and stable. The frequency of blood glucose levels in the well baby varies between institutions. The most conservative regimen tests blood glucose levels at 1 hour, 2 hours and 4 hours of age, then every 4 hours for 24 hours until normal and stable. Any unwell or symptomatic baby should have their blood glucose level checked immediately.

REFERENCES

1. Magann EF, Chauhan SP, Doherty DA, et al. A Review of Idiopathic Hydramnios and Pregnancy Outcomes. *Obstet Gynecol Surv.* 2007;62(12):795–802.
2. Dashe JS, McIntire DD, Ramus RM, et al. Hydramnios: anomaly prevalence and sonographic detection. *Obstet Gynecol.* 2002;100:134.
3. Beloosesky R, Ross MG. Polyhydramnios (UpToDate, 2011).
4. Hill LM, Breckle R, Thomas ML, et al. Polyhydramnios: ultrasonically detected prevalence and neonatal outcome. *Obstet Gynecol.* 1987;69:21.
5. Underwood MA, Gilbert WM, Sherman MP. Amniotic fluid: not just fetal urine anymore. *J Perinatol.* 2005;25:341.
6. Chamberlain MB, Manning FA, Morrison I, et al. Ultrasound evaluation of amniotic fluid II. The relationship of increased amniotic fluid volume to perinatal outcome. *Am J Obstet Gynecol.* 1984;150:250–254.
7. Idris N, Wong SF, Thomae M, et al. Influence of polyhydramnios on perinatal outcome in pregestational diabetic pregnancies. *Ultrasound Obstet Gynecol.* 2010;36:338.
8. Golan A, Wolman I, Sagi J, et al. Persistence of polyhydramnios during pregnancy—its significance and correlation with maternal and fetal complications. *Gynecol Obstet Invest.* 1994;37:18.
9. Senat M, Deprest J, Boulvain M, et al. Endoscopic laser surgery versus serial amnioreduction for severe twin-to-twin transfusion syndrome. *N Eng J Med.* 2004;351(2):136–144.
10. Moise KJ. Management of rhesus alloimmunization in pregnancy. *Obstet Gynecol.* 2008 Jul;112(1):164–176.
11. Moise Jr KJ. Polyhydramnios. *Clin Obstet Gynecol.* 1997;40:266.
12. Touboul C, Boileau P, Picone O, et al. Outcome of children born out of pregnancies complicated by unexplained polyhydramnios. *BJOG.* 2007;114:489.

CHAPTER 13

Hydrops

Paul Woodgate, Carol Portmann

Hydrops fetalis is a clinical condition affecting the fetus in which there is excessive fluid accumulation in the extravascular compartments. This results in generalised oedema and fluid accumulation in various body cavities. The diagnosis is made on fetal ultrasound when there is accumulation of fluid in two or more extravascular compartments: pleural effusions, pericardial effusion, ascites, skin oedema (skin thickness of >5 mm) or placental enlargement.

Hydrops fetalis is generally described as either immune or non-immune. Immune hydrops is caused by red blood cell alloimmunisation haemolytic disease (see Chapter 26). All other causes are grouped together as non-immune hydrops.

Hydrops fetalis may result from a large number of conditions. A diagnosis is frequently not available antenatally or postnatally and the condition is associated with a high mortality rate. Careful assessment and a multidisciplinary approach are essential. Therapies are limited and have variable success depending on the underlying aetiology.

PREVALENCE
Hydrops occurs in 1 in 1500–1 in 3750 pregnancies. Non-immune hydrops fetalis occurs in approximately 1 in 3000 pregnancies. The ratio of non-immune to immune hydrops is about 9:1. The prevalence of hydrops fetalis is falling in regions where there is pre-screening for associated conditions; e.g., haemoglobinopathies, blood group antibodies and aneuploidy, and with the availability of intra-uterine transfusions.

PATHOPHYSIOLOGY AND AETIOLOGY
Hydrops is a non-specific finding associated with many different fetal, placental and maternal diseases. Most cases arise from similar pathological mechanisms and these are summarised in Figure 13.1.

Immune hydrops is a result of significant persistent anaemia due to transplacental allo-antibody destruction of fetal blood cells. The condition is becoming progressively less common since the introduction of blood group antibody screening, anti-D administration, assessment of risk of fetal anaemia through ultrasound evaluation of middle cerebral artery peak systolic velocity and intrauterine transfusion prior to the development of hydrops.

For non-immune hydrops, the direct link between the suspected or known cause and the development of non-immune hydrops is not always

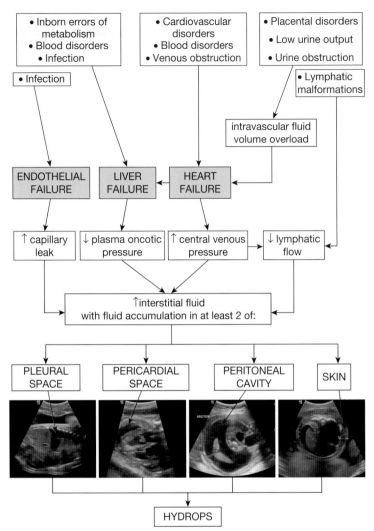

Figure 13.1 Pathophysiological mechanisms in the development of hydrops fetalis.
Modified after Bellini.[1]

clear, but the end result of any pathophysiology is the development of generalised oedema. This may be caused by conditions that lead to congestive heart failure, decreased plasma oncotic pressure, increased capillary permeability and/or obstructed lymphatic flow.

Non-immune hydrops may result from a heterogeneous group of conditions which can be categorised as:

◗ chromosomal (13–19%);
◗ cardiovascular (10–20%);
◗ haematological (10%);
◗ infection (6–13%);
◗ thoracic (6–12%);
◗ lymphatic (4–18%);
◗ syndromic/genetic (4–12%);
◗ inborn storage disorders (1–2%);
◗ extra thoracic tumours (<1%);
◗ placental (including twin-to-twin transfusion syndrome);
◗ miscellaneous structural conditions; and
◗ idiopathic (20%).

Specific conditions are detailed in Table 13.1. Despite these multiple possible aetiologies, there is no identified mechanism or disorder in about 30–40% of cases. The cause may remain unknown even after birth in 20% of cases.

Gestational age at presentation impacts on likely aetiology. Aneuploidy and parvovirus are the most common aetiologies under 24 weeks gestation; hydrothorax and tachyarrhythmias are more common after 24 weeks.

CONSEQUENCES

Non-immune hydrops fetalis has a significant perinatal mortality rate which depends upon the severity of the hydrops and its cause. The mortality ranges from 50–75%, but approaches 100% when hydrops fetalis is associated with structural cardiac disease, other major congenital anomalies or twin-to-twin transfusion syndrome.

Outcomes of pregnancies in prenatal studies shows a live birth rate of 40–60%, termination of pregnancy in 17–37% and intrauterine death rate of 17–23%. Survival to 28 days ranges from 27–48%.[2]

Mortality and morbidity are dependent upon the cause and gestational age at diagnosis. Hydrops fetalis is often a presentation of a lethal condition or a lethal complication of an underlying disorder; e.g., skeletal dysplasia, metabolic disease or inborn error of metabolism, congenital myotonic dystrophy, aneuploidy or cardiac anomalies. Pleural effusions may cause severe pulmonary hypoplasia and pericardial effusions may impair cardiac function.

On the other hand, hydrops fetalis may also be a presentation of a treatable condition; e.g., transient or immune anaemia, tachyarrhythmia or chylothorax.

Table 13.1 Specific causes of non-immune hydrops

Category	Causes
Primary cardiac failure	Arrhythmia • tachyarrhythmias • bradyarrhythmias Cardiomyopathies Cardiac rhabdomyoma Cardiac malformation (40% of cases) • left ventricular hypoplasia • endocardial fibroelastosis
Secondary cardiac failure	High-output cardiac failure • arterio-venous malformation • large haemangiomas • placental chorioangiomas • teratomas—sacrococcygeal/cervical Twin-to-twin transfusion syndrome • "recipient" twin Non-immune haematological causes of fetal anaemia • glucose-6-phosphate dehydrogenase deficiency • pyruvate kinase deficiency • alpha-thalassaemia
Chromosomal causes	Turner syndrome—45X Trisomy 13, 18 or 21
Thoracic and pulmonary causes	Primary chylothorax/hydrothorax Lung masses • congenital cystic adenomatoid malformation • sequestration • tumour • other fetal intrathoracic masses Congenital diaphragmatic hernia
Infection	Parvovirus Cytomegalovirus Coxsackievirus Toxoplasmosis
Genetic Disorder	Fetal dyskinesias • skeletal dysplasias • congenital myopathies Inborn errors of metabolism • lysosomal storage diseases • mucopolysaccharidoses
Gastrointestinal abnormalities	Tracheo-oesophageal fistula Small bowel volvulus Meconium peritonitis

If live born, normal developmental outcome is seen in 60% of babies, but the proportion is greater with some specific causes; e.g., immune hydrops, parvovirus and tachyarrhythmia.

Hydrops fetalis is one of the few congenital fetal conditions that may have significant implications for maternal welfare. Maternal mirror syndrome may arise as a result of placental and fetal hydrops. This may present as maternal nephrotic syndrome or severe pre-eclampsia requiring delivery. Polyhydramnios, often associated with hydrops, predisposes to preterm labour, premature rupture of membranes and placental abruption.

MANAGEMENT—ANTENATAL

Hydrops fetalis may present with clinical symptoms such as reduced fetal movements, increased fundal height (polyhydramnios) or, more commonly, on routine ultrasound. A thorough investigation to determine the cause should occur if any fetal oedema or effusions are detected on ultrasonography. All cases should be referred to a tertiary hospital with maternal fetal medicine specialists (or high level obstetric imaging). A multidisciplinary approach involving maternal fetal medicine specialists, neonatologists, geneticists and other relevant specialists is often required.

Antenatal investigations should include:

- a detailed tertiary-level fetal morphology ultrasound scan:
  - identify structural fetal or placental anomalies,
  - assess fetal movements,
  - assess fetal middle cerebral artery peak systolic velocity (increased systolic velocity in the middle cerebral artery may indicate fetal anaemia), and
  - assess fetal Dopplers for current wellbeing (this is described in detail in Chapter 25);
- fetal echocardiography, especially if a cardiac aetiology suspected;
- maternal investigations:
  - blood group and blood group antibody screen,
  - serology for parvovirus, cytomegalovirus, toxoplasmosis and coxsackievirus,
  - Kleihauer test for maternal fetal haemorrhage, and
  - other tests as indicated—e.g., anti-SSA and anti-SSB antibodies if bradyarrhythmia identified, haemoglobin electrophoresis if haemoglobinopathy suspected;
- amniocentesis:
  - fetal karyotype,
  - viral polymerase chain reaction (PCR)—cytomegalovirus, parvovirus and coxsackievirus,
  - biochemical assays if indicated,
  - genetic studies if indicated, and
  - DNA storage (for later investigation); and
- fetal blood sampling—primarily indicated if fetal anaemia is suspected.

The management of non-immune hydrops will depend on the primary aetiology or pathophysiology of the condition, the gestational age and the assessment of fetal well being (assessed by ultrasound and/or cardiotocography). Antenatal treatment will depend on the specific cause for the hydrops. Such treatments may include:

- intrauterine transfusion if hydrops is associated with fetal anaemia;
- transplacental anti-arrhythmic medication may be used to treat fetal tachyarrhythmias (e.g., maternal digoxin, flecainide or sotolol);
- pulmonary hypoplasia is a significant issue with long standing hydrops associated with large pleural effusions. Drainage of the effusions may prevent pulmonary hypoplasia if the lungs are still able to grow. Repeated drainage or insertion of thoraco-amniotic shunts may be needed, especially if primary pleural effusion/chylothorax is the cause of the hydrops;
- amniodrainage may be required to prevent preterm labour in the presence of significant polyhydramnios; and
- hydrops in the recipient twin complicating twin-to-twin transfusion syndrome may resolve after selective laser photocoagulation of placental anastomoses.

Delivery may be required if maternal welfare is considered at risk. The method of delivery is dependent upon many factors including maternal condition, fetal condition, the likely prognosis and the safety of vaginal delivery.

Elective preterm delivery is often considered after 34 weeks gestation. Ultimately it is best to consider the difference between doing nothing (i.e., continuing the pregnancy) and delivering early, with regard to the ultimate outcome for the baby including not only mortality but also long-term neurodevelopmental outcome, disability and quality of life. If it is not known that the ultimate outcome will be improved by early delivery (or any intervention) then the fetus should remain *in utero* until it is known.

Termination of pregnancy is often considered an option, particularly for untreatable or idiopathic conditions at less than 24 weeks gestational age.

DELIVERY

Any baby known or suspected to have hydrops fetalis should be delivered in a tertiary level centre with an intensive care nursery and other paediatric subspecialist support (especially paediatric cardiology and/or paediatric surgery if relevant).

MANAGEMENT—POSTNATAL

Babies with severe hydrops will frequently require resuscitation in the delivery room which may involve intubation and mechanical ventilation, and drainage of the pleural and/or peritoneal cavities. All should be admitted to an intensive care nursery.

Once admitted to the nursery the initial management will focus on continued respiratory and circulatory support, as needed, and will involve investigations such as:

- X-rays—chest and abdomen;
- ultrasound scans—chest and abdomen;
- echocardiography;

▶ haematology—full blood count and film, red blood cell enzymes and haemoglobin electrophoresis;
▶ testing for inborn errors of metabolism; and
▶ other tests as indicated to confirm or identify the cause of the hydrops (e.g., lymphoscintigraphy).

A prolonged stay in a hospital may be required before resolution of the effects of generalised oedema. Consultation with other specialists such as cardiologists, nephrologists and haematologists may be required. The longer-term management and recurrence risks will depend upon the identified cause of the hydrops. Review by a geneticist is recommended where genetic or syndromic cases are suspected or, in idiopathic cases, to guide relevant genetic or biochemical testing and to provide advice for future pregnancies.

REFERENCES

1. Santo S, Mansour S, Thilaganathan B, et al. 2011 Prenatal diagnosis of non-immune hydrops fetalis: what do we tell the parents? *Prenat Diagn.* 2011;31:186–195.
2. Bellini C, Hennekam RC, Bonioli E. A diagnostic flow chart for non-immune hydrops fetalis. *Am J Med Genet Part A.* 2009;149A:852–853.

Further Reading

Bellini C, Hennekam RCM, Fulcheri E, et al. Etiology of nonimmune hydrops fetalis: A systematic review. *Am J Med Genet Part A.* 2009;149A:844–851.
de Haan TR, Oepkes D, Beersma MFC, et al. Aetiology, diagnosis and treatment of hydrops foetalis. *Current Pediatric Reviews.* 2005;1:63–72.
Forouzan I. Hydrops fetalis: Recent advances. *Obstet Gynecol Surv.* 1997;52(2):130–138.
Maternal-Fetal Medicine. In: Brodsky D, Martin C, ed. Neonatology Review. Philadelphia: Hanley and Belfus; 2003:1–41.
Sohan K, Carroll SG, De La Fuente S, et al. Analysis of outcome of hydrops fetalis in relation to age at diagnosis, cause and treatment. *Acta Obstet Gynecol Scand.* 2001;80:726–730.

CHAPTER 14
Maternal Diabetes Mellitus

Karen Lust, Luke A Jardine

Diabetes mellitus in pregnancy can be either pre-existing (Type 1 or 2 diabetes mellitus) or gestational diabetes mellitus. The relevant factors are set out below.

Pre-existing diabetes mellitus (type 1 or 2):

- in the presence of symptoms of hyperglycaemia, a single fasting venous glucose ≥7 mmol/L or random venous glucose of ≥11.1 mmol/L is diagnostic of diabetes;
- in the absence of symptoms, an abnormal plasma glucose level requires laboratory confirmation on a subsequent day; and
- an oral glucose tolerance test (GTT) is only needed when the plasma glucose is equivocal on two occasions.

Gestational diabetes mellitus:

- gestational diabetes is glucose intolerance resulting in hyperglycaemia (of variable severity), with the onset or first recognition occurring during pregnancy, which resolves after delivery;
- all pregnant women should undergo testing for gestational diabetes between 26 and 28 weeks of gestation; and
- pregnant women with previously undiagnosed type 2 diabetes mellitus are often mistakenly diagnosed as having gestational diabetes.

PREVALENCE
According to the Australian Bureau of Statistics, the prevalence of diabetes in Australia is:

- type 1–0.4% of the whole population and 0.4% in women of child bearing age;
- type 2–3.5% of the whole population and 1% in women of child bearing age; and
- gestational diabetes—5% of the obstetric population but higher in some ethnic groups (e.g., Asian, Indian).

PRECONCEPTION COUNSELLING
Preconception review and counselling should be offered to all women with pre-existing diabetes. Studies have shown this to be associated with

improvements in diabetic control with fewer maternal and fetal complications associated with pregnancy.

MANAGEMENT—ANTENATAL

Evidence suggests that outcomes are improved if women with pre-existing diabetes mellitus are managed jointly by obstetricians and physicians with expertise in the management of pregnant women with diabetes.[1]

An early dating and viability scan should be offered, as well as a nuchal translucency scan. Regular fetal ultrasounds for growth and liquor volume assessment are generally recommended.

PHYSIOLOGY OF GLUCOSE METABOLISM IN PREGNANCY

Glucose is transported across the placenta and fetal glucose values are approximately 80% of maternal values. Amino acids are actively transported across the placenta.

Pregnancy is normally associated with pancreatic beta cell hyperplasia and increased serum insulin levels in the fasting and fed state. This results in a doubling of the insulin production from the first to the third trimester. Fasting blood glucose levels are 10–15% lower compared to the non-pregnant state and post-prandial blood glucose levels are elevated.

Insulin resistance develops as pregnancy continues due to placental production of hormones (e.g., cortisol, growth hormone, human placental lactogen). This explains the increased insulin requirements in pre-existing diabetes mellitus and the development of gestational diabetes where there is insufficient insulin production to account for the increasing insulin resistance.

Pregnancy is a state of "accelerated starvation"; fasting is associated with a switch from the use of hepatic glycogen for energy production to lipolysis and ketone body formation. Thus, there is an increased risk of diabetic ketoacidosis throughout pregnancy.

FETAL AND NEONATAL EFFECTS OF PRE-EXISTING DIABETES

Poor maternal diabetic control in the first trimester, as evidenced by elevated glycosylated haemoglobin (HbA1C) values, is associated with an increased incidence of congenital abnormalities and spontaneous abortion. Later in pregnancy there is an increased risk of polyhydramnios and pre-eclampsia. The rate of pre-eclampsia is increased in the presence of hypertension with or without nephropathy. The exact molecular mechanisms involved in the development of these complications are uncertain.

Maternal hyperglycaemia is associated with fetal hyperglycaemia. This then results in fetal pancreatic beta cell hyperplasia causing fetal hyperinsulinaemia. Chronic fetal hyperinsulinaemia leads to increased activity of hepatic enzymes, glycogen accumulation in the liver and fat accumulation in adipose tissue. The increased metabolic rate leads to increased oxygen consumption and fetal hypoxaemia. Fetal hypoxaemia stimulates the synthesis of erythropoietin, which can result in polycythaemia and promotes catecholamine production, which can lead to hypertension and cardiac hypertrophy.

Approximately half of all pregnancies will have an uneventful course.

Early Pregnancy Effects

The overall risk of one or more major congenital malformations is 6–7%, which is double the risk compared to the general obstetric population. Infants of women with diabetes appear to be at significantly higher risk of renal agenesis/caudal dysgenesis syndrome, congenital heart defects and neural tube defects. The congenital heart defects which increase in diabetic pregnancy include heterotaxia, tetralogy of Fallot, transposition of the great arteries, septal defects, anomalous pulmonary venous return and various defects causing left or right outflow tract obstruction. Central nervous system defects include anencephaly, spina bifida, encephalocele, hydrocephaly and anotia/microtia. The risks of limb deficiencies, hypospadias and orofacial clefts are also increased.

Late Pregnancy Fetal and Neonatal Effects

Macrosomia is a frequent complication, particularly if there has been poor maternal control. The most serious potential complication of macrosomia is an obstructed delivery. This may result in any or all of the following: traumatic delivery, fractured clavicles, brachial plexus injury, hypoxic ischaemic encephalopathy (HIE) and death. Macrosomia also increases the likelihood that a caesarean delivery will be performed (up to 60% in some studies).

Intrauterine growth restriction (IUGR) can occur in some pregnancies. This carries its own risks and complications (see Chapter 25).

Infants of diabetic mothers have a greater risk of developing respiratory distress syndrome. This is not just related to prematurity. It occurs in term babies as well. Proposed mechanisms include delayed lung maturation, polycythaemia and surfactant inactivation by insulin.

Pregnant women with pre-existing diabetes mellitus have significantly higher rates of both spontaneous preterm delivery (16% for diabetes versus 11% for healthy controls) and preterm delivery for some specific indications (22% for diabetes versus 3% for healthy controls).[2]

Polycythaemia can occur in up to 40% of babies. Hyperviscosity syndrome secondary to polycythaemia occurs more rarely. Hypocalcaemia, hypomagnesaemia and hyperbilirubinaemia are also more common in infants of diabetic mothers.

Hypertrophic cardiomyopathy predominantly affects the intraventricular septum and may cause outflow tract obstruction. Severe cases have been associated with neonatal death. However, in most cases it is transient and resolves over the first few months of life.

Neonatal hypoglycaemia is a frequent finding in babies and often requires management in the neonatal period. Hypoglycaemia has been associated with increased risk of neurodevelopmental impairment; however, the lower limit of blood glucose and/or duration of hypoglycaemia before damage occurs are controversial.

Long-Term Effects
Long-term neurodevelopmental outcome may be difficult to predict. It may be adversely affected by the presence of congenital anomalies or perinatal complications. In general, babies born to mothers with well controlled diabetes in pregnancy have a good neurodevelopmental outcome.

There is a risk of diabetes mellitus developing in the child in later life:[3]
▶ the risk of type 1 diabetes mellitus developing by 20 years of age:
  • if the mother has type 1 diabetes mellitus is 1.3%, and
  • if the father has type 1 diabetes mellitus is 6.1%; and
▶ the risk of type 2 diabetes mellitus (if the mother has type 2 diabetes mellitus) depends on multifactorial inheritance. There is an increased relative risk of offspring developing type 2 diabetes mellitus later in life. The risk also depends on the presence of classical clinical risk factors for diabetes mellitus.

FETAL AND NEONATAL EFFECTS OF GESTATIONAL DIABETES MELLITUS
Babies who are born to mothers with gestational diabetes mellitus can have any of the late complications outlined above but generally have a lower incidence. The risk of complications relates to the adequacy of blood glucose control. Maternal obesity also increases the risk of these complications but independently of the diabetes.[4]

Children born to mothers with gestational diabetes mellitus have nearly double the risk of developing childhood obesity and/or metabolic syndrome compared to children born to non-diabetic mothers.[5]

There is a growing body of evidence suggesting that the risk of many of these consequences can be significantly reduced or eliminated by aggressive treatment of gestational diabetes mellitus.

DELIVERY
If a major abnormality has been detected, the baby should be delivered at a hospital which has the required facilities (e.g., paediatric cardiology).

Each maternity centre should have protocols for the management of maternal diabetes in labour. Management protocols differ depending on the mode of delivery. Maternal blood glucose levels (BGL) should be checked regularly (hourly to second hourly depending on the type of maternal diabetes mellitus) in labour to maintain normoglycaemia as this is associated with improved fetal oxygenation and acid–base balance.

POSTNATAL CARE

The basic principles of management in the neonate include:

◗ prevention of hypoglycaemia;

◗ detection of those babies who become hypoglycaemic; and

◗ treatment of the babies that are hypoglycaemic.

If the baby is well, the baby should initially receive routine care. Early initiation of feeding within 30–60 minutes of birth is recommended. There is no evidence to suggest improved outcome with any of the following: "routine" admission to a neonatal unit, "routine" supplementation or replacement of breast feeds with formula, delayed skin-to-skin contact and first feed, or testing the blood glucose level too soon after delivery.[6]

The baby should be examined for signs of macrosomia and monitored for hypoglycaemia. Reported signs and symptoms of hypoglycaemia include tremors/jitteriness, pallor, poor feeding/feed intolerance, irritability, hypothermia, high pitched cry, sweating, temperature instability, tachycardia, apnoea with cyanosis, hypotonia, changes in level of consciousness and seizures.

The blood glucose level should be checked shortly after birth and regularly thereafter until normal and stable. The frequency of blood glucose levels in the well baby varies between institutions. The most conservative regimen tests blood glucose levels at 1 hour, 2 hours and 4 hours of age, then every 4 hours for 24 hours until normal and stable.

Any unwell or symptomatic baby should have their blood glucose level checked immediately.

If the infant of a diabetic mother is symptomatic or has hypoglycaemia then admission to the nursery is usually required for intravenous dextrose and possibly other medications (e.g., glucagon, diazoxide).

REFERENCES

1. McElduff A, Cheung N, McIntyre D, et al. Position Statement: The Australasian Diabetes in Pregnancy Society consensus guidelines for the management of type 1 and type 2 diabetes in relation to pregnancy. *MJA*. 2005;183(7):373–377.

2. Sibai B, Caritis S, Hauth J, et al. Preterm delivery in women with pregestational diabetes mellitus or chronic hypertension relative to women with uncomplicated pregnancies. The National institute of Child health and Human Development Maternal-Fetal Medicine Units Network. *Am J Obstet Gynecol*. 2000;183:1520.

3. Powrie R, Green MF, Cammann W, eds. de Swiet's Medical Disorders in Obstetric Practice. 5th ed. Melbourne: Wiley-Blackwell; 2010.

4. Reece EA. The fetal and maternal consequences of gestational diabetes mellitus. *Journal of Maternal-Fetal and Neonatal Medicine*. 2010;23(3):199–203.

5. Vohr BR, Boney CM. Gestational diabetes: the forerunner for the development of maternal and childhood obesity and metabolic syndrome? *J Matern Fetal Neonatal Med*. 2008;21:149–157.

6. Hawdon JM. Babies born after diabetes in pregnancy: what are the short- and long-term risks and how can we minimise them? *Best Practice & Research Clinical Obstetrics and Gynaecology*. 2011;25(1):91–104.

Further Reading

Australian Institute of Health and Welfare 2010. Diabetes in pregnancy: its impact on Australian women and their babies. Diabetes series no. 14. Cat. no. CVD 52. Canberra: AIHW; 2010.

De Luca AKC, Nakazawa CY, Azevedo BC, et al. Influence of glycemic control on fetal lung maturity in gestations affected by diabetes or mild hyperglycemia. *Acta Obstetricia et Gynecologica Scandinavica.* 2009;88(9):1036–1040.

Deshpande S, Platt MW. The investigation and management of neonatal hypoglycaemia. *Seminars in Fetal and Neo Med.* 2005;10(4):351–361.

Greene M. Spontaneous abortions and major malformations in women with diabetes mellitus. *Semin Reprod Endocrinol.* 1999;17:127.

Hoffman L, Nolan C, Wilson JD, et al. Gestational diabetes mellitus: management guidelines. The Australasian Diabetes in Pregnancy Society. *Med J Aust.* 1998;169(2):93–97.

Kitzmiller J. Sweet success with diabetes. The development of insulin therapy and glycemic control for pregnancy. *Diabetes Care.* 1993;16(Suppl 3):107.

Levene M, Tudehope D, Sinha S. Endocrine and Metabolic Disorders. In: Levene M, Tudehope D, Sinha S, eds. *Essential Neonatal Medicine.* 4th ed. Carlton: Blackwell Publishing; 2008:157–175.

Standards of medical care in diabetes-2010. American Diabetes Association. *Diabetes Care.* 2010 January;33(suppl 1):S11–S61.

Widness JA, Teramo KA, Clemons GK, et al. Direct relationship of antepartum glucose control and fetal erythropoietin in human type 1 (insulin-dependent) diabetic pregnancy. *Diabetologia.* 1990;33(6):378–383.

World Health Organization. Definition, diagnosis and classification of diabetes mellitus and its complications. Report of a WHO consultation. Part 1: Diagnosis and classification of diabetes mellitus. Geneva: World Health Organization; 1999. WHO/NCD/NCS/99.2.

CHAPTER 15

Maternal Thyroid Disease

Sarah McMahon, Zsuzsoka Kecskes

Maternal thyroid disease can cause abnormalities of thyroid function in newborn infants. This can be due to maternal antithyroid antibodies transferred to the fetus (thyroid stimulating antibodies or thyroid blocking antibodies or both), the state of maternal thyroid function during the pregnancy or any treatment the mother has had for her thyroid disease during the pregnancy.

MATERNAL HYPERTHYROIDISM
Definition
Women with hyperthyroidism have subnormal thyroid stimulating hormone (TSH) concentration and elevated free thyroxine (T4) and free triiodothyronine (T3) concentrations.

Maternal symptoms and signs of hyperthyroidism, with or without Graves' disease, include tachycardia, warm moist skin, tremor, goitre and/or ophthalmopathy.

Aetiology
Graves' disease, mediated by anti-TSH receptor antibodies (TRAb), accounts for 85% of cases of maternal hyperthyroidism.[1] Other causes include single toxic adenomas, multinodular toxic goitres and thyroiditis.

Prevalence
Maternal hyperthyroidism occurs in 0.1–0.4% of pregnancies.[1]

Differential Diagnosis
Gestational thyrotoxicosis is a self-limiting condition sometimes seen in the first half of pregnancy (<15% of pregnancies). It is not due to thyroid disease and resolves spontaneously by 20 weeks. Gestational thyrotoxicosis is associated with hyperemesis gravidarum. The hyperthyroidism will rarely require treatment.[2]

Associated Abnormalities
Other autoimmune diseases in the mother need to be considered whenever hyperthyroidism is found.

Consequences
The effects of maternal hyperthyroidism on the fetus include intrauterine growth restriction, fetal goitre, tachycardia, hydrops associated with heart

failure, preterm delivery or fetal death.[1,3] The risk of fetal death can be as high as 50% if the mother has hyperthyroidism that is not treated; this risk decreases to normal if she is adequately treated.[4]

Up to 5% of babies born to mothers with hyperthyroidism can have neonatal hyperthyroidism due to transplacental transfer of stimulating anti-TSH receptor antibodies. Babies with hyperthyroidism can have warm moist skin, tachycardia, arrhythmias, hyperphagia, poor weight gain, diarrhoea, irritability and/or craniosynostosis. The risk of hyperthyroidism is increased:

▶ in women currently requiring anti-thyroid drug treatment or with anti-TSH receptor antibody levels greater than 150–500% of control values;
▶ if there is a previously affected baby;[1,5] and
▶ in infants of currently euthyroid mothers who have previously been treated with thyroidectomy or radio-iodine, but who are positive for anti-TSH receptor antibodies.[1]

The risk of neonatal hyperthyroidism is decreased if mothers are negative for anti-TSH receptor antibodies and do not require anti-thyroid medication.

Transient hypothyroidism in the neonate is possible due to transplacental transfer of inhibitory anti-TSH receptor antibodies. Transient hypothalamic-pituitary hypothyroidism has also been described in infants of mothers with poorly controlled Graves' disease.[6]

Management—Antenatal
All pregnant women with hyperthyroidism should have their anti-TSH receptor antibodies measured in early pregnancy.

For mothers on anti-thyroid drug treatment, the aim is to decrease free thyroxine levels to the upper end of the normal range. A potential side effect is fetal hypothyroidism and goitre.[7]

The anti-thyroid drugs used include:
▶ propylthiouracil (first line); and
▶ carbimazole (or methimazole, a metabolite of carbimazole)—its use is associated with teratogenicity: aplasia cutis, choanal atresia, oesophageal atresia and situs inversus.[1,5]

If the mother is anti-TSH receptor antibody positive or is on anti-thyroid drugs, the fetus should be monitored with a monthly ultrasound for goitre, heart rate and growth parameters.[1]

Management—Labour / Delivery / Immediate Postnatal Management
Delivery should be planned according to the usual considerations of maternal and fetal well being. Delivery should be planned in a regional centre that has a paediatrician.

The newborn infant should be examined soon after birth for goitre (may be due to neonatal Graves' disease, or hypothyroidism from maternal anti-thyroid drugs), and signs of hyperthyroidism (fever, tachycardia, vomiting). The baby should also be observed in hospital for a few days for the development of these signs.

Postnatal Management

The risk of neonatal hyperthyroidism is based on the presence of anti-TSH receptor antibodies; i.e., past or present Graves' disease (even if the mother has had a thyroidectomy or radioiodine treatment). This does not apply if there is a history of hyperthyroidism secondary to Hashimoto's thyroiditis with negative anti-TSH receptor antibodies. Therefore, if the maternal anti-TSH receptor antibody levels were high at 30 weeks gestation, then the baby's thyroid function tests should be done at six hours of age.[3] Repeat thyroid function tests should be done after several days and after two weeks as neonatal Graves' disease may initially be masked by transplacental transfer of anti-thyroid drugs.[3] Hyperthyroidism has been diagnosed as late as the third week of life in infants whose mothers were treated with anti-thyroid drugs.[6]

The normal newborn screening test should be collected as usual.

If any of these tests are abnormal the baby should be referred to a paediatric endocrinologist. If the neonate is found to be hyperthyroid, treatment with carbimazole should be commenced. Propylthiouracil has been associated with liver failure in children and should therefore be avoided.

Neonatal Graves' disease will usually resolve after approximately 3–12 weeks, but occasionally may last up to 6 months.[2]

Monitor thyroid function tests intermittently in breastfed neonates whose mothers are treated with anti-thyroid drugs; although the risk of hypothyroidism is very low.[3] Breast feeding is not contraindicated as long as the doses of carbimazole, methimazole or propylthiouracil can be kept moderate (propylthiouracil <250–300 mg/day, methimazole <20 mg/day).[8]

Recurrence

Any of the problems noted above may recur with subsequent pregnancies.

MATERNAL HYPOTHYROIDISM
Definition

It is very important to use gestational age-specific reference ranges to interpret maternal thyroid function tests.

Pregnant women can have varying degrees of hypothyroidism:

▶ overt hypothyroidism—elevated thyroid stimulating hormone (TSH), i.e., >2.5 micro-units/mL in first trimester or >3.0 micro-units/mL in the second or third trimesters, and low free thyroxine level;

▶ subclinical hypothyroidism—elevated thyroid stimulating hormone (TSH) with a normal free thyroxine level; and

▶ hypothyroxinaemia—normal thyroid stimulating hormone (TSH) with a free thyroxine level at the lower end of the normal range.

Maternal symptoms and signs of hypothyroidism are only present in around 20% of cases. These include a firm, painless goitre and any of the typical signs of hypothyroidism.

Aetiology

In developed countries, the leading causes of hypothyroidism are autoimmune and these are associated with elevated thyroid peroxidase and thyroglobulin antibodies (TPO-Ab and Tg-Ab).[1]

Hypothyroidism can also be secondary to treatment of hyperthyroidism (i.e., radio-iodine or surgery).

Hypothalamic-pituitary causes are less common (note: TSH will be low in these cases).

Worldwide, iodine deficiency is the most common cause of hypothyroidism.[1]

Prevalence

Overt hypothyroidism occurs in 0.3–0.5% of pregnancies.[1] Subclinical hypothyroidism is more common, occurring in 2–3% of pregnancies.

Associated Abnormalities

Other autoimmune conditions in the mother need to be considered.

Consequences

The consequences of untreated cases of overt hypothyroidism include:

- obstetric complications, e.g., breech presentation;
- fetal complications, e.g., preterm delivery, intrauterine growth restriction, respiratory distress, fetal or perinatal death (the increased risk of fetal or perinatal death has not been seen in all studies);[1] and
- maternal thyroid hormone is necessary for early fetal brain development and there is an increased risk of developmental delay and learning disabilities.[1]

If there is suboptimal treatment of overt hypothyroidism then some areas of intelligence may be affected.[1]

In cases of subclinical hypothyroidism, there is an increased risk of adverse obstetric outcomes (e.g., abruption, preterm delivery, intrauterine growth restriction, hypertension—similar risks but less frequent than in overt hypothyroidism) and impaired neurodevelopmental outcome.[2]

Prolonged hypothyroxinaemia may also result in developmental problems in infancy and/or mild expressive language delay.[9]

Autoimmune thyroid disease can result in transient hypothyroidism in the neonate (2–3% may require thyroxine treatment).[10]

Hashimoto's thyroiditis is a very common autoimmune disease. In the presence of maternal Hashimoto's thyroiditis, there are usually no consequences for the fetal thyroid.

Management—Antenatal

Ideally, maternal hypothyroidism should be treated prior to pregnancy aiming for a thyroid stimulating hormone (TSH) level of ≤2.5 micro-units/mL.[1]

Pregnant women usually require an increase in thyroxine dose of 30–50% by 4–6 weeks of gestation.[1] They should be monitored more frequently (e.g., every 8 weeks).[2]

The thyroid stimulating hormone (TSH) level should be maintained at <2.5 micro-units/mL in the first trimester and <3.0 micro-units/mL in the second and third trimesters.

If the hypothyroidism is diagnosed after the first trimester, then thyroid function should be optimised as soon as possible and the parents advised regarding the possible intellectual problems.[1]

The treatment of subclinical hypothyroidism may improve obstetric outcomes.[1]

Management—Labour / Delivery / Immediate Postnatal Management

There is an increased risk of pre-eclampsia and chronic hypertension. Delivery should be planned according to the usual considerations of maternal and fetal well being. Delivery should be planned in a regional centre that has a paediatrician.

Management—Postnatal

The normal newborn screening test should be collected as usual. This will include a thyroid stimulating hormone (TSH) level.[10]

Thyroid function tests should be done at 2–4 weeks of age.[10] If thyroid function is persistently abnormal, the baby will require thyroxine treatment.[10]

If any of these tests are abnormal, the baby should be referred to a paediatric endocrinologist.

Infants of mothers with untreated or undertreated hypothyroidism in pregnancy should have long-term follow-up by a paediatrician for developmental problems. If the baby has transient hypothyroidism that is treated appropriately, they should not need developmental follow-up.

Recurrence

The mother is likely to require ongoing thyroxine following pregnancy and in subsequent pregnancies.

REFERENCES

1. Abalovich M, Amino N, Barbour LA, et al. Management of thyroid dysfunction during pregnancy and postpartum: an Endocrine Society Clinical Practice Guideline. *J Clin Endocrinol Metab.* 2007;92:S1–S47.
2. Rashid M, Rashid MH. Obstetric management of thyroid disease. *Obstet Gynecol Surv.* 2007;62:680–688.

3. Marx H, Amin P, Lazarus JH. Hyperthyroidism and pregnancy. *BMJ*. 2008;336:663–667.

4. LeBeau SO, Mandel SJ. Thyroid disorders during pregnancy. *Endocrinol Metab Clin N Am*. 2006;35:117–136.

5. Clementi M, Di Gianantonio E, Cassina M, et al. Treatment of hyperthyroidism in pregnancy and birth defects. *J Clin Endocrinol Metab*. 2010;95:E337–E341.

6. Papendieck P, Chiesa A, Prieto L, et al. Thyroid disorders of neonates born to mothers with Graves' disease. *J Pediatr Endocrinol Metab*. 2009;22:547–553.

7. Rosenfeld H, Ornoy A, Shechtman S, et al. Pregnancy outcome, thyroid dysfunction and fetal goitre after in utero exposure to propylthiouracil: a controlled cohort study. *Br J Clin Pharmacol*. 2009;68:609–617.

8. Muller AF, Drexhage HA, Berghout A. Postpartum thyroiditis and autoimmune thyroiditis in women of childbearing age: recent insights and consequences for antenatal and postnatal care. *Endocrine Reviews*. 2001;22:605–630.

9. Henrichs J, Bongers-Schokking JJ, Schenk JJ, et al. Maternal thyroid function during early pregnancy and cognitive functioning in early childhood: the generation R study. *J Clin Endocrinol Metab*. 2010;95:4227–4234.

10. Rovelli R, Vigone MC, Giovanettoni C, et al. Newborn of mothers affected by autoimmune thyroiditis: the importance of thyroid function monitoring in the first months of life. *Italian Journal of Pediatrics*. 2010;36:24.

Meryta May, Maureen Dingwall

Cytomegalovirus (CMV) is a herpes virus which can be transmitted transplacentally from an infected mother to her fetus.

EPIDEMIOLOGY

The seroconversion rate for cytomegalovirus in the general population is approximately 2–3% per annum. This rate is higher in childcare workers (11% per annum), teachers and parents with a child in daycare (20–30% per annum).

Transmission is by close physical contact; e.g., sexual contact, sharing drinks or food, transplacental, changing soiled nappies, contact with saliva or through breast milk.

The risk of reactivation of cytomegalovirus and transmission to the fetus is increased by maternal immunocompromise, including maternal human immunodeficiency virus (HIV).

Congenital Cytomegalovirus

In Australia, congenital cytomegalovirus affects 0.3–2% of live births or 3–6 in 1000 births per annum.

If infection occurs during pregnancy:

‣ the risk of fetal infection is greatest with primary maternal infection—the mean transmission rate is 50% (ranging from 30–40% in first trimester to 70–80% in the third trimester); and

‣ reactivation or reinfection in the mother has a risk of fetal infection of 1% and these infants are rarely symptomatic.

If infection occurs pre-conception:

‣ the risk of congenital cytomegalovirus following documented cytomegalovirus seroconversion is about 13% (this risk declines to background levels, about 1%, over the 2–4 years following seroconversion, the risk being highest in the first 2 years); and

‣ routine screening for cytomegalovirus antibodies in pregnancy is not advisable due to the asymptomatic nature of most cytomegalovirus infections, and the frequency of non-specific cytomegalovirus IgM titres in the general population—without a documented clinical illness, it is usually impossible to determine if a cytomegalovirus infection has occurred in the previous few years.

OUTCOME

Fetal damage is highest during primary maternal infection in the first 20 weeks of pregnancy. Infection in the first half of pregnancy is more likely to lead to neurological sequelae. Infection in the second half of pregnancy is more likely to lead to visceral disease (e.g., hepatitis, pneumonia, thrombocytopaenia).

At delivery, 90% of infected babies are asymptomatic at birth and 10% are symptomatic at birth.

Of those babies that are asymptomatic at birth, 10% will develop symptoms:

▶ chorioretinitis (2%); and
▶ sensorineural hearing loss (5%)—this can be bilateral or unilateral, and is progressive in 57% (up to five years of age)—sensorineural hearing loss due to congenital cytomegalovirus **cannot** be excluded by a normal newborn hearing screening test.

For those babies that are symptomatic at birth, the severity of the disease varies from transient hepatomegaly, jaundice and thrombocytopaenia, to severe mental retardation, blindness and death. Features can include:

▶ 10–30% mortality;
▶ neurological sequelae—microcephaly (30–50%), seizures (10%), chorioretinitis (10–20%), mental retardation (60–70%), sensorineural hearing loss (25–50%);
▶ ascites, hydrops, oligo- or polyhydramnios, pseudomeconium ileus, hydrocephalus, intrauterine growth restriction, pleural or pericardial effusions;
▶ intracranial calcification; and
▶ intra-abdominal calcification.

DIAGNOSIS

Maternal

Cytomegalovirus infection is diagnosed in the mother when there is a significant rise or a seroconversion in paired serological samples taken at least 2 weeks apart. Caution is needed in interpreting single serological samples as low levels of cytomegalovirus IgM may persist for months or years after primary infection.

Fetal

Fetal cytomegalovirus infection can be diagnosed with a polymerase chain reaction (PCR) test of amniotic fluid obtained after 20 weeks gestation. Testing earlier is associated with false negatives. A negative result after 20 weeks gestation generally excludes fetal infection. If there is a positive result a quantitative polymerase chain reaction (PCR) test should be done. A higher cytomegalovirus viral load in the amniotic fluid is associated with a higher risk of symptomatic disease in the infant.

A normal antenatal ultrasound does not exclude abnormalities. The signs on fetal ultrasound are not predictive of the degree of fetal damage. Possible findings include:

◗ microcephaly;
◗ intracranial calcification;
◗ intrauterine growth restriction;
◗ hydrocephalus;
◗ hydrops;
◗ oligohydramnios; and
◗ polyhydramnios.

Postnatal

Infection can be diagnosed with urine cytomegalovirus polymerase chain reaction (PCR) test within 21 days of delivery. The serum can be tested for cytomegalovirus polymerase chain reaction (PCR) or cytomegalovirus IgM (there is a significant rate of false negatives with IgM).

If the baby is older than 21 days, the diagnosis can be confirmed by cytomegalovirus polymerase chain reaction (PCR) test of blood collected on the neonatal screening test card that is routinely collected on all infants at about five days of age.

MANAGEMENT
Antenatal

Cytomegalovirus infection is best prevented in the first place. Transmission in an occupational setting is usually prevented by strict adherence to universal precautions, especially hand hygiene. Transmission within the home (often by an older toddler to the expectant mother) is less easily avoided.

There is a non-randomised, case-controlled study where it was suggested that cytomegalovirus immunoglobulin given during an affected pregnancy may ameliorate or even prevent fetal damage.[1] A large trial in the USA is currently ongoing to investigate this more fully.

Currently in Australia, cytomegalovirus immunoglobulin (CSL) is available (via the Australian Red Cross Blood Bank Service) on a case-by-case compassionate-use basis for treatment of proven intrauterine cytomegalovirus infection. This should not be considered as routine treatment.

Currently there is no role for the use of ganciclovir in the fetus due its toxicity.

Postnatal

Resuscitation should proceed as for any baby. The initial management is supportive especially for any thrombocytopaenia, hepatitis and pneumonia. These conditions generally improve spontaneously within the first few weeks of life.

If the baby is well it should stay with the mother in the postnatal ward. The following investigations should be done:

▶ urine cytomegalovirus polymerase chain reaction (PCR) test;
▶ send serum for cytomegalovirus polymerase chain reaction (PCR) and cytomegalovirus IgM;
▶ full blood count film examination—10–50% have haemolytic anaemia, 50% have thrombocytopaenia;
▶ liver function tests, including serum bilirubin;
▶ ophthalmology review;
▶ audiology assessment—at birth, 6 months and annually until 5 years old;
▶ head ultrasound scan—especially looking for hydrocephalus; and
▶ also consider a computed tomography (CT) scan and/or magnetic resonance imaging (MRI) of the brain—head ultrasounds are not sensitive for detecting intracranial calcification and cerebral atrophy.

Evidence for the definitive benefit of ganciclovir treatment in congenital cytomegalovirus is lacking. Ganciclovir use in congenital cytomegalovirus is currently restricted to the treatment of cytomegalovirus retinitis or severe, life-threatening multi-organ disease in the newborn. Treatment requires a 6-week course of intravenous therapy followed by oral valganciclovir for up to 12 months. Ganciclovir is associated with marrow suppression (neutropenia) and renal impairment. Studies in this area are ongoing.

Long-term developmental follow-up by a general paediatrician is required.

RISK OF RECURRENCE
As discussed above, the risk of fetal infection with primary maternal infection occurring during pregnancy is about 50%. The risk of congenital cytomegalovirus in a subsequent pregnancy in the years following documented cytomegalovirus seroconversion is about 13%:

▶ this risk declines to background levels (1%) over the 2–4 years following seroconversion; and
▶ the risk is highest in the first 2 years following seroconversion.

For parents of a child who is known to have congenital cytomegalovirus (symptomatic or asymptomatic), follow-up counselling regarding subsequent pregnancies should occur as part of the mother's postnatal obstetric review.

REFERENCE
1. Nigro G, Adler SP, LaTorre R, et al. Passive immunisation during pregnancy for congenital cytomegalovirus infection. Congenital Cytomegalovirus Collaborating Group. *N Engl J Med*. 2005;353:1350–1362.

Further Reading
Adler S, Nigro G, Pereira L. Recent advances in the Prevention and Treatment of Congenital Cytomegalovirus Infections. *Semin Perinatol*. 2007; 31:10–18.
Palasanthiran P, Starr M, Jones C, eds. Management of Perinatal Infections. Sydney: Australasian Society for Infectious Diseases; 2002 (Emendations 2006):1–4.

CHAPTER 17

Toxoplasma

Clare Nourse, Fiona Hutchinson

Toxoplasmosis is caused by the parasitic protozoa *Toxoplasma gondii*. Infection is asymptomatic or unremarkable in immunocompetent individuals, but leads to a lifelong antibody response. During pregnancy, toxoplasma can be transmitted across the placenta and may cause fetal infection.

Fetal infection is diagnosed if the following criteria are met:

▶ confirmation of acute infection during pregnancy—i.e., seroconversion and/or serology which is IgM positive, IgA positive, low IgG avidity (with or without symptoms of infection);
AND

▶ confirmation of infection in the fetus—i.e., positive toxoplasma polymerase chain reaction (PCR) from amniotic fluid (with or without abnormalities on fetal ultrasound).

AETIOLOGY

Toxoplasma gondii infection is acquired by pregnant women primarily through ingestion of cysts in infected, undercooked meat or ingestion of oocysts that may contaminate soil, water and food. Transmission to the fetus occurs predominantly in women who acquire their primary infection during pregnancy. In rare cases, congenital transmission has occurred in chronically infected women whose infection was reactivated because of their immunocompromised state (e.g., from acquired immunodeficiency syndrome (AIDS) or treatment with corticosteroids for an underlying disease).

PREVALENCE

In Australia, primary infection with toxoplasma during pregnancy is rare and congenital toxoplasmosis is very rare; there are no conclusive data on the rate of fetal infection. There have only been one or two confirmed congenital cases per year.

In Europe, the overall rate of fetal infection in mothers infected during pregnancy is about 17%.

It is likely that there are asymptomatic cases that may develop retinitis later in life.

CONSEQUENCES OF INFECTION AND ASSOCIATED ABNORMALITIES

The risk of abnormalities related to congenital infection depends on the gestation at the time of maternal infection and the duration of follow-up and treatment of the infant.

Table 17.1 *Toxoplasma gondii* congenital infection risk and the proportion of infants with clinical signs by gestational age at the time of maternal infection

Gestational Age of Fetus at the Time of Maternal Infection (Weeks)	Proportion with Congenital Infection %	Proportion of those Infected with Clinical Signs by Age 3 Years %
13	6	61
26	40	25
36	72	9

Source: Data are from Montoya and Remington 2008; 603 women with *Toxoplasma gondii* infection during pregnancy (84% had anti-toxoplasma treatment).

The frequency of vertical transmission increases with the gestational age but severely affected fetuses are more commonly seen in women whose infection was acquired early in gestation. The approximate risks according to gestation at the time of maternal infection were studied by Montoya and Remington.[1] The congenital infection rate and the proportion of infants with clinical signs are shown in Table 17.1.

The majority of congenitally infected infants are asymptomatic at birth. Features of symptomatic congenital infection include:
▶ chorioretinitis or retinal scarring;
▶ intracranial calcification;
▶ hydrocephalus;
▶ hepatospenomegaly;
▶ pneumonia;
▶ thrombocytopaenia;
▶ lymphadenopathy; and
▶ myocarditis.

The presentation of those clinically affected can vary and ranges from mild ocular damage to severe intellectual and physical disability. Congenital toxoplasmosis may present as subclinical disease, which may evolve and lead to neurological or ophthalmological disease later in life.

In large European cohorts:
▶ most women are treated if infected during pregnancy;
▶ if the fetus has a cerebral ultrasound abnormality, consideration is usually given to termination of pregnancy (the presence of a brain abnormality on fetal ultrasound usually results in an abnormal postnatal brain ultrasound and the risk of poor neurodevelopmental outcome is very high);
▶ infected babies are treated postnatally; and
▶ approximately three-quarters of infected newborns will have normal neurodevelopmental follow-up and a quarter will develop chorioretinitis

(the overwhelming majority will have normal vision). Significantly adverse neurodevelopmental outcomes occur in less than 2% (given that most pregnancies with abnormal fetal brain scans are terminated).[2–4]

The proportion of children with poor neurodevelopmental outcomes is increased if the mother is not treated.[5, 6]

ANTENATAL MANAGEMENT

Investigations to be considered following confirmation of recent maternal toxoplasmosis include:
- fetal ultrasound to detect abnormalities; and
- amniocentisis at 18–20 weeks gestation for toxoplasma polymerase chain reaction (PCR) testing—ideally PCR should be done ≥4 weeks after maternal infection.

If the amniocentesis PCR is positive, the parents should be counselled regarding continuing the pregnancy.

Treatment of maternal infection is complex and specialist infectious disease input is recommended. The medications used include pyrimethamine, sulfadiazine and spiramycin. Different doses, regimens and agents are indicated at different gestations.

If the fetus is severely affected, and the parents opt to continue the pregnancy, then the option of not initiating advanced life support at birth should be considered and discussed in advance with the parents. Comfort care would be provided for the baby under these circumstances.

OTHER CONSULTS REQUIRED

The mother should be seen by a paediatric infectious diseases specialist.

PERINATAL MANAGEMENT

Delivery should be planned in a regional centre that has a paediatrician. If there are abnormalities seen on a fetal ultrasound, then a member of the paediatric staff should attend the delivery.

The placenta should be examined and sent for pathology including histology and polymerase chain reaction (PCR) testing.

The baby should be assessed for clinical evidence of congenital toxoplasmosis (see above).

POSTNATAL MANAGEMENT

The majority of babies, including infected babies, will be asymptomatic but require careful assessment.

If well, the baby can be nursed with its mother with standard precautions. (The parasites can be excreted in urine and other bodily fluids.) Breast feeding is safe.

The following tests should be done:
- whole blood for toxoplasma polymerase chain reaction (PCR) testing;
- serology for toxoplasma—IgM, IgA, IgG;

▶ cerebro-spinal fluid for toxoplasma polymerase chain reaction (PCR) testing; and
▶ cerebral ultrasound.

An ophthalmologist should see the baby soon after birth. The eyes will need to be followed up for at least 10 years.

If the clinical assessment is normal, and all of the above investigations are negative and the baby is deemed to be uninfected, then repeat the toxoplasma IgG at 6 months of age (by 6 months maternal IgG in the baby is no longer detectable). If negative, no further follow-up is required.

If any of the above investigations suggest infection (i.e., IgM positive, polymerase chain reaction (PCR) positive, baby's IgG titre is significantly higher than mother's at birth or IgG is positive at 6 months of age) then anti-toxoplasma treatment should be considered.

Treatment has not been proven beneficial in clinical trials but is generally recommended. The usual recommendation is 12 months treatment with pyrimethamine and sulphadoxine (plus folinic acid) either continuously or alternating with spiramycin.

The baby should be seen by a paediatric infectious diseases specialist.

RECURRENCE RISK
Recurrence in future pregnancies is unlikely as antibody responses provide long-term protection. Reactivation and recurrence can occur in immunosuppressed pregnant women.

ETHICS
Ethical issues arise following confirmation of fetal infection. Fetal infection in early pregnancy is associated with a high risk of sequelae in the infant. The option of terminating of pregnancy needs to be discussed.

REFERENCES
1. Montoya JG, Remington JS. Management of *Toxoplasma gondii* Infection during Pregnancy. *Clinical Infectious Diseases*. 2008;47(4):554–566.
2. Berrebi A, Bardou M, Bessieres MH, et al. Outcome for children infected with congenital toxoplasmosis in the first trimester and with normal ultrasound findings: a study of 36 cases. *European Journal of Obstetrics, Gynecology, & Reproductive Biology*. 2007;135(1):53–57.
3. Berrebi A, Assouline C, Bessieres MH, et al. Long-term outcome of children with congenital toxoplasmosis. *American Journal of Obstetrics & Gynecology*. 2010. 203(6):552.e1–e6.
4. Freeman K, Tan HK, Prusa A, et al. European Multicentre Study on Congenital Toxoplasmosis. Predictors of retinochoroiditis in children with congenital toxoplasmosis: European, prospective cohort study. *BMC Pediatrics*. 2008;121(5):e1215–e1222.
5. Cortina-Borja M, Tan HK, Wallon M, et al. European Multicentre Study on Congenital Toxoplasmosis (EMSCOT). Prenatal treatment for serious neurological sequelae of congenital toxoplasmosis: an observational prospective cohort study. *PLoS Medicine*. 2010;7(10).

6. Gras L, Wallon M, Pollak A, et al. The European Multicenter Study On Congenital Toxoplasmosis. Association between prenatal treatment and clinical manifestations of congenital toxoplasmosis in infancy: A cohort study in 13 European centres. *Acta Pædiatrica*. 2005;94:1721–1731.

Further Reading

Cortina-Borja M, Tan HK, Wallon M, et al. European Multicentre Study on Congenital Toxoplasmosis (EMSCOT). Prenatal treatment for serious neurological sequelae of congenital toxoplasmosis: an observational prospective cohort study. *PLoS Medicine*. 2010;7(10).

Dunn D, Wallon M, Peyron F, et al. Mother-to-child transmission of toxoplasmosis: risk estimates for clinical counselling. *Lancet*. 1999;353:1829–1833.

Palasanthiran P, Starr M, Jones C, eds. Management of Perinatal Infections. Sydney: Australasian Society for Infectious Diseases; 2002 (Emendations 2006):39–41.

CHAPTER 18

Herpes Simplex Virus

Clare Nourse, Fiona Hutchinson

Neonatal herpes simplex virus infection is an infection with a high morbidity and mortality which is most commonly acquired by babies at or near the time of delivery. The clinical illness is classified into three subgroups:
- disease localised to skin, eye and mouth;
- local central nervous system (CNS) disease (encephalitis alone); and
- disseminated infection with multiple organ involvement.

AETIOLOGY

Neonatal herpes virus infection may be caused by herpes simplex virus type 1 (HSV-1) or herpes simplex virus type 2 (HSV-2). Either viral type can cause genital herpes (HSV-2 is more likely) and be transmitted via maternal genital secretions to infant. Either type can cause non-genital infection and be transmitted via skin and mucous membrane contact. The risk of perinatal transmission to the neonate may be higher with HSV-1 than with HSV-2.[1]

Neonatal infection occurs most commonly at the time of delivery via contact with infected maternal genital secretions (85% of neonatal herpes simplex virus infections). Infection can also occur *in utero* (1–5%), i.e., congenital herpes; or postnatally via contact with an infected caregiver (10–15%).

The risks of maternal to neonatal transmission are greatest (30–50%) when a woman acquires a new infection (primary genital herpes) in the third trimester, particularly within six weeks of delivery, as viral shedding may persist and the baby is likely to be born before the development of protective maternal antibodies.[1,2]

Recurrent maternal genital herpes is associated with a very low risk of neonatal herpes infection (1–3% if shedding virus at time of delivery; <1% if not shedding). Recurrent maternal herpes infection at the time of delivery is commonly asymptomatic or unrecognised but may cause localised forms of neonatal herpes infection such as central nervous system or skin, eye and mouth disease.[1,2] Disseminated herpes infection is more common in preterm infants and occurs almost exclusively as a result of primary infection in the mother.

Risk factors for transmission include the following:[1,2]
- primary maternal genital infection, particularly in late pregnancy (30–50% transmission rates);
- low level transplacental maternal neutralising antibodies—high titres of type-specific neutralising antibody in the neonate convey some, albeit not

total, protection and are associated with a lower risk of neonatal infection. The likelihood of neonatal herpes may be a function of the time it takes to elicit a mature antibody response; if the mother develops primary genital herpes during the third trimester, maternal or neonatal antibodies to herpes simplex virus may not develop rapidly enough to protect the infant against infection. The titre is also related to disease presentation with the highest levels seen in skin, eye, mouth disease, lower levels in central nervous system disease and very low levels detected in disseminated disease;

▶ prolonged rupture of membranes before delivery;

▶ invasive obstetric procedures such as electronic fetal monitoring scalp electrodes, early artificial rupture of the fetal membranes, forceps or vacuum extraction; and

▶ vaginal (compared with caesarean) delivery—Brown et al[1] provided the first demonstration that caesarean delivery may protect against herpes simplex virus transmission which occurred in 1 (1.2%) of 85 caesarean deliveries *versus* 9 (7.7%) of 117 vaginal deliveries (odds ratio (OR) 0.14, 95% CI 0.02–1.08, P = 0.047).

INCIDENCE

The reported incidence in Australia of neonatal herpes simplex virus infection is 3.5 in 100,000 live births.

Data from the USA suggest that approximately 2% of women acquire genital herpes simplex virus infection in pregnancy.[2]

CONSEQUENCES OF NEONATAL HERPES SIMPLEX VIRUS INFECTION

Australian data[3] suggest that neonatal herpes simplex virus infection results in:

▶ skin, eye, mouth disease in 45%—neurological and/or ocular morbidity following skin, eye, mouth disease is less than 2%;

▶ disseminated disease in 28%—this has a mortality of about 30% with 17% having long-term neurological sequelae and disability;

▶ central nervous system disease alone in 21%—this has a mortality of about 6% with 70% having long-term neurological sequelae and disability; and

▶ congenital herpes simplex virus in 3%—the manifestations include microcephaly, hydrocephalus and chorioretinitis with or without skin lesions.[4]

The long-term neurological sequelae include developmental delay, cognitive impairment and cerebral palsy.

DIAGNOSIS

Diagnosis in the neonate is made most commonly by polymerase chain reaction (PCR) detection of viral DNA from lesions or from cerebrospinal fluid.

For skin or mucous membrane lesions, specimens from ulcerated lesions should be sampled by swabbing the base of the ulcer, vesicular lesions should be de-roofed and the fluid sampled. A swab for viral detection should be used. Viral culture is not widely available. Although type-specific herpes simplex virus serological testing (immunoglobulin G antibodies to HSV-1 and HSV-2) is now widely available, its use for the management of herpes in pregnancy has not been fully evaluated.

ANTENATAL/LABOUR MANAGEMENT

Recommendations for antenatal management are summarised in the algorithm shown in Figure 18.1.

Women With a Primary Episode of Genital Herpes at the Time of Delivery

For these women, the following apply:

▶ Caesarean section should be recommended to all women presenting with a primary episode of genital herpes lesions at the time of delivery, or within 6 weeks of the expected date of delivery.

▶ For women who develop primary genital herpes lesions within 6 weeks of delivery and who elect to attempt vaginal birth, rupture of membranes should be avoided and invasive procedures such as internal fetal monitoring or fetal blood sampling should not be used. Intravenous aciclovir given intrapartum to the mother and subsequently to the neonate (20 mg/kg/dose 8 hourly) may be considered. The neonatal staff should be informed.

▶ Aciclovir prophylaxis should be considered for women at or beyond 36 weeks gestation who had a first episode of herpes simplex virus occurring during the current pregnancy, and could be considered for women at risk for recurrent disease.[5] Aciclovir may be administered orally to pregnant women who have first-episode genital herpes or severe recurrent herpes, and should be administered intravenously to pregnant women who have severe herpes simplex virus infection. It is important to recognise that primary herpes simplex virus cannot be distinguished from non-primary first-episode disease unless serology is performed.

Women With Recurrent Episodes of Genital Herpes at the Onset of Labour

For these women, the following apply:

▶ Women presenting with recurrent genital herpes lesions at the onset of labour should be advised that the risk to the baby of herpes infection is very small (≤1%).[6]

▶ Caesarean section is not routinely recommended for women with recurrent genital herpes lesions at the onset of labour. The mode of delivery should be discussed with the woman and individualised according to the clinical circumstances and the woman's preferences.

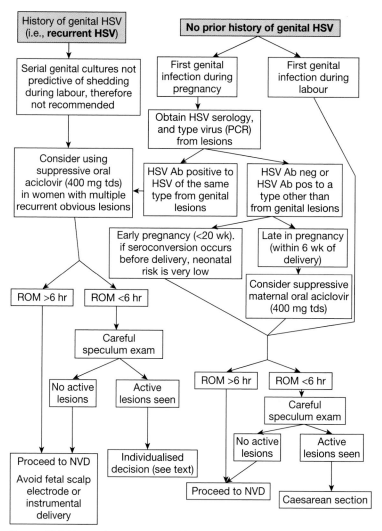

Figure 18.1 Maternal management of herpes simplex virus (adapted from *Management of Perinatal Infections*).[7]

Key: Ab—antibodies, HSV—herpes simplex virus, NVD—normal vaginal delivery, ROM—rupture of membranes.

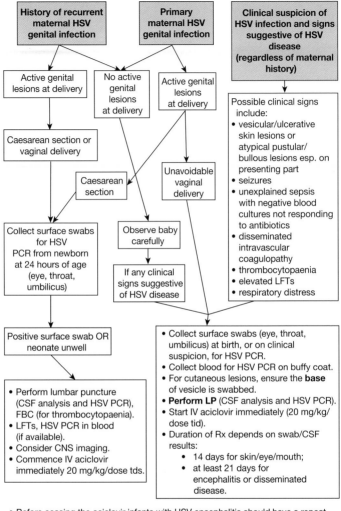

History of recurrent maternal HSV genital infection

Primary maternal HSV genital infection

Clinical suspicion of HSV infection and signs suggestive of HSV disease (regardless of maternal history)

Active genital lesions at delivery

No active genital lesions at delivery

Active genital lesions at delivery

Caesarean section or vaginal delivery

Caesarean section

Unavoidable vaginal delivery

Collect surface swabs for HSV PCR from newborn at 24 hours of age (eye, throat, umbilicus)

Observe baby carefully

If any clinical signs suggestive of HSV disease

Possible clinical signs include:
- vesicular/ulcerative skin lesions or atypical pustular/bullous lesions esp. on presenting part
- seizures
- unexplained sepsis with negative blood cultures not responding to antibiotics
- disseminated intravascular coagulopathy
- thrombocytopaenia
- elevated LFTs
- respiratory distress

Positive surface swab OR neonate unwell

- Perform lumbar puncture (CSF analysis and HSV PCR), FBC (for thrombocytopaenia).
- LFTs, HSV PCR in blood (if available).
- Consider CNS imaging.
- Commence IV aciclovir immediately 20 mg/kg/dose tds.

- Collect surface swabs (eye, throat, umbilicus) at birth, or on clinical suspicion, for HSV PCR.
- Collect blood for HSV PCR on buffy coat.
- For cutaneous lesions, ensure the **base** of vesicle is swabbed.
- **Perform LP** (CSF analysis and HSV PCR).
- Start IV aciclovir immediately (20 mg/kg/dose tid).
- Duration of Rx depends on swab/CSF results:
    - 14 days for skin/eye/mouth;
    - at least 21 days for encephalitis or disseminated disease.

- Before ceasing the aciclovir infants with HSV encephalitis should have a repeat LP towards the end of the 21 day treatment course to confirm that the CSF is negative for HSV PCR. Continue IV aciclovir until CSF HSV PCR is negative.
- Survivors should be monitored closely for signs of relapse or reactivation of HSV. A LP should always be performed on relapsed infants to exclude CNS involvement.
- Current recommendation is for 6 months of suppressive oral aciclovir following initial treatment of neonatal HSV disease (see text).

Figure 18.2 Neonatal management herpes simplex virus (adapted from *Management of Perinatal Infections*).[7]
Key: CSF—cerebrospinal fluid, CNS—central nervous system, FBC—full blood count, HSV—herpes simplex virus, IV—intravenous, LFT—liver function tests, LP—lumbar puncture, NVD—normal vaginal delivery, PCR—polymerase chain reaction, ROM—rupture of membranes.

▶ Women with recurrent genital herpes lesions and confirmed rupture of membranes at term should be advised to have delivery expedited by the appropriate means.

▶ Invasive procedures in labour should be avoided for women with recurrent genital herpes lesions.

▶ The neonatal staff should be informed of babies born to mothers with recurrent genital herpes lesions at the time of labour.

NEONATAL MANAGEMENT

Postnatal management is summarised in the algorithm shown in Figure 18.2.

Note: A recent study supports the use of suppressive therapy with aciclovir for 6 months after initial treatment of neonatal herpes simplex virus disease (oral aciclovir 300 mg per square metre per dose administered three times daily). Babies with skin, eye and mouth disease can benefit because this therapy helps to prevent skin recurrences, whereas babies with central nervous system disease may have additional benefit with respect to neurodevelopmental outcomes. There are no controlled data that suggest that suppressive therapy administered longer than six months or with the use of higher doses of oral aciclovir is beneficial. An extemporaneously compounded oral solution of valaciclovir has not been sufficiently studied in neonates and young infants to warrant its use instead of oral aciclovir for antiviral suppression.[8]

Prevention of Postnatal Herpes Simplex Virus Transmission to the Neonate

For neonates, the following apply:

▶ Mothers, family members and healthcare workers should be aware of the risk of neonatal transmission from any active herpes simplex virus lesions (including orolabial herpes and herpetic whitlows) and measures should be taken to avoid transmission of the virus to the neonate.

▶ Breast feeding is only contraindicated in the event of a herpetic lesion on the breast.

Babies who have had neonatal herpes with central nervous system involvement should be referred to a general paediatrician and/or developmental paediatrician for long-term follow-up.

REFERENCES

1. Brown ZA, Wald A, Morrow RA, et al. Effect of serologic status and cesarean delivery on transmission rates of herpes simplex virus from mother to infant. *JAMA.* 2003;289:203–209.

2. Brown ZA, Selke S, Zeh J, et al. The acquisition of herpes simplex virus during pregnancy. *N Engl J Med.* 1997;337:509–515.

3. Jones CA, Isaacs D, McIntyre P, et al. Neonatal herpes simplex virus infection. In: Ridely G, Zurynski Y, Elliott EJ, eds. Australian Paediatric Surveillance Unit Research Report. Sydney: Australian Paediatric Surveillance Unit; 2007;24.

4. Marquez L, Levy M, Munoz F, et al. A Report of Three Cases and Review of Intrauterine Herpes Simplex Virus Infection. *Pediatr Infect Dis J.* 2011;30:153–157.
5. American College of Obstetricians and Gynecologists. Management of herpes in pregnancy. ACOG practice bulletin Number 8. Washington (DC)7 American College of Obstetricians and Gynecologists; 1999.
6. Randolph AG, Washington E, Prober CG. Cesarian delivery for women presenting with genital herpes lesions. *JAMA.* 1993;270:77–82.
7. Jones C. Herpes simplex virus. In: Palasanthiran P, Starr M, Jones C, eds. Management of Perinatal Infections. Sydney: Australasian Society for Infectious Diseases; 2002 (Emendations 2006):16–18.
8. Kimberlin D, Whitley R, Wan W, et al. Oral Acyclovir Suppression and Neurodevelopment after Neonatal Herpes. *N Engl J Med.* 2011;365:1284–1292.

CHAPTER 19

Varicella

Meryta May, Maureen Dingwall

Varicella zoster virus is a herpes virus which causes chickenpox and herpes zoster (shingles). The virus can be transmitted transplacentally.

EPIDEMIOLOGY

Varicella zoster virus is usually acquired during childhood and 90% of adults in western countries are immune.

The current Australian Immunisation Program Schedule includes vaccination for varicella zoster virus. Vaccination of adults with two doses of vaccine is generally considered protective. Those who have been previously infected by the wild-type virus usually remain seropositive for life.

Primary varicella zoster virus infection is highly contagious and is spread by direct contact with lesions, aerosolised secretions and bodily fluids. Infected individuals are contagious during the prodromal phase of their illness (usually 1–2 days of fever and/or non-specific upper respiratory tract symptoms) before the rash appears. Significant exposure of a susceptible individual is defined as: 1) five minutes or more of face-to-face contact with a confirmed case; or 2) one hour or more in the same room as a confirmed case.

Reactivation of latent varicella zoster virus infection is known as shingles or herpes zoster.

FETAL/PERINATAL OUTCOMES

Almost all (98%) fetal infections are asymptomatic. Miscarriage, intrauterine fetal death and premature labour have been reported as rare complications following maternal varicella zoster virus infection. Other complications include severe clinical varicella and congenital varicella syndrome.

Severe Clinical Varicella

Severe clinical varicella occurs when there is maternal primary varicella zoster virus infection **<7 days prior to delivery or up to 28 days after delivery**. In these circumstances there is a high risk of severe clinical varicella zoster virus infection in the neonate as transmission of maternal antibodies may not have occurred. The mortality rate if untreated is 30%.

Congenital Varicella Syndrome

The risk of the fetus developing congenital varicella syndrome depends on the gestation when infected:

- <12 weeks gestation—0.4%;
- 12–20 weeks gestation—2%;
- >20 weeks gestation: negligible risk (case reports only); and
- reactivation of varicella zoster virus carries no risk to the fetus.
  The signs of congenital varicella syndrome include:
- skin scars (78%);
- eye abnormalities—cataracts, chorioretinitis, microphthalmia (60%);
- limb hypoplasia of bones, muscles or digits (68%);
- cortical atrophy, microcephaly and mental retardation (46%); and
- autonomic—neurogenic bladder, oesophageal dilatation, gastro-oesophageal reflux.

Overall, the prognosis for babies with congenital varicella syndrome is poor, with approximately 30% mortality in early infancy. Death is usually due to recurrent, severe aspiration pneumonia.

DIAGNOSIS
Maternal
The diagnosis is usually made clinically but it can be confirmed by polymerase chain reaction (PCR) test of a swab taken from the base of a vesicular lesion. Serology can be used to differentiate herpes zoster from varicella when this is not clinically obvious.

Fetal
If the diagnosis is suspected then serial fetal ultrasounds are recommended. Amniocentesis is not routinely recommended. A positive varicella zoster virus polymerase chain reaction (PCR) test does not confirm that the fetus has congenital varicella syndrome; a negative test will confirm that the fetus does not have congenital varicella syndrome.

Neonatal
A varicella zoster virus polymerase chain reaction (PCR) test can be done on a swab of any zoster lesion, or a mucosal swab.

MANAGEMENT[1,2]
Maternal
Zoster immunoglobulin (ZIG) is recommended for any pregnant woman who is seronegative for varicella zoster virus IgG and who has a confirmed exposure. The immunoglobulin should be given within the first 72 hours after exposure, but it can be given up to 96 hours following exposure, although with less efficacy.

If a pregnant woman is symptomatic with active varicella, she should be treated with aciclovir if:
- it has been <24 hours since the onset of the rash;
- if she is immunocompromised;

❯ if there is evidence of severe disease; or
❯ if she is in the latter half of pregnancy (when there is a greater risk for varicella pneumonitis).

Due to the low incidence of congenital varicella syndrome, it is not known if treatment of maternal varicella infection with aciclovir decreases the risk of fetal damage. There is no role for prophylactic aciclovir in an attempt to prevent fetal infection. Treatment of varicella zoster virus in pregnancy is aimed at preventing severe maternal infection.

Neonatal

If the baby is born at ≤28 weeks gestational age, zoster immunoglobulin (ZIG) should be administered. Give intravenous aciclovir if clinical varicella develops.

If the baby is born at >28 weeks gestational age then the timing of maternal infection guides therapy:

❯ maternal infection >7 days prior to delivery—no specific intervention or isolation of the baby from its mother is required, the baby is able to breast feed; or
❯ maternal infection <7 days prior to delivery or up to 28 days after delivery—give zoster immunoglobulin (ZIG) immediately. **The baby is at high risk of severe clinical varicella which has a mortality rate of 30% if untreated.** No specific intervention or isolation of the baby from its mother is required, the baby is able to breast feed.

If the baby has clinical varicella, treatment is determined by the severity of baby's illness and the timing of zoster immunoglobulin (ZIG) administration:

❯ if the baby has mild symptoms and zoster immunoglobulin (ZIG) was given <24 hours from birth:
   • observe,
   • give intravenous aciclovir if respiratory symptoms develop;
❯ if the baby has mild symptoms and zoster immunoglobulin (ZIG) was given between 24 and 72 hours of birth:
   • clinical judgment is required—it is acceptable to observe the infant and to progress to intravenous aciclovir if there is any clinical deterioration.
❯ if the baby has severe disease **or** zoster immunoglobulin (ZIG) was given >72 hours after birth, give intravenous aciclovir;
❯ there is no role for outpatient management with oral aciclovir in neonates due to its poor efficacy; and
❯ long-term developmental follow-up by a general paediatrician is required.

RECURRENCE

There is no risk of recurrence in subsequent pregnancies. Babies exposed to varicella zoster virus *in utero* or perinatally have a higher incidence of herpes zoster (shingles) in early childhood.

REFERENCES

1. Heuchan AM, Isaacs D, on behalf of the Australasian Subgroup in Paediatric Infectious Diseases of the Australasian Society for Infectious Diseases. The management of varicella-zoster virus exposure and infection in pregnancy and the newborn period. *MJA*. 2001;174:288–292.
2. Palasanthiran P, Starr M, Jones C, eds. Management of Perinatal Infections. Sydney: Australasian Society for Infectious Diseases; 2002 (Emendations 2006):1–4.

CHAPTER 20

Human Immunodeficiency Virus

Jonathan W Davis, Michael Nissen

Human immunodeficiency virus (HIV) infection in pregnancy is a potential threat to the fetus and newborn infant. The virus can be transmitted from the infected mother to her fetus or child (vertical transmission).

AETIOLOGY AND PATHOPHYSIOLOGY

While HIV infection is associated with perinatal acquisition, the precise mechanism of transmission remains speculative. Vertical transmission of HIV can occur *in utero*, during labour or after delivery, generally through breast feeding. Most (50–80%) of the vertical transmission of HIV occurs around birth. Prevention strategies are based on the variation in the timing and mode of transmission. Currently it is not possible to accurately diagnose HIV in the fetus.

PREVALENCE

The incidence of HIV infection among women giving birth in the United Kingdom increased steadily through the 1990s and early 2000s but has since stabilised. In 2006, the prevalence of HIV infection in women giving birth was 1 in 238 (0.42%) in London and 1 in 705 (0.14%) in the rest of England.[1] In Australia, the prevalence is much lower—the perinatal exposure rate in infants born from 2003–2006 was 0.008%, or about 1 in 12,000.[2]

RISK

Maternal viral load appears to be the strongest predictor of vertical HIV transmission. In pregnancy, the risk of transmission increases when plasma HIV load peaks. Little or no viral transmission occurs when the plasma viral load is less than 1000 copies/mL.

HIV levels in maternal genital tract secretions may also affect the vertical transmission risk. The transmission risk increases when the fetus comes into contact with maternal blood or genital tract secretions; for example:

- ruptured membranes, longer than four hours;
- placental abruption;
- amniocentesis;
- chorionic villous sampling;
- fetal scalp electrode monitoring;
- episiotomy;

▶ vaginal lacerations; and
▶ preterm delivery associated with prolonged rupture of membranes.

Postnatally, a HIV-infected mother can transmit the virus to her baby through breast feeding. HIV is detectable in breast milk, with breast milk viral loads correlating with plasma viral loads. The risk of HIV transmission from breast feeding is about 15%. The risk is highest if the maternal CD4$^+$ T-cell count is low, if she has mastitis or with prolonged breast milk exposure. Most breast milk HIV transmission occurs in the first 6 weeks of life.

Low maternal CD4$^+$ T-cell levels are a measure of poor immune function and have been associated with enhanced HIV transmission. Vitamin A deficiency and malnutrition also cause immune deficiency and may increase vertical transmission risk. Other maternal risk factors include recreational drug use and cigarette smoking. There is a near linear relationship between increasing infant prematurity and vertical transmission.

Figure 20.1 summarises an approach to risk assessment based on major risk factors and Table 20.1 provides estimates of the risk according to various risk-modification strategies.

CONSEQUENCES

Infants with HIV infection usually have no clinical signs at birth. Signs are usually non-specific and can include lymphadenopathy, failure to thrive, persistent diarrhoea, recurrent infections, oral thrush and parotitis. HIV tends to be more rapidly progressive in children than in adults.

ANTENATAL MANAGEMENT

The aim of antenatal management is to minimise vertical HIV transmission while avoiding neonatal or maternal morbidity.

Antiretroviral therapy during pregnancy decreases perinatal HIV transmission by up to 70%. Combination therapy is more effective than monotherapy. Treatment is best started after the first trimester (due to teratogenic risk) and no later than 28 weeks gestation. Side effects of treatment, as well as the risks of not treating, must be discussed with the parents.

An infectious diseases physician should be involved in maternal management. Monitoring at least every four weeks during pregnancy includes HIV RNA viral load, CD4$^+$ T-cell levels, full blood count, urea and electrolytes, liver function tests and additional serology (syphilis, hepatitis B and C, *Toxoplasma* and cytomegalovirus).

INTRAPARTUM MANAGEMENT

Delivery should be planned in a centre that has a special care nursery attended by paediatricians. The delivery plan should be made in consultation with a paediatric infectious diseases/HIV specialist.

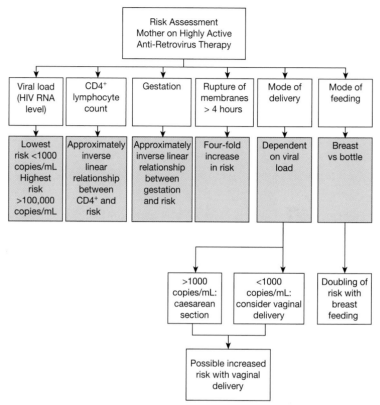

Figure 20.1 Assessment of the risk of transmission of human immunodeficiency virus (HIV) dependent on antenatal and postnatal factors.[3]

For mothers with a viral load of ≥1000 copies/mL, caesarean section at 38 weeks is recommended. For mothers with a viral load of <1000 copies/mL, caesarean section should be considered, based on other relevant factors, but is not compulsory.

If labour starts before a planned caesarean section and the membranes are ruptured for less than four hours, urgent caesarean section should be considered. Wherever possible, avoid fetal scalp electrodes, episiotomy and instrumentation.

Intravenous zidovudine (previously known as azidothymidine or AZT), 2 mg/kg over one hour should be given at the onset of labour or 4 hours

Table 20.1 Quantification of risk of transmission[3]

	ART in Pregnancy	Intra-partum ART	Infant ART	Delivery	Feeding	Transmission Risk %
Dunn et al, 1992	×	×	×	Vaginal	Breast	40
Nduati et al, 2000	×	×	×	Vaginal	Breast	36
Baseline	×	×	×	Vaginal	Formula	20
Connor et al, 1994 (Full course AZT, 076 Study)	✓	✓	✓	Vaginal	Formula	8
The international Perinatal HIV Group, 1998	✓	✓	✓	Caesarean	Formula	2

Key: ART—antiretroviral therapy. Baseline—based on the observed risk of transmission before the introduction of intervention strategies.

before caesarean delivery. This is followed by a continuous infusion of 1 mg/kg/hr until the cord is clamped.

On delivery of the head, the obstetrician or midwife should clean the baby's eyes with sterile water.

IMMEDIATE POSTNATAL MANAGEMENT

The infant should be assessed and washed as soon as possible after delivery. Do not break the skin (e.g., for blood sampling, vitamin K injection) unless it has been thoroughly cleaned first. Take blood samples for HIV polymerase chain reaction (PCR), HIV antibodies and full blood count.

Post-exposure prophylaxis with antiretroviral medication should be started within 12 hours of birth. Monotherapy is usually sufficient. Combination therapy should be considered in the following circumstances:

‣ the mother did not receive adequate antepartum or intrapartum treatment which may have been due to:
  • HIV being diagnosed late in pregnancy,
  • HIV being diagnosed after delivery,
  • poor compliance with treatment,
  • unexpected preterm delivery; and
‣ persistent or rebound high maternal viral load.

Combination therapy will usually consist of zidovudine, nevarepine and lamivudine, but is dependent on factors such as the maternal medications, HIV genotype and resistance profile. It is essential to seek the advice of a paediatric HIV specialist if combination therapy is being considered.

Monotherapy usually consists of zidovudine for 6 weeks. Consult your own local guidelines and paediatric HIV specialist. It must be started within 12 hours of birth (the sooner the better).

The dose of zidovudine is:

‣ oral—2 mg/kg; or
‣ intravenous—1.5 mg/kg.

The dosing interval of zidovudine is:

‣ <30 weeks gestation—every 12 hours for four weeks, then every 8 hours;
‣ 30–35 weeks gestation—every 12 hours for two weeks, then every 8 hours;
‣ >35 weeks gestation—every 6 hours.

OTHER POSTNATAL MANAGEMENT

Following post-exposure prophylaxis, co-trimoxazole (0.5 mL/kg daily until three months of age) should be considered, especially in infants at higher risk of HIV transmission. Again, consult your local paediatric HIV specialist.

Infants should be tested according to the schedule shown in Table 20.2. Also, monitor for antiretroviral drug side effects such as neutropaenia, electrolyte imbalance and liver dysfunction.

Table 20.2 Testing schedule for infants born at risk of human immunodeficiency virus (HIV)[3]

Time	PCR	HIV Antibody	T Cell Subsets
Day 1	✓	—	—
Week 1	✓	—	✓
Week 6	✓	—	✓
Week 12	✓	—	—
6 months	✓	—	—
12 months	—	✓	✓
18–24 months (if still seropositive at 12–18 months)	—	✓	✓
Key: PCR—polymerase chain reaction			

In developed countries, breast feeding should be avoided as it substantially increases the risk of HIV transmission.

Arrange for follow-up with your local paediatric infectious diseases team or HIV specialist, who will monitor the infant until the HIV status is determined. This may take up to 18–24 months, and is confirmed by a negative HIV polymerase chain reaction and negative HIV antibody test.

Immunisations

The standard immunisation schedule should be followed, except for BCG which, if indicated, should be withheld until the infant is confirmed to be uninfected.

Inactivated poliomyelitis vaccine (IPV) should be used to prevent loss of viral attenuation in the recipient and viral shedding to household members. Oral poliomyelitis vaccine (OPV) should not be used and it is no longer available in Australia.

OTHER CONSULTS REQUIRED

A paediatric infectious diseases/HIV specialist should be consulted. Liaise with the maternal infectious diseases team regarding the mother's therapy and viral load measurements, as this will influence management of the infant.

Refer to social work and/or HIV management teams for family support and long-term family planning.

REFERENCES

1. The UK Collaborative Group for HIV and STI Surveillance. A Complex Picture. HIV and other Sexually Transmitted Infections in the United Kingdom: 2006. London: Health Protection Agency, Centre for Infections. November 2006. Available at http://www.hpa.org.uk/Publications/InfectiousDiseases/HIVAndSTIs /0611ComplexPictureUKHIVSTI/ [accessed 1 June 2011].

2. McDonald AM, Zurynski YA, Wand HC, et al. Perinatal exposure to HIV among children born in Australia, 1982–2006. *Med J Aust.* 2009;190(8):416–420.

3. Palasanthiran P. Human immunodeficiency Virus. In: Palasanthiran P, Starr M, Jones C, eds. *Management of Perinatal Infections.* Sydney: Australasian Society for Infectious Diseases; 2002:19–23.

Further Reading

Anonymous. The mode of delivery and the risk of vertical transmission of human immunodeficiency virus type 1—a meta-analysis of 15 prospective cohort studies. The International Perinatal HIV Group. *N Engl J Med.* 1999;340:977–987.

Connor EM, Sperling RS, Gelber R, et al. Reduction of maternal-infant transmission of human immunodeficiency virus type 1 with zidovudine treatment. Pediatric AIDS Clinical Trials Group Protocol 076 Study Group. *N Eng J Med.* 1994;331(18):1173–1180.

de Ruiter A, Mercey D, Anderson J, et al. British HIV Association and Children's HIV Association guidelines for the management of HIV infection in pregnant women 2008. *HIV Medicine.* 2008;9(7):452–502.

Dickover RE, Garratty EM, Herman SA, et al. Identification of levels of maternal HIV-1 RNA associated with risk of perinatal transmission. Effect of maternal zidovudine treatment on viral load. *JAMA.* 1996;275(8):599–605.

Dunn DT, Newell ML, Ades AE, et al. Risk of human immunodeficiency virus type 1 transmission through breastfeeding. *Lancet.* 1992;340(8819):585–588.

Kreiss J. Breastfeeding and vertical transmission of HIV-1. *Acta Paediatrica Supplement.* 1997;421:113–117.

Kuhn L, Steketee RW, Weedon J, et al. Distinct risk factors for intrauterine and intrapartum human immunodeficiency virus transmission and consequences for disease progression in infected children. Perinatal AIDS Collaborative Transmission Study. *J Infect Dis.* 1999;179(1):52–58.

Landesman SH, Kalish LA, Burns DN, et al. Obstetrical factors and the transmission of human immunodeficiency virus type 1 from mother to child. The Women and Infants Transmission Study. *N Engl J Med.* 1996;334(25):1617–1623.

Leroy V, Newell ML, Dabis F, et al. International multicentre pooled analysis of late postnatal mother-to-child transmission of HIV-1 infection. Ghent International Working Group on Mother-to-Child Transmission of HIV. *Lancet.* 1998 Aug 22;352(9128):597–600.

Mofenson LM. Interaction between timing of perinatal human immunodeficiency virus infection and the design of preventive and therapeutic interventions. *Acta Paediatrica Supplement.* 1997;421:1–9.

Mofenson LM. Centers for Disease Control and Prevention, US Public Health Service Task Force. US Public Health Service Task Force recommendations for use of antiretroviral drugs in pregnant HIV-1-infected women for maternal health and interventions to reduce perinatal HIV-1 transmission in the United States. Morbidity and Mortality Weekly Report. *Recommendations and Reports.* 2002 Nov 22;51(RR-18):1–38.

Mofenson LM, Lambert JS, Stiehm ER, et al. Risk factors for perinatal transmission of human immunodeficiency virus type 1 in women treated with zidovudine. Pediatric AIDS Clinical Trials Group Study 185 Team. *N Engl J Med.* 1999;341(6):385–393.

Nduati R, John G, Mbori-Ngacha D, et al. Effect of breastfeeding and formula feeding on transmission of HIV-1: a randomized clinical trial. *JAMA.* 2000;283(9):1167–1174.

Panel on Treatment of HIV-Infected Pregnant Women and Prevention of Perinatal Transmission. Recommendations for Use of Antiretroviral Drugs in Pregnant HIV-1-Infected Women for Maternal Health and Interventions to Reduce Perinatal HIV Transmission in the United States. May 24, 2010:1–117. Available at http://aidsinfo.nih.gov/ContentFiles/PerinatalGL.pdf. [Accessed 2 June 2011].

Stringer JS, Vermund SH. Prevention of mother-to-child transmission of HIV-1. *Curr Opin Obstet Gynecol.* 1999;11(5):427–434.

CHAPTER 21

Hepatitis B and Hepatitis C

Richard Muir, Pieter J Koorts

Maternal infection with hepatitis B virus (HBV) or hepatitis C virus (HCV) carries a substantial risk of perinatal transmission. HBV and HCV are the most common causes of chronic hepatitis, cirrhosis, liver failure and hepatocellular carcinoma worldwide.

Screening for both these viruses is usual for all pregnant women at booking-in or first antenatal clinic visit.

HEPATITIS B
Prevalence
The prevalence of hepatitis B infection in Australia is reported to be 0.49–0.87%;[1] perinatal transmission rates have not been reported.

Pathophysiology
The hepatitis B virus is a double-shelled DNA virus. The incubation period varies from 60–150 days. The virus is transmitted by parenteral or mucosal exposure to hepatitis B surface antigen (HBsAg) positive body fluids from infected people. The highest concentrations are in blood or serous fluids. It is also present in saliva but saliva is thought to be an unlikely mode of transmission given low concentration rates.

Consequences
Perinatal infection in the absence of post-exposure prophylaxis is 70–90% if the mother is positive for both hepatitis B e-antigen (HBeAg) and HBsAg. The risk of transmission is 10–40% if HBsAg positive only.[2] Maternal HBV DNA viral loads of $>10^8$ copies per mL are another risk factor for perinatal infection.[3]

The importance of routine post-exposure prophylaxis of hepatitis B must be emphasised. Post-exposure prophylaxis decreases the infection rate in infants of HBeAg positive mothers to 5–10%.[4]

Hepatitis B vaccination and one dose of hepatitis B immunoglobulin (HBIG) administered within 24 hours of delivery are 85–95% effective in preventing acute or chronic hepatitis B virus infection.

Fulminant hepatitis B has been reported in the infant period, usually in infants of HBeAg negative mothers. The incidence is exceedingly rare (<1%) and it usually only occurs in endemic areas.

If hepatitis B virus is acquired perinatally there is a 95% risk of chronic hepatitis B virus infection. Chronic hepatitis B virus infection is responsible for most of the morbidity and mortality and 15–25% of chronic hepatitis B virus carriers will die from hepatitis B virus related liver disease in adulthood.[5]

Management—Antenatal
The hepatitis B vaccine is safe in all trimesters of pregnancy. Any pregnant woman who is non-immune and in a high risk group should be administered the standard hepatitis B vaccination series.

There is currently limited data on the safety of antiviral treatment of pregnant women with chronic hepatitis B. However, potential benefits may outweigh potential risks to the fetus in select cases (e.g., maternal liver disease, perinatal HBV transmission in prior pregnancy) and treatment can be considered in consultation with an adult hepatologist.

Management—Delivery
Caesarean section does not appear to reduce the rate of perinatal transmission of hepatitis B. Universal precautions should be undertaken.

Management—Immediate Postnatal
All infants born to HBsAg positive women should receive hepatitis B vaccine and HBIG within 12 hours of delivery (regardless of birth weight or gestational age).

Management—Postnatal
Prophylaxis (as above) should be followed by repeat doses of hepatitis B vaccine at 2, 4 and 6 months of age (as for all babies according to the Australian Immunisation Schedule).

Routine hepatitis B virus vaccination for preterm infants with a birthweight of <2000 grams born to HBsAg negative mothers can be delayed as they have a decreased vaccination response if given before one month of chronological age.

Breast feeding is not contraindicated as it does not pose a risk of hepatitis B virus transmission to the infant.

Hepatitis B virus is not considered to be a cause of neonatal hepatitis (onset <1 month of age) and is a rare cause of infant icteric hepatitis. Fulminant hepatitis B infection should prompt immediate specialist hepatologist review.

Infants who acquire HBV from HBsAg positive women do not manifest serological evidence of hepatitis B virus infection until 1–3 months of age.

Post Vaccination Serological Testing
The current U.S. Centers for Disease Control (CDC) Hepatitis B Guidelines recommend that infants born to HBsAg positive women should

be tested for HBsAg and antibody to HBsAg (anti-HBs) after completion of the vaccination series between 9 and 18 months of age. If HBsAg is not present and anti-HBs antibody levels are adequate (≥10 mIU/mL), the child can be considered protected.

If levels are inadequate and HBsAg is negative, a repeat immunisation course should be performed.

Perinatal transmission can still occur despite active and passive immunisation.

HEPATITIS C
Prevalence
Hepatitis C is thought to affect 3% of the world's population.

Pathophysiology
The hepatitis C virus is a single-stranded ribonucleic acid (RNA) virus with an incubation period of around 40–50 days. The virus is transmitted via hepatitis C infected blood.

The risk of hepatitis C virus (HCV) transmission from mother to infant has been shown to be 6% in anti-HCV antibody positive mothers and 10% in hepatitis C virus RNA positive mothers.[6] In general, studies indicate that high levels of hepatitis C virus RNA (e.g., 10^5 to 10^6 copies per mL) confer increased risk of maternal–fetal transmission.[7] Maternal co-infection with Human Immunodeficiency Virus (HIV) increases the risk of transmission.

Consequences
Approximately 5–10% of infants with vertically acquired hepatitis C will progress to significant hepatic fibrosis or cirrhosis.[8]

Management—Antenatal
There are no effective measures to reduce the risk of vertical transmission and antiviral treatment is contraindicated due to teratogenicity.

Management—Delivery
Routine caesarean delivery for HCV-infected mothers is not currently recommended. Minimisation of possible blood exposure during delivery is a prudent precaution (e.g., no use of scalp electrodes for fetal monitoring, no fetal blood sampling, minimal use of forceps or ventouse).

Management—Immediate Postnatal
Vertically acquired HCV is usually asymptomatic in the infant period.

Breast feeding is not considered a risk factor in mother-to-infant transmission of HCV, although data is limited. It may be prudent to stop breast feeding if the mother's nipples are cracked or bleeding.

Management—Postnatal

Generally, HCV disease of the newborn is not seen and fulminant hepatitis secondary to HCV is not reported in children.

Blood test results should be interpreted with caution in the neonate given their capacity to spontaneously clear infection.

When screening for perinatal transmission, be aware that maternal anti-HCV antibodies will persist until around 12–18 months of age.

Testing can be delayed until 1 year of age, at which time a qualitative polymerase chain reaction (PCR) for hepatitis C virus should be performed. If positive, it should be repeated when the child is 18–24 months of age.[9]

If consistently positive, the child has chronic hepatitis C virus and should be referred to a paediatric hepatologist.

REFERENCES

1. O'Sullivan BG, Gidding HF, Law M, et al. Estimates of chronic hepatitis B virus infection in Australia, 2000. *Aust N Z J Public Health*. 2004;28:212–216.
2. Alter MJ. Epidemiology of hepatitis B in Europe and worldwide. *J Hepatol*. 2003;39(Suppl 1):S64–S69.
3. Wiseman E, Fraser MA, Holden S, et al. Perinatal transmission of hepatitis B virus: an Australian experience. *Med J Aust*. 2009;190:489–492.
4. Jonas M. Hepatitis B and pregnancy: an underestimated issue. *Liver Int*. 2009;29(Suppl 1):133–139.
5. Centers for Disease Control (CDC). Recommendations for Identification and Public Health Management of Persons with Chronic Hepatitis B. *Infection*. 2008;57(RR08);1–20. MMWR.
6. Ohto H, Terazawa S, Sasaki N, et al. Transmission of hepatitis C virus from mothers to infants. *N Engl J Med*. 1994;330:744–750.
7. Roberts EA, Yeung L. Maternal-infant transmission of hepatitis C virus infection. *Hepatology*. 2002;36:S106–S113.
8. Garcia-Monzon C, Jara P, Fernandez-Bermejo M, et al. Chronic hepatitis C in children: A clinical and immunohistochemical comparative study with adult patients. *Hepatology*. 1998;28:1696–1701.
9. Slowik MK, Jhaveri R. Hepatitis B and C viruses in infants and young children. *Seminars in Pediatric Infectious Diseases*. 2005 Oct;16(4):296–305.

Further Reading

Beasley RP, Hwang LY, Lee GC, et al. Prevention of perinatally transmitted hepatitis B virus infections with hepatitis B immune globulin and hepatitis B vaccine. *Lancet*. 1983;2(8359):1099–1102.

Keeffe EB, Dieterich DT, Han SB, et al. A treatment algorithm for the management of chronic hepatitis B virus infection in the United States: 2008 update. *Clin Gastroenterol Hepatol*. 2008;6(12):1315–1341.

CHAPTER 22

Parvovirus

Jeremy D Robertson, Garry DT Inglis

Parvovirus B19 is a small DNA virus. Infection causes a common viral exanthem, known as erythema infectiosum, or fifth disease, in children and adults. It causes non-specific symptoms such as fever, malaise, myalgia and headache, followed later by rash and arthralgia. About 25% of those infected, including pregnant women, have asymptomatic viraemia. Infection during pregnancy may lead to non-immune hydrops from either severe anaemia or cardiomyopathy.[1]

Acute infection is confirmed serologically (IgM positive). A polymerase chain reaction (PCR) test for viral DNA (from maternal blood and/or amniotic fluid) is the confirmatory test of choice.

AETIOLOGY/PATHOPHYSIOLOGY/EMBRYOLOGY

The virus has marked tropism for erythroid precursors, in which it is cytotoxic. This can result in severe anaemia, which in turn can cause high output cardiac failure.

The virus also infects hepatic cells causing hypoalbuminaemia, and myocardial cells causing cardiomyopathy which may contribute to the severity of hydrops. It may also infect megakaryocytes, causing thrombocytopaenia.

PREVALENCE AND EPIDEMIOLOGY[2–4]

About 30–50% of pregnant women are susceptible to parvovirus B19 infection (i.e., they have had no past infection/immunity). The virus is usually acquired from household contacts, particularly school-aged children, and transmitted via droplet spread and the respiratory route. The highest incidence is in winter to early spring.

If the mother is acutely infected in pregnancy, the risk of vertical transmission to the fetus is about 30%. The fetus is at highest risk if infection occurs at 8–20 weeks gestation. Typically, the onset of fetal symptoms is about 6 weeks after maternal exposure.

DIFFERENTIAL DIAGNOSIS

The differential diagnosis is basically that of fetal anaemia and non-immune hydrops, including:

▶ other fetal infections;
▶ primary haematologic disorders;

▶ chromosomal abnormalities and major malformation syndromes;
▶ congenital heart disease and cardiomyopathies;
▶ vascular malformations;
▶ lymphatic dysplasia;
▶ thoracic anomalies; and
▶ twin anaemia-polycythaemia sequence (TAPS).

CONSEQUENCES[2-4]

Following maternal infection, 70–80% of fetuses are either not infected or asymptomatic. Fetal anaemia occurs in 10–25% and this can resolve spontaneously.

Non-immune hydrops occurs in 3–12% of infected fetuses. Intrauterine fetal death, which may occur without hydrops, occurs in 5–10% of infected fetuses. The highest risk is in second trimester.

There are rare reports of myocarditis and fetal arrhythmia and of brain injury.

MANAGEMENT—ANTENATAL

There is no vaccine and no specific treatment available for the mother or fetus.

Weekly fetal surveillance by ultrasound scan for assessment of fetal well being is prudent (including assessment of fetal size and growth, heart rate, movements, amniotic fluid volume and Doppler waveform of the umbilical or middle cerebral artery (MCA) blood flow). Fetal blood sampling for measurement of haemoglobin may be indicated if there is evidence of hydrops or significant elevation of peak MCA velocity.

Seek parental permission to give blood products (antenatally or postnatally) to the baby. Intrauterine transfusion may be used for fetal anaemia and usually no more than one transfusion is needed in the pregnancy.

Transfusion of red blood cells into the fetus can be either intravascular (usually into an umbilical vessel at the placental end of the cord or the intrahepatic portion of the umbilical vein) or intraperitoneal.

MANAGEMENT—LABOUR/DELIVERY/IMMEDIATE POSTNATAL

If there is evidence of hydrops or other significant complications, the baby should be delivered at a hospital with a neonatal intensive care unit.

If hydrops is severe, the baby will usually require intubation and ventilation from immediately after birth. The baby will be transferred to the neonatal intensive care unit and most likely have umbilical catheters inserted. Drainage of any pleural or peritoneal fluid may be required.

On day 1, baby will have haemoglobin and platelet count checked. If these are low, then transfusions of blood products (red cells/platelets) may be required.

OTHER CONSULTS REQUIRED

Depending on the findings and complications that arise, other antenatal consults may be sought from:

▶ clinical haematologist;
▶ paediatric cardiologist; and
▶ neurologist.

MANAGEMENT—POSTNATAL

Ongoing intensive care may be required for any cardio-respiratory compromise.

Occasional blood counts will need to be checked until the anaemia or thrombocytopaenia has resolved.

If there is concern about organ damage (heart or brain), follow-up may be arranged with a general paediatrician or the relevant sub-specialist.

RECURRENCE

Infection results in lifelong immunity so there is no recurrence risk to the mother (i.e., future pregnancies) or the affected child.

ETHICS

Ethical dilemmas may arise where:

▶ there is concern about fetal viability and there is an opportunity to terminate the pregnancy; and
▶ the parents have a moral or religious objection to blood product transfusions.

REFERENCES

1. Bellini C, Hennekam RCM, Fulcheri E, et al. Etiology of non-immune hydrops fetalis: a systematic review. *Am J Med Genet Part A*. 2009;149A:844–851.
2. Lamont RF, Sobel JD, Vaisbuch E, et al. Parvovirus B19 infection in human pregnancy. *BJOG*. 2011;118:175–186.
3. Ramirez MM, Mastrobattista JM. Diagnosis and management of Parvovirus B19 infection. *Clin Perinatol*. 2005 Sep;32(3):697–704.
4. Tolfvenstam T, Broliden K. Parvovirus B19. *Semin Fetal Neonatal Med*. 2009 Aug;14(4):218–221.

CHAPTER 23
Multiple Pregnancy

Glenn J Gardener, Luke Jardine

Multiple pregnancies account for a disproportionate share of major adverse perinatal outcomes. In addition to the increased rates of perinatal mortality and morbidity attributed to preterm delivery, multiple pregnancies are also at higher risk of miscarriage, fetal abnormality, stillbirth, fetal growth restriction, delivery complications and neurodevelopmental impairment.

The rates of multiple pregnancy vary worldwide with dizygous twinning and high order multiple rates affected by maternal age, parity, ethnicity and the use of assisted reproductive techniques. The incidence of monozygous twinning is relatively constant. In developed countries, multiple gestation rates have increased over the last 40 years and account for up to 2% of all births. In Australia, multiple births have increased by 43% from 1990 to 2010 and account for approximately 1.5% of births.[1]

PATHOPHYSIOLOGY—ZYGOSITY, CHORIONICITY AND AMNIONICITY

Zygosity describes the number of separate fertilised ova. Chorionicity refers to the number of chorions which corresponds to the number of placentae. Amnionicity refers to the number of amniotic sacs. Multiple pregnancies are normally classified by the number of placentas and the number of amniotic sacs.

A multiple pregnancy may arise through the fertilisation of more than one oocyte (multizygotic) or from the spontaneous splitting of a single zygote (monozygotic). One-third of twins are monozygotic and two-thirds are dizygotic. Higher order multiples usually arise from multiple ova but very rarely can arise from zygotic splitting and then re-splitting.

If the pregnancy is multizygotic or if monozygotic division occurs before implantation, they will have separate placentas (i.e., **dichorionic**) and separate amniotic cavities. If the division occurs after implantation, they will share the placenta (i.e., **monochorionic**) and either share the amniotic cavity (i.e., **monoamniotic**) or have their own (i.e., **diamniotic**). The

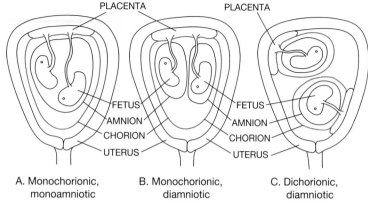

A. Monochorionic,
monoamniotic

B. Monochorionic,
diamniotic

C. Dichorionic,
diamniotic

Figure 23.1 Chorionicity and amnionicity.

majority of monozygotic twins will be **monochorionic-diamniotic** (MCDA). Some monozygotic twins (approximately 1 in 7) will have separate placentae and be **dichorionic-diamniotic** (DCDA). Hence, in same sex **dichorionic-diamniotic** twins, zygosity cannot be determined without DNA testing.

Chorionicity and amnionicity can be accurately established in the first trimester using ultrasound. It is important to establish chorionicity to enable the risk stratification of a multiple pregnancy.

SIGNIFICANCE
Monoamniotic Pregnancies
Monoamniotic twins account for approximately 1% of twins and are confirmed on ultrasound when there is a single placenta, two fetuses and no inter-twin dividing membrane. Umbilical cord entanglement is a major complication. The majority of fetal deaths in **monoamniotic** twins are due to cord entanglement. The risk of fetal death increases by 2–5% every week from 15 weeks gestation and totals 30–40% by 30 weeks gestation.

Twin-To-Twin Transfusion Syndrome
Twin-to-twin transfusion syndrome (TTTS) complicates 10–15% of **monochorionic** pregnancies (see Chapter 24).

Selective Fetal Growth Restriction
Selective fetal growth restriction (sFGR) complicates 10–15% of **monochorionic** pregnancies. The underlying cause of selective fetal growth

restriction is unequal placental sharing and this is often associated with a velamentous cord insertion. There are usually placental vascular anastomoses present in **monochorionic** twins with selective fetal growth restriction. Three different types can be identified on the basis of the umbilical artery Doppler waveforms:

❱ type 1—normal umbilical artery Doppler waveform;
❱ type 2—persistent absent or reversed end-diastolic flow; and
❱ type 3—intermittent absent or reversed end-diastolic flow.

In most cases, these Doppler types are apparent from early in pregnancy and do not change once the diagnosis is established. Type 1 is associated with a good prognosis. Type 2 is associated with a greater risk of fetal death (30–40%) of the smaller twin and the mean gestation at delivery is 30 weeks. For type 2, the overall risk of neurological injury for survivors (either small or normal size) is 15%. Type 3 is associated with a risk of unexpected fetal death of the smaller twin of 10–20% and there is an increased risk of neurological injury for the normally grown twin (10–20%).

The mainstay of management of selective fetal growth restriction in **monochorionic** twins is appropriately timed delivery balancing the risks of fetal death and its co-twin consequences with the risks of prematurity if delivered. Ultrasound assessment and monitoring of twin pregnancies with selective fetal growth restriction should be undertaken in tertiary facilities with appropriate multidisciplinary support. The effects of intrauterine growth restriction are discussed in Chapter 25.

Twin Anaemia-Polycythaemia Sequence

Twin anaemia-polycythaemia sequence (TAPs) is characterised by large inter-twin haemoglobin differences in the absence of amniotic fluid discordance. Twin anaemia-polycythaemia sequence may occur spontaneously in up to 5% of **monochorionic** twins and in 2–13% of cases of twin-to-twin transfusion syndrome treated by laser photocoagulation.

The underlying cause of twin anaemia-polycythaemia sequence is the presence of small arteriovenous vascular anastomoses which allow a slow transfusion of blood over time from the donor to the recipient twin.

The antenatal diagnosis of twin anaemia-polycythaemia sequence is based on discordant Doppler ultrasound velocities of the middle cerebral artery (MCA) flows in each twin. For timely diagnosis of twin anaemia-polycythaemia sequence, routine middle cerebral artery Doppler ultrasound surveillance is recommended in all **monochorionic** twins, and in particular in those following laser surgery for twin-to-twin transfusion syndrome.

Postnatal diagnosis of twin anaemia-polycythaemia sequence is based on a haemoglobin discordance between twins (<11 g/dL in the anaemic twin and >20 g/dL in the polycythaemic twin).[2]

Reports on the management and perinatal outcome in twin anaemia-polycythaemia sequence are limited. The incidence of neurodevelopmental impairment is unknown. Treatment options for twin anaemia-polycythaemia sequence include:

▶ expectant management;
▶ intrauterine transfusion;
▶ delivery;
▶ fetoscopic laser surgery; and
▶ selective fetocide via an occlusive cord procedure.

Further studies are required to determine optimal treatment strategies and prognosis in twin anaemia-polycythaemia sequence.

Discordant Fetal Abnormality

Multiple pregnancy is associated with an increased incidence of structural and chromosomal abnormalities compared to singleton pregnancies (although in dizygotic twins the rate of abnormalities is not increased per twin). Anomaly rates are higher in monozygotic twins compared with dizygotic twins. Discordant fetal abnormality increases the likelihood of an adverse outcome for the normal co-twin. Detection rates of fetal abnormalities in twins are similar to those reported in singleton pregnancies.

Twin Reversed Arterial Perfusion (TRAP)

The twin reversed arterial perfusion sequence (TRAP), or acardiac twinning, occurs in 1% of **monochorionic** pregnancies. The acardiac twin is haemodynamically dependent on the co-twin which is designated as the 'pump twin'. The growth of the acardiac twin threatens the pump twin exposing it to the risk of cardiac failure, polyhydramnios, ruptured membranes, preterm delivery, hydrops and death. Perinatal mortality rates for the pump twin of 35–55% have been reported.

The acardiac twin is usually severely malformed to the extent that it may not resemble a fetus. Management strategies for twin reversed arterial perfusion sequence include:

▶ expectant observation with planned preterm delivery;
▶ termination; and
▶ surgical interventions aimed at interrupting the blood flow to the acardiac twin.

Adverse neurological outcomes have been reported in the surviving twins of pregnancies with twin reversed arterial perfusion but the true risk of this outcome has not been defined. Further studies are needed to define optimal management strategies to reduce perinatal mortality and morbidity in the pump twin.

Single Twin Death

The death of one of the twins occurs in up to 6.2% of all twin pregnancies. Risks to the co-twin include fetal death, preterm delivery and neurodevelopmental impairment with outcome influenced by the underlying cause and gestational age at delivery. Causes of single fetal death in a multiple pregnancy include:

- infection;
- fetal abnormality;
- cord abnormality or event (e.g. entanglement);
- growth restriction; and
- vascular anastomoses (e.g., twin-to-twin transfusion syndrome, twin anaemia-polycythaemia sequence).

The surviving co-twin is potentially at risk from the same condition that led to the death of the other twin. The main features that affect outcome are the chorionicity and the timing of fetal death. **Monochorionic** pregnancies are at greater risk due to shared placental vessels. Following the death of one twin, the risk of death to the co-twin is 12% in **monochorionic** pregnancies and 4% in **dichorionic** pregnancies. First trimester loss does not usually impact on the surviving co-twin. Fetal loss in the second and third trimester can cause preterm delivery in both **dichorionic** and **monochorionic** pregnancies.

Management of the surviving co-twin following single twin demise depends upon the gestation and the chorionicity of the pregnancy. In **monochorionic** pregnancies, conservative management is recommended prior to 34 weeks gestation to avoid additional risks of prematurity. Doppler ultrasound assessment of the middle cerebral artery velocity to examine for fetal anaemia in the surviving twin should be done as soon as possible after the death of a twin is noted. Fetal brain magnetic resonance imaging (MRI) should be considered following single twin death in **monochorionic** twins with an interval of at least 3 weeks from the event. In **dichorionic** pregnancies, delivery is not indicated prior to term unless indicated for obstetric reasons.

Conjoined Twins

Conjoined twins are a rare complication of multiple pregnancy. The classification of conjoined twins is typically based on the description of the fused anatomical region followed by the Greek suffix 'pagus' which means fastened (e.g., craniopagus twins are joined at the head). Conjoined twins can be reliably diagnosed on routine antenatal ultrasound in the late first and early second trimester. Fetal magnetic resonance imaging (MRI) can also be used to more precisely determine the extent of fusion and to assist with counselling of the parents about prognosis. Survival after birth is difficult to predict antenatally and each set of conjoined twins is unique.

Preterm Birth and Multiple Pregnancy

The association between multiple pregnancy and spontaneous preterm birth is well established. Preterm birth in multiple pregnancy may also result from obstetric intervention for maternal medical reasons. More than 50% of twin pregnancies deliver <37 weeks gestation and 10% deliver before 32 weeks. The rate of preterm delivery in triplet and higher order multiples is almost 100%.

The neonatal mortality rate of twins is 6–7 times that of singletons at 18 in 1000 live births. For triplets and higher order multiples, the neonatal mortality rate reaches 40 per 1000 births. More than 50% of neonatal deaths among multiple births are attributable to prematurity.

The risks of prematurity are detailed in Chapters 3–10.

Fetal Growth Restriction and Multiple Pregnancy

Fetal growth discordance of at least 20% affects approximately 16% of all twin pregnancies. Discordance is defined using the larger twin as the standard of growth. Due to lack of international consensus, the range of 15–25% difference in weight between the twins is considered significant and associated with an increased risk of morbidity and mortality. The effects of intrauterine growth restriction are discussed in Chapter 25.

MANAGEMENT—ANTENATAL

Early ultrasound assessment to establish chorionicity is essential for the management of multiple pregnancy so as to permit identification and treatment of certain complications.

First trimester nuchal translucency assessment can be used for aneuploidy risk assessment in multiple pregnancies. Discordant nuchal translucency in **monochorionic** twins can predict an increased risk of twin-to-twin transfusion syndrome.

Detailed morphology ultrasound is recommended at 20 weeks gestation. Ultrasound surveillance of **monochorionic** twins every 2–3 weeks from 16 weeks gestation is recommended for early recognition of twin-to-twin transfusion syndrome and twin anaemia-polycythaemia sequence.

Regular fetal growth assessment every 4 weeks from 24 weeks gestation is recommended in both **monochorionic** and **dichorionic** twins.

Cervical length as measured by transvaginal ultrasound shows a correlation with risk of preterm birth with the shorter the cervix, the higher the risk. The clinical usefulness of cervical length assessment however is predominantly associated with its negative predictive value so as to avoid unnecessary hospitalisation and intervention.

There are no proven treatments to prevent preterm delivery in multiple pregnancy. Randomised trials showing that antenatal progesterone therapy may prevent preterm birth in singleton pregnancies have not demonstrated similar benefits in multiple pregnancies. Cervical cerclage for cervical shortening has also been found to have no beneficial effect on rates of preterm birth in multiple pregnancy.

The type and frequency of fetal monitoring in **monoamniotic** twins remains controversial with cardiotocography and ultrasound imaging used variably.

LABOUR AND DELIVERY

Consideration of early delivery in multiple pregnancies occurs commonly because one or more of the fetuses may be at risk if they remain *in utero*. Usually the options to be considered are either do nothing (i.e., continue the pregnancy) or deliver early. Each option should be explored with regard to the ultimate outcome for the babies including not only mortality but also long-term neurodevelopmental outcome, disability and quality of life. If it is not known that the ultimate outcome will be improved by early delivery (or any intervention) then the fetuses should remain *in utero* until it is known.

The perinatal mortality rate for twins increases after 37–38 weeks and delivery is usually recommended at this gestation in the absence of an earlier indication.

Recent guidelines published by the National Institute for Health and Clinical Excellence (UK),[3] recommend that elective delivery be offered from 36 weeks gestation for uncomplicated **monochorionic** twins and from 37 weeks gestation for uncomplicated **dichorionic** twins. For triplet pregnancies, elective birth from 35 weeks gestation is recommended. A course of antenatal steroids is recommended for deliveries undertaken prior to 37 weeks gestation.

The timing of delivery remains controversial for **monoamniotic** twins. Elective delivery by caesarean section is generally recommended at 32–34 weeks gestation in otherwise uncomplicated cases.

The safest mode of delivery of twins when the presenting twin is cephalic remains uncertain.

When the presenting twin is breech, then delivery by caesarean section is usually undertaken.

If delivery is threatened at <36 weeks gestation, it should be planned at a hospital that has a paediatrician. If delivery is threatened at <32 weeks gestation, it should be planned at a hospital that has an intensive care nursery.

POSTNATAL MANAGEMENT

In same sex **dichorionic-diamniotic** twins, zygosity cannot be determined without DNA testing. Parent support groups recommend that this testing be routinely performed to determine whether or not the twins are identical.

Both twins should be carefully assessed after birth for structural and chromosomal abnormalities.

A full blood count and film examination in each twin may be required to check haemoglobin levels. The blood count is useful in cases of twin-to-twin transfusion syndrome and twin anaemia-polycythaemia sequence.

A cranial ultrasound scan is often recommended in cases of twin-to-twin transfusion syndrome, twin anaemia-polycythaemia sequence and twin reversed arterial perfusion sequence. These children should also be referred to a general or developmental paediatrician for long-term neurodevelopmental follow-up because of their high risk of disability.

ETHICS

In higher order multiples, selective fetal reduction may be considered.

Management strategies for twin reversed arterial perfusion sequence include expectant observation with planned preterm delivery, termination and surgical interventions aimed at interrupting the blood flow to the acardiac twin.

In conjoined twins, management options may include termination of pregnancy or pregnancy continuation with a view to detailed assessment after birth.

REFERENCES

1. Australian Bureau of Statistics. Births, Australia. 2010. (3301.0). Australian Bureau of Statistics. www.abs.gov.au. Accessed online 26.10.11.
2. Lewi L, Jani J, Blickstein I, et al. The outcome of monochorionic diamniotic twin gestations in the era of invasive fetal therapy: a prospective cohort study. *American Journal of Obstetrics & Gynecology.* 2008;199:514–518.
3. National Institute of Health and Clinical Excellence (NICE). NICE Clinical Guideline 129 Multiple Pregnancy. www.nice.org.uk/guidance/CG129. Accessed online 26.10.11.

Further Reading

Chalouhi GE, Stirnemann JJ, Salomon LJ, et al. Specific complications of monochorionic twin pregnancies: twin-twin transfusion syndrome and twin reversed arterial perfusion sequence. *Seminars in Fetal and Neonatal Medicine.* 2010;15:349–356.

Dickinson JE. Monoamniotic twin pregnancy: a review of contemporary practice. *Australian and New Zealand Journal of Obstetrics and Gynaecology.* 2005;45:474–478.

Hillman SC, Morris RK, Kilby MD. Single twin demise: consequence for survivors. *Seminars in Fetal and Neonatal Medicine.* 2010;15:319–326.

Valsky DV, Eixarch E, Martinez JM, et al. Selective intrauterine growth restriction in monochorionic twins: pathophysiology, diagnostic approach and management dilemmas. *Seminars in Fetal & Neonatal Medicine.* 2010;15:342–348.

Blickstein I, Keith L. Prenatal assessment of multiple pregnancy. London: Informa Healthcare; 2007.

Neilson JP, Kilby MD. Management of monochorionic twin pregnancy. London: Royal College of Obstetricians and Gynaecologists, UK; 2008. Green-top Guideline No 51.

Miller J, Chauhan SP, Abuhamad AZ. Discordant Twins: Diagnosis, Evaluation and Management. *American Journal of Obstetrics and Gynecology.* 2011; doi:10.1016/j.ajog.2011.06.075.

CHAPTER 24

Twin-To-Twin Transfusion Syndrome

Rob Cincotta, Peter H Gray

Twin-to-twin transfusion syndrome (TTTS) is the major complication of monochorionic pregnancies where twins share a single placenta. It is characterised by the development of polyhydramnios in one twin sac, whilst the other develops oligohydramnios. Untreated, the polyhydramnios usually results in premature delivery and the loss of both twins.

PATHOPHYSIOLOGY
Monochorionic twins have a shared placenta and have anastomoses on the surface that join the two twins' circulations. These anastomotic patterns are generally balanced, but in about 10–15% of monochorionic pregnancies, there is an unbalanced transfusion of blood from one twin to the other resulting in the development of twin-to-twin transfusion syndrome. The donor twin loses its blood volume and decreases its urine output, which results in the development of oligohydramnios. The recipient twin increases its urine production resulting in the development of polyhydramnios.

Twin-to-twin transfusion syndrome is diagnosed on ultrasound when the deepest pocket of amniotic fluid around the donor twin is ≤2 cm and the deepest pocket around the recipient is ≥8 cm. There can be abnormalities in fetal Doppler flow patterns with absent or reversed flow in the umbilical arteries and, in the more severe form of twin-to-twin transfusion syndrome, hydrops can develop in the recipient with cardiomegaly, ascites, oedema and abnormal Doppler flow patterns in the ductus venosus.[1]

SIGNIFICANCE
Twin-to-twin transfusion syndrome is the commonest cause of increased mortality and morbidity in monochorionic twin pregnancies. Untreated, twin-to-twin transfusion syndrome will result in loss of up to 90% of the pregnancies, with major risk of preterm delivery and long-term morbidity in the survivors.

ASSOCIATED COMPLICATIONS
Intrauterine growth restriction (IUGR) can occur in up to 20% of twins with twin-to-twin transfusion syndrome. Brain injuries can be detected in severe cases, with ventriculomegaly at the time of presentation occasionally being seen.

Death of one monochorionic twin *in utero* may occur with twin-to-twin transfusion syndrome. If this occurs prior to intervention, then the loss of one twin may result in an acute transfusion from one twin to the other. About half of these transfusions will be minor with survival of the co-twin. The other half will have a major transfusion leading to loss of the co-twin (about 25%). In the remaining 25%, the twin survives but with significant long-term neurodevelopmental disability.[2]

MANAGEMENT

Pregnancies managed conservatively have a very poor outcome, apart from mild (stage 1) twin-to-twin transfusion syndrome, when the condition may stabilise and resolve.

Serial amnioreduction of the polyhydramniotic sac has been used but is associated with poorer short- and long-term outcomes in comparison to fetoscopic laser ablation, which is now the treatment of choice.

Antenatal

Fetoscopic laser ablation of the placental communicating vessels interrupts the twin-to-twin transfusion process and allows the twins to recover, with urine production recommencing in the donor twin and both the oligo- and polyhydramnios normalising after the procedure. Laser ablation may be performed from 16 weeks gestation up until 28 weeks. The median gestational age at the time of treatment has been reported as 21 weeks, whilst the median gestational age at delivery is 31 weeks.[3]

The risks of surgery are preterm premature rupture of membranes and/or preterm delivery in about 10–15% of pregnancies within 2 weeks of the procedure. There is the potential for loss of one (usually the smaller donor) or both twins. Reported outcomes following laser show survival of both twins of up to 66%, of at least one twin of up to 85%, with overall survival of up to 75%.

In cases of hydrops, the cardiac failure generally resolves over the course of a few weeks following laser ablation. Long-term cardiac function normalises although there are cases of pulmonary stenosis described.[4]

Labour and Delivery

Once fetal laser ablation is performed and the twin-to-twin transfusion syndrome process resolves, the twins may progress normally. However, there is still the risk of intrauterine growth restriction (if there is unequal placental sharing). There is also the risk that neurological damage may have occurred either before or about the time of surgery and so close surveillance of the brains of both twins is indicated and fetal magnetic resonance imaging (MRI) may be considered. If the recipient was hydropic, assessment of the fetal heart of the recipient is indicated post-delivery. Laser ablation is not an indication, *per se*, for delivery by caesarean section. However, there needs to be close monitoring and management as for other multiple pregnancies.

NEONATAL AND LONG-TERM OUTCOMES

During the neonatal period, infants affected by twin-to-twin transfusion syndrome have an increased risk of:

- respiratory distress syndrome;
- the need for ventilatory assistance;
- chronic lung disease;
- hypotension requiring inotropic support; and
- oliguric renal failure.

These neonatal morbidities are largely related to the preterm delivery and occur less frequently with twin-to-twin transfusion syndrome pregnancies treated with laser ablation. The consequences of preterm delivery are discussed in Chapters 3 to 9.

Neurodevelopmental disability in the survivors of twin-to-twin transfusion syndrome is considerable. With serial amnioreduction (without laser ablation) as the mode of management, cerebral palsy and severe cognitive impairment occurs in 19–26% of survivors. Following treatment with laser ablation, long-term outcome is somewhat better with cerebral palsy rates of 4–14% and overall neurodevelopmental disability rates of 12–18% having been reported. The severity of the twin-to-twin transfusion syndrome at diagnosis is an independent risk factor for adverse long-term outcome. It is recommended that all survivors of severe twin-to-twin transfusion syndrome pregnancies should receive detailed follow-up.

ETHICS

There is a high incidence of loss and long-term major morbidity in surviving babies with this condition. The optimal treatment for twin-to-twin transfusion syndrome is fetoscopic laser ablation, but other options include termination of pregnancy, or selective reduction if one twin is found to have a major anomaly or neurological damage either at the time of diagnosis or after treatment with laser. As these diagnoses may be made late in the second trimester, this may raise difficult ethical issues and the laws and practices regarding late terminations vary between various states and countries.

REFERENCES

1. Cincotta RB, Gray PH, Gardener G, et al. Selective fetoscopic laser ablation in 100 consecutive pregnancies with severe twin–twin transfusion syndrome. *Australian and New Zealand Journal of Obstetrics and Gynaecology*. 2009;49:22–27.
2. Fisk NM, Duncombe GJ, Sullivan MHF. The basic and clinical science of twin–twin transfusion syndrome. *Placenta*. 2009;30:379–390.
3. Gray PH, Poulsen L, Gilshenan K, et al. Neurodevelopmental outcome and risk factors for disability for twin-twin transfusion syndrome treated with laser surgery. *American Journal of Obstetrics and Gynecology*. 2011;204:159.e1–e6.
4. Gray PH, Ward C, Chan FY. Cardiac outcomes of hydrops as a result of twin-twin transfusion treated with laser surgery. *Journal of Paediatrics and Child Health*. 2009;45:48–52.

CHAPTER 25

Intrauterine Growth Restriction

Joseph Thomas, Elizabeth Hurrion

Intrauterine growth restriction (IUGR) is a term used to describe the condition of a fetus that has failed to reach its genetically determined growth potential. It is also known as fetal growth restriction.

Small for gestational age (SGA) is a term used when a baby's birth weight is below the 10th percentile for their gestational age.

A fetus may be small for gestational age because of intrauterine growth restriction, but this is not always the case. Some small for gestational age infants are constitutionally small (i.e., their growth is appropriate for their genetic or ethnic background).[1]

Not all growth-restricted infants are small for gestational age. An infant may be on the 25th percentile, but have fallen from the 75th percentile earlier in pregnancy, and hence is considered to have intrauterine growth restriction. One study found that 47% of pregnancies with intrauterine growth restriction resulted in a baby with a birthweight above the 10th percentile.[2]

For these reasons, growth is best assessed by serial growth scans using population-specific weight and gestational age percentile charts (see Figure 25.1) and must take into consideration parental anthropometrics. In addition, assessment includes evidence of fetal compromise.

Historically, a distinction was made between symmetric intrauterine growth restriction (all growth parameters are affected equally; i.e., weight, length and head circumference are on similar percentiles) or asymmetric intrauterine growth restriction (length and head circumference relatively preserved compared with weight). This distinction was used to help distinguish cause. However, these terms are no longer used as there is a great deal of overlap between the two, making the distinction unhelpful.

CAUSES OF INTRAUTERINE GROWTH RESTRICTION

The causes of intrauterine growth restriction can be categorised as fetal, placental, maternal or environmental:

▶ fetal causes:
- chromosomal abnormalities, particularly aneuploidy—trisomy 13, 18, 21 and triploidy,
- fetal malformations—gastroschisis,

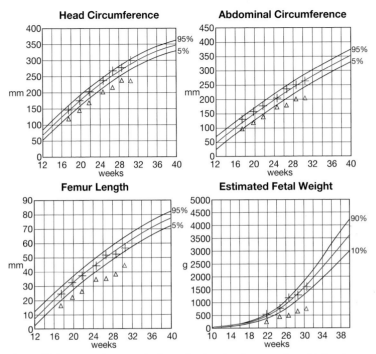

Figure 25.1 Intrauterine growth chart of twins showing growth restriction in fetus 2 (triangle) compared with fetus 1 (cross).

- multiple pregnancy, and
- intrauterine infection—toxoplasmosis, rubella, cytomegalovirus, herpes;
- placental causes:
  - chronic placental insufficiency,
  - placenta praevia,
  - placental tumours—chorioangiomas, and
  - placental mosaicism;
- maternal causes:
  - hypertension—pre-existing or pregnancy-induced,
  - diabetes,
  - renal disease,
  - connective tissue disorders—systemic lupus erythematosus (SLE), antiphospholipid syndrome,
  - inflammatory bowel disease,

- thrombophilias—heterozygote for Factor 5 Leiden, prothrombin gene mutation G20210A,
- hypoxia—cardiorespiratory disease,
- anaemia, and
- maternal uterine malformations—myomas, bicornuate or septate uterus; and
▶ environmental causes:
  - low socioeconomic status,
  - poor nutrition,
  - smoking,
  - alcohol,
  - drug dependence—cocaine, heroin, methadone,
  - therapeutic drugs—anti-cancer, and
  - living at high altitude.

Placental Insufficiency

The presence of oligohydramnios (indicating decreased fetal renal perfusion) and/or increased resistance to flow in the umbilical artery, as assessed by Doppler studies, is suggestive of intrauterine growth restriction due to placental insufficiency. Notching or poor flow in diastole in the uterine arteries may add to the diagnosis.

CONSEQUENCES

Short-Term Risks to the Fetus or Infant

Intrauterine growth restriction is reported to increase the risk of intrauterine fetal death (IUFD). It is very difficult to provide a figure for the risk of IUFD because epidemiological studies are extremely heterogeneous in terms of the definition of the group studied (i.e., severity of fetal compromise) and the approach to management in pregnancy (fetal surveillance and decisions to deliver). As an example, two studies of consecutive singleton pregnancies with absent/reversed end-diastolic flow in the umbilical artery that received intensive fetal surveillance in a tertiary institution and were delivered between 24 and 32/34 completed weeks of gestation give an incidence of intrauterine fetal death of 11–27%.[3,4] In a less severely affected cohort (30% of which had normal umbilical artery Dopplers) the incidence of intrauterine fetal death was only 2%.[5]

The growth-restricted fetus is at risk of iatrogenic preterm delivery because of concerns about imminent fetal death. Prematurity adds to the risks of mortality and morbidity for the growth-restricted fetus in the following ways:
▶ there is an increased risk of mortality and morbidity due to prematurity, according to gestational age (see Chapters 3–10);
▶ preterm infants with severe intrauterine growth restriction have an increased risk of mortality beyond that predicted by their gestation—for example, in the study by Hartung et al,[3] the mortality for liveborn infants

was 16%, compared with 2–3% for gestational-age-matched appropriately-grown controls. Another study found a similar figure for the subgroup of infants with absent or reversed end-diastolic flow.[6] Preterm infants with intrauterine growth restriction who are liveborn weighing <500 g have a particularly high mortality, at around 60%;[6,7] and

▶ preterm infants with intrauterine growth restriction have an increased risk of necrotising enterocolitis and chronic neonatal lung disease.[3,6]

Long-Term Risks Following Intrauterine Growth Restriction

There is an increased risk of cerebral palsy, which is most clearly the case for infants born at 32–42 weeks gestation. The rate of cerebral palsy among small for gestational age term/near-term singletons is 5–7 times that of normally grown term/near-term singletons.[8,9] For infants born below 32 weeks gestation, the risk of cerebral palsy seems to be swamped by the risk attributable to prematurity. There may be an additional independent increased risk associated with intrauterine growth restriction, but this is difficult to quantify because of marked heterogeneity of epidemiological studies. As an example, in a study of small for gestational age infants born at 24–32 weeks of gestation, the rate of moderate/severe disability for those who had absent or reversed end-diastolic flow was 17%.[6]

The child may remain small. The vast majority of small for gestational age children achieve catch-up growth during the first year of life. Of those that do not, approximately 50% catch up slowly throughout childhood, but a significant proportion of children will remain small into adulthood.[10,11] Babies who are born preterm and small for gestational age appear to do worse with limited or no catch-up growth during the first year.[11]

There is considerable debate as to whether or not children affected by intrauterine growth restriction are at increased risk of developing the "metabolic syndrome". The metabolic syndrome includes combinations of the following: central obesity, insulin resistance / raised fasting blood glucose / type 2 diabetes, hypertension, dyslipidaemia. This is associated with an increased incidence of cardiovascular disease.[12] Evidence is emerging that being small for gestational age may not be an independent predictor of obesity and the metabolic syndrome, but only becomes a risk factor if there is subsequent over-nutrition in infancy, suggested by accelerated growth in early childhood.[13,14] This is consistent with the "thrifty phenotype" hypothesis, which proposes that when the intrauterine nutritional environment is poor there is a fetal adaptive response designed to enhance survival in an expected postnatal environment of poor nutrition.[15] When there is abundant postnatal nutrition, these metabolic adaptations become maladaptive (incongruent with the postnatal environment) with adverse metabolic consequences. Research suggests that the metabolic pathway for this effect is via initial insulin sensitivity.[13] By 48 hours of age, small for gestational age infants are insulin-sensitive and have higher plasma free fatty acid levels than their appropriate for gestational age counterparts. They then undergo a period of accelerated postnatal growth that is associated with the increased sensitivity. The early period of increased insulin sensitivity and accelerated growth precedes the subsequent emergence of insulin resistance in later life.[13]

MANAGEMENT—ANTENATAL

The pregnancy should be investigated to establish the cause for any intrauterine growth restriction. This includes an assessment of maternal health (blood pressure, renal disease, etc) and lifestyle factors such as smoking and drug use. Investigations for viral infections (especially toxoplasmosis, rubella, cytomegalovirus, herpes) should be done. Depending on the aetiology, management of the underlying cause is important (such as treatment of hypertension, smoking cessation, etc)

A detailed morphological ultrasound scan should be done and an amniocentesis for fetal karyotype should be considered.

Pregnancy interventions have been shown to be ineffective in preventing or improving intrauterine growth restriction.

Fetal surveillance is indicated to inform the decision about when to deliver.

Fetal Surveillance

Fetal surveillance consists of various ultrasound and Doppler assessments and other assessments of fetal well being.

Fetal growth is monitored to determine the velocity of growth.

Doppler studies are done on various vessels. Placental and fetal Doppler flow studies represent a major advance in management of intrauterine growth restriction since the 1980s. These include the following vessels:

▶ Umbilical artery (UA) flow velocity assesses blood flow from the fetus to the placenta representing placental vessel resistance. When there is increased resistance to flow an increased systolic/diastolic ratio ($\uparrow$S/D ratio) or increased resistance index ($\uparrow$ RI) is seen first, followed by absent end-diastolic flow velocity (AEDV), and finally reversed end-diastolic flow velocity (REDV), at which point nearly 70% of the placental bed is non-functional. The S/D (systolic/diastolic) ratio is the simplest of the Doppler ratios. The RI (resistance index) and PI (pulsatility index) are also used.

▶ Middle cerebral artery (MCA) flow velocity assesses cerebral blood flow. A decreased resistance to flow in diastole ($\downarrow$S/D ratio or $\downarrow$ RI) represents redistribution of blood flow towards the brain and heart and away from visceral organs. However, when placental insufficiency becomes severe, this compensatory redistribution is lost ($\uparrow$S/D ratio or $\uparrow$RI).

▶ Ductus venosus (DV) flow velocity assesses cardiac preload (right heart failure). A deep or reversed "a" wave in the ductus venosus is seen when there is reversed flow during atrial systole. This is a sign of raised central venous pressure and congestive cardiac failure. Ductus venosus flow waveforms become abnormal only when fetal compromise is severe. These changes define a subgroup of infants at extremely high risk of intrauterine fetal death and neonatal death.[4,16]

The fetal biophysical profile (BPP) is favoured in some centres. The biophysical profile is a score derived from amniotic fluid volume, fetal tone, fetal movements, fetal breathing movements and fetal heart rate monitoring.[17]

Fetal heart rate monitoring (cardiotocography, CTG) can also be used. A loss of heart rate variability has been shown to correlate well with fetal metabolic acidaemia and the risk of intrauterine death.[18,19]

With worsening intrauterine growth restriction there is a recognised sequence of abnormalities. These include:[16]

1. decreased amniotic fluid volume;
2. increased resistance in the umbilical artery;
3. middle cerebral artery flow changes;
4. ductus venosus flow changes; and
5. decreased heart rate variability (cardiotocography changes).

Decision to Deliver

Recommendations for delivery are an evolving area of active research. The reports by Baschat,[20] Bachat et al,[21] Baschat,[22] Hecher et al[23] and Ferrazzi et al[24] are some of the many that are relevant to this topic.

Below 32 weeks of gestation the decision to deliver is based on maternal health (e.g., severe pre-eclampsia) or signs of fetal deterioration suggesting imminent fetal death.

The European GRIT study (Growth Restriction Intervention Trial) was a randomised trial of immediate or delayed delivery for pregnancies between 24 and 36 weeks gestation with evidence of fetal compromise and clinical uncertainty about whether delivery was indicated. About 30% had normal umbilical artery Doppler flows. The delayed delivery group were delivered according to the treating obstetrician based on other clinical indicators. This study showed no difference in perinatal mortality or developmental outcome at 2 years between the immediate and delayed delivery groups. There was a trend to reduced disability (5% *versus* 13%) in the delayed delivery group for the subgroup of infants born below 31 weeks gestation. At school-age follow-up (age 6–13 years), this trend had narrowed (6% *versus* 10% severe disability) and there was actually a trend towards a higher rate of the composite outcome of death or severe disability in the delayed delivery group born below 31 weeks gestation (37% *versus* 25%).[5,25,26]

Perinatal mortality is significantly increased in fetuses with reversed end-diastolic flow, compared with absent end-diastolic flow, and this is often used by obstetricians to indicate the necessity for delivery.[27] Ductus venosus changes and loss of heart rate variability on cardiotocography identify a group at extremely high risk of imminent fetal demise.[16] Fetal deterioration does not appear to increase the risk of adverse neurodevelopmental outcome and hence delivery should not be recommended to prevent this outcome. Since adverse neurodevelopmental outcome is heavily influenced by gestational age at birth, every effort should be made to prolong the pregnancy. Nevertheless, the decision to deliver remains a difficult balance between complications of extreme prematurity and prolonged intrauterine exposure to hypoxia, malnutrition and the risk of fetal death.

Above 32 weeks gestation, significant complications of prematurity are much less of a risk (see Chapter 10) and so delivery is recommended before fetal compromise becomes severe. Reversed umbilical artery end-diastolic flow velocities after 32 weeks of gestation and absent end-diastolic flow velocities at more than 34 weeks are considered by many clinicians as an indication for prompt delivery.

DELIVERY

If the decision to deliver has been made, and the gestation is preterm, then antenatal steroids should be administered and consideration given to magnesium sulphate infusion for neuroprotection (see Chapters 3–10.)

The location for delivery should be considered to ensure that neonatal services appropriate for the gestation and estimated fetal weight are available. If the gestation is <32 weeks or the estimated fetal weight is <1500 g then delivery should be planned at a hospital with an intensive care nursery.

There is no clear evidence to support the need for an operative mode of delivery, though it is common practice to deliver severely compromised infants by caesarean section in the belief that fetal hypoxia may be worsened by labour. Certainly absent or reversed umbilical artery Dopplers or a non-reassuring fetal heart rate trace is generally considered a contra-indication for attempting vaginal delivery. If the fetus is extremely small with oligohydramnios then the lower segment may not be well developed and classical caesarean section may be required, with consequent risks for subsequent pregnancies.

POSTNATAL MANAGEMENT

Depending on the condition of the baby when it is born, and its gestational age, varying degrees of resuscitation and respiratory support may be required. Chapters 5–9 discuss these issues for babies born from 24–32 weeks gestational age.

The baby should be closely examined for other abnormalities. Chromosomal studies may be indicated (if they have not been done antenatally).

A full blood count and film examination should be done to check for thrombocytopaenia which is common in placental insufficiency and some of the congenital infections.

If intrauterine infection is suspected, a cranial ultrasound scan should be done to look for intracranial calcifications.

An ophthalmology assessment may be indicated in some cases. Auditory assessment should be done before hospital discharge.

Long-term neurodevelopmental follow-up by a general paediatrician will be required in most cases.

RECURRENCE RATE

The risk of recurrence will ultimately depend upon the cause of the intrauterine growth restriction. Pre-eclampsia is likely to recur in subsequent pregnancies. Low dose aspirin given before 16 weeks in women at risk of pre-eclampsia decreases the risk of intrauterine growth restriction by 15%.[28]

Some chromosomal abnormalities will have increased risk of recurrence. Cases of intrauterine growth restriction due to intrauterine infections are unlikely to recur but this may depend on the timing of primary maternal infection (see Chapters 16–20).

Intrauterine growth restriction due to lifestyle factors (e.g., maternal smoking) may be modifiable prior to conception or early in a future pregnancy.

REFERENCES

1. Gardosi J. Clinical strategies for improving the detection of fetal growth restriction. *Clin Perinatol.* 2011;38(1):21–31.
2. Marconi AM, Ronzoni S, Bozzetti P, et al. Comparison of fetal and neonatal growth curves in detecting growth restriction. *Obstet Gynecol.* 2008;112(6): 1227–1234.
3. Hartung J, Kalache KD, Heyna C, et al. Outcome of 60 neonates who had ARED flow prenatally compared with a matched control group of appropriate-for-gestational age preterm neonates. *Ultrasound Obstet Gynecol.* 2005;25:566–572.
4. Schwarze A, Gembruch U, Krapp M, et al. Qualitative venous Doppler flow waveform analysis in preterm intrauterine growth-restricted foetuses with ARED flow in the umbilical artery—correlation with short-term outcome. *Ultrasound Obstet Gynecol.* 2005;25:573–579.
5. The GRIT Study Group. A randomised trial of timed delivery for the compromised preterm fetus: short term outcomes and Bayesian interpretation. *BJOG.* 2003;110(1):27–32.
6. Shand AW, Hornbuckle J, Nathan E, et al. Small for gestational age preterm infants and relationship of abnormal artery Doppler blood flow to perinatal mortality and neurodevelopmental outcomes. *Aust N Z J Obstet Gynecol.* 2009;49:52–58.
7. Petersen SG, Wong SF, Urs P, et al. Early-onset, severe fetal growth restriction with absent or reversed end-diastolic flow velocity waveform in the umbilical artery: Perinatal and long-term outcomes. *Aust N Z J Obstet Gynaecol.* 2009;49:45–51.

8. Surveillance of cerebral palsy in Europe (SCPE). Collaborative Group Surveillance of Cerebral Palsy in Europe; a collaboration of cerebral palsy surveys and registers. *Dev Med Child Neurol*. 2000;42:816–824.

9. Jacobsson B, Ahlin K, Francis A, et al. Cerebral Palsy and restricted growth status at birth: population-based case-control study. *BJOG*. 2008;115(10): 1250–1255.

10. Karlberg J, Albertsson-Wikland K. Growth in full-term small-for-gestational-age infants: from birth to final height. *Pediatr Res*. 1995;38:733–739.

11. Hediger ML, Overpeck MD, Maurer KR, et al. Growth of infants and young children born small or large for gestational age. *Arch Pediatr Adolesc Med*. 1998;152: 1225–1231.

12. Ford ES. Risks for all-cause mortality, cardiovascular disease and diabetes associated with the metabolic syndrome. *Diabetes Care*. 2005;28:1769–1778.

13. Morrison JL, Duffield JA, Muhlhausler BS, et al. Fetal growth restriction, catch-up growth and the early origins of insulin resistance and visceral obesity. *Pediatr Nephrol*. 2010;25:669–677.

14. Neitzke U, Harder T, Plagemann A. Intrauterine growth restriction and developmental programming of the metabolic syndrome. *Microcirculation*. 2011; 18(4):304–311.

15. Hales CN, Barker DJP. The thrifty phenotype hypothesis. *Br Med Bull*. 2001;60:5–20.

16. Bamfo JE, Odibo AO. Diagnosis and Management of Fetal Growth Restriction. *J Pregnancy*. Epub 2011; Apr 13.

17. Manning FA, Morrison I, Lange IR, et al. Fetal assessment based on fetal biophysical profile scoring: experience in 12,620 referred high-risk pregnancies. I. Perinatal mortality by frequency and etiology. *Am J Obstet Gynecol*. 1985;151(3): 343–350.

18. Pardey J, Moulden M, Redman CWG. A computer system for the numerical analysis of nonstress tests. *Am J Obstet Gynecol*. 2002;186(5):1095–1103.

19. Visser GHA, Sadovsky G, Nicolaides KH. Antepartum heart rate patterns in small-for-gestational-age third-trimester fetuses: correlations with blood gas values obtained at cordocentesis. *Am J Obstet Gynecol*. 1990;162(3):698–703.

20. Baschat AA. Opinion and Review; Doppler application in the delivery timing of the preterm growth-restricted fetus: another step in the right direction. *Ultrasound Obstet Gynecol*. 2004;23(2):111–118.

21. Baschat AA, Cosmi E, Bilardo CM, et al. Predictors of neonatal outcome in early-onset placental dysfunction. *Obstet Gynecol*. 2007;109(2 Pt 1):253–261.

22. Baschat AA. Neurodevelopment following fetal growth restriction and its relationship with antepartum parameters of placental dysfunction. *Ultrasound Obstet Gynecol*. 2011;37(5):501–514.

23. Hecher K, Bilardo CM, Stigter RH, et al. Monitoring of fetuses with intrauterine growth restriction: a longitudinal study. *Ultrasound Obstet Gynecol*. 2001;18(6): 564–570.

24. Ferrazzi E, Bozzo M, Rigano S, et al. Temporal sequence of abnormal Doppler changes in the peripheral and central circulatory systems of the severely growth-restricted fetus. *Ultrasound Obstet Gynecol*. 2002;19(2):140–146.

25. Thornton JG, Hornbuckle J, Vail A, et al. GRIT study group. Infant wellbeing at 2 years of age in the Growth Restriction Intervention Trial (GRIT): multicentred randomised controlled trial. *The Lancet*. 2004;364(9433):513–520.

26. Walker DM, Marlow N, Upstone L, et al. The Growth Restriction Intervention Trial: long-term outcomes in a randomised trial of timing of delivery in fetal growth restriction. *Am J Obstet Gynecol.* 2011;204:34.e1–e9.

27. Vasconcelos RP, Brazil Frota Aragao JR, Cosat Carvalho FH, et al. Differences in neonatal outcome in fetuses with absent versus reverse end-diastolic flow in umbilical artery Doppler. *Fetal Diagn Ther.* 2010;28(3):160–166.

28. Bujold E, Roberge S, Lacase Y, et al. Prevention of preeclampsia and intrauterine growth restriction with aspirin started in early pregnancy: a meta-analysis. *Obstet Gynaecol.* 2010;116(1):402–414.

CHAPTER 26

Red Cell Alloimmunisation Haemolytic Disease

Bronwyn Williams, Garry DT Inglis

Haemolytic disease of the fetus and newborn occurs when:
- fetal red cells express an antigen which is not present on maternal cells; and
- the mother forms an antibody which can cross the placenta (IgG); and
- the antibody binds to fetal or neonatal red cells causing premature destruction.

AETIOLOGY
Antibodies which cause haemolytic disease develop following exposure of the mother to red cell antigens that she lacks. This results from transfusion of red cells or passage of fetal cells across the placenta in the current or a prior pregnancy. The antibodies associated with haemolytic disease are:
- antibodies which cause haemolytic disease are Anti D, c, E, e, C, K, k; anti D, c and K are associated with moderate to severe haemolytic disease;
- antibodies that are occasionally associated with haemolytic disease are anti Cw, Fya, Fyb, Jka, Jkb, Lua, Lub, S, s, M; usually the IgG titre is high if these antibodies are implicated; and
- antibodies which are not associated with haemolytic disease are anti P1, N, H, Lea, Leb, Sda, Bga, Bgb and HLA.

PREVALENCE
Red cell antibodies occur in approximately 57 in 10,000 pregnancies. Clinically significant antibodies occur in approximately 24 in 10,000 pregnancies.

DIFFERENTIAL DIAGNOSIS
The differential diagnoses include:
- haemolytic disease due to ABO incompatibility;
- genetic and acquired haemolytic anaemia;

> haemorrhage; and
> red cell aplasia (parvovirus B19 or genetic) may need exclusion.

ASSOCIATED ABNORMALITIES

There are no associated abnormalities.

CONSEQUENCES

Fetus

Clinically significant antibodies may cause fetal anaemia. If severe and untreated, hydrops (~25% in Rhesus haemolytic disease) and *in utero* fetal death may result.

Neonate

Hyperbilirubinaemia is the main cause of morbidity (~30% in Rhesus haemolytic disease). Phototherapy is required. Exchange transfusion may occasionally be warranted.

Anaemia is common and a simple "top-up" red cell transfusion is often required. Recurrent or late anaemia may occur up to 6 months of age in severe cases.

Inadequately treated hyperbilirubinaemia can lead to brain injury. Initially this causes acute bilirubin encephalopathy. The baby is at first obtunded and hypotonic with poor primitive reflexes; this soon progresses to irritability with a high-pitched cry, hypertonia and opisthotonus. The long-term consequences include choreoathetosis, sensorineural deafness and cognitive impairment.

MANAGEMENT

Antenatal—Detection of Pregnancies at Risk

Maternal blood group and antibody screening should be performed early in pregnancy (~12 weeks) with follow-up at 28 weeks in Rh-positive women and at 28 and 36 weeks in Rh-negative women if no antibody is detected.

If clinically significant antibodies are present, the following course of action is advised:

> seek advice from a maternal fetal specialist;
> assess severity with serial ultrasound for fetal growth, liver size, signs of hydrops and middle cerebral artery flow rates;
> use middle cerebral artery Doppler to reliably detect fetal anaemia from 18 weeks gestation—the sensitivity for diagnosing moderate to severe anaemia is approximately 100%;
> fetal blood sampling and transfusion may be required in severe cases; and
> amniocentesis, if indicated, can be performed from 15 weeks gestational age to determine the fetal genotype and assess levels of bilirubin (delta-OD450).

Laboratory Testing

Titration of antibody is done about every 4 weeks to 36 weeks gestational age and then every 2 weeks until delivery. Antibody quantitation and assays of functional potency provide additional prognostic information when available.

Note: The antibody titre is unreliable in assessing severity of Kell haemolytic disease; fetal monitoring is indicated (i.e., serial ultrasound as described above).

If paternity can be guaranteed, paternal blood group and genotype assists in determining the fetal risk. Fetal genotyping (Rh and Kell) on cells from maternal blood or amniotic fluid can assist in risk analysis.

MANAGEMENT—LABOUR AND DELIVERY

Timing and method of delivery will be influenced by:

◗ severity of disease;
◗ gestation; and
◗ maternal factors.

OTHER CONSULTS REQUIRED

A maternal fetal medicine specialist will be required in the antenatal management phase.

MANAGEMENT—POSTNATAL

Cord blood should be collected immediately after birth and the following tests done: blood group, Direct Coombs test, haemoglobin level and serum bilirubin. Advise the parents that these results should be available within hours of the baby's birth.

Bilirubin levels should be monitored closely. Check another serum bilirubin in the first few hours to determine the rate of rise; depending on the initial results, bilirubin levels should be checked frequently in the first 24–48 hours.

The baby will therefore need either frequent heel-prick samples or an arterial line inserted.

Affected infants will be treated with phototherapy. Phototherapy may need to be intensive—i.e., numerous lights placed around the baby with banks of overhead and side lights plus a biliblanket below the baby. This will dictate that the baby may not be allowed out of phototherapy for feeding. The baby may have bottle feeds of formula or expressed breast milk while receiving phototherapy. Likewise, baths should be avoided until the bilirubin level is safely controlled.

Exchange transfusion will be considered if there is:

◗ severe anaemia;
◗ cord bilirubin > 70 umol/L; or
◗ rapidly rising bilirubin despite intensive phototherapy.

Affected babies will be anaemic and simple red cell transfusion is often required for treatment of anaemia. Recurrent anaemia requiring repeated red cell transfusion may last for up to 6 months. Affected infants will clear the antibody within 6 months of age. The haemoglobin levels should be monitored in all infants until there is evidence that transfusion is no longer required. Erythropoietin administration may minimise the need for transfusion and may be considered in severe cases.

RECURRENCE

There is a risk of recurrence which may be more severe in subsequent pregnancies.

ETHICS

Failure to provide RhIG therapy to a Rh-negative woman, which results in maternal alloimmunisation that affects offspring, has a very high potential for medicolegal litigation.

Risks of an alloimmunised gestation irrespective of its severity should be clearly explained to the parent including fetal loss, prematurity and risk and effects of bilirubin encephalopathy.

Further Reading

1. ACOG Practice Bulletin No 75: Management of alloimmunization. *Obstet Gynecol.* Aug 2006;108(2):457–464.
2. American Academy of Pediatrics. Clinical Practice Guideline. Subcommittee on Hyperbilirubinaemia: Management of hyperbilirubinaemia in the newborn infant 35 or more weeks of gestation. *Pediatrics.* 2004;114:297–316.
3. http://www.ranzcog.edu.au/womenshealth/pdfs/ANZSBT-antenatal-guidelines.pdf
4. Madan A, MacMahon JR, Stevenson DK. Neonatal hyperbilirubinemia. In: Taeusch HW, Ballard RA, eds. *Avery's Diseases of The Newborn.* 8th ed. Philadelphia, PA: Elsevier Saunders; 2005:1226–1256.
5. Maisels MJ, Watchko JF. Treatment of jaundice in low birthweight infants. *Arch Dis Child Fetal Neonatal Ed.* 2003;88:F459–F463.
6. Moise KJ Jr. Management of rhesus alloimmunization in pregnancy. *Obstet Gynecol.* Jul 2008;112(1):164–176.
7. Moise KJ. Fetal anemia due to non-Rhesus-D red-cell alloimmunization. *Semin Fetal Neonatal Med.* Aug 2008;13(4):207–214.
8. Moise KJ. Hemolytic disease of the fetus and newborn. In: Creasy RK, Resnik R, eds. *Maternal-fetal Medicine: Principles and Practice.* 6th ed. Philadelphia: WB Saunders; 2008:477–503.
9. Murray NA, Roberts IA. Haemolytic disease of the newborn. *Arch Dis Child Fetal Neonatal Ed.* Mar 2007;92(2):F83–F88.
10. Oepkes D, Seaward PG, Vandenbussche FP, et al. Doppler ultrasonography versus amniocentesis to predict fetal anemia. *N Engl J Med.* Jul 13 2006;355(2):156–164.
11. Van der Schoot CE, Tax GH, Rijnders RJ, et al. Prenatal typing of Rh and Kell blood group system antigens: the edge of a watershed. *Transfus Med Rev.* Jan 2003;17(1):31–44.

CHAPTER 27

Fetomaternal Alloimmune Thrombocytopaenia (FMAIT)

Jeremy D Robertson, Mark W Davies

Alloimmune thrombocytopaenia occurs when there is destruction of fetal platelets by maternal allo-antibodies directed against paternally inherited human platelet antigens. This leads to fetal thrombocytopaenia. The condition is known as fetomaternal alloimmune thrombocytopaenia (FMAIT) in the fetus and neonatal alloimmune thrombocytopaenia (NAIT) in the newborn baby. FMAIT/NAIT is the most common cause of severe thrombocytopaenia in the fetus and in otherwise healthy term infants.

The diagnosis is confirmed serologically using blood from both parents: maternal serum and EDTA whole blood from both parents. Such testing requires a high level of expertise, and should be performed by a specialised platelet reference laboratory.

PATHOPHYSIOLOGY

Human platelet antigens (HPA) are epitopes on platelet surface glycoproteins; each is biallelic ("a" for high frequency, "b" for low frequency), and inherited in an autosomal co-dominant fashion.

HPA-1a incompatibility is the most common cause in Caucasians. HPA-4a incompatibility is more common in Asians. HPA-5a incompatibility accounts for ~5–10% cases but is typically less severe. The involvement of other antigens is rare.

Maternal IgG antibodies are produced following sensitisation by fetal platelet antigens. Transplacental passage of these antibodies results in platelet destruction and thrombocytopaenia. This situation is analogous to the pathogenesis of anaemia in Rhesus disease.

Due to the greater ability of platelets to cross the placenta (relative to red cells), maternal sensitisation to fetal platelet antigens can occur as early as the second trimester, and a first pregnancy can be severely affected (in contrast to Rh disease). The severity of FMAIT increases with each subsequent pregnancy and this is known as anamnesis (immunologic memory).

The maternal anti-platelet antibody titre during pregnancy correlates with the severity; however, currently no non-invasive biomarker of fetal platelet count exists.

EPIDEMIOLOGY

About 2% of the Caucasian population is HPA-1a negative (homozygous 1b). Only 5–15% of "at risk" mothers produce anti-HPA antibodies.

The incidence of FMAIT (from prospective screening studies) is about 1 in 1000–1 in 2000 pregnancies. Severe FMAIT occurs much less frequently, in around 1 in 8000–1 in 15,000 pregnancies.

Without appropriate management, the risk of intracranial haemorrhage in the current pregnancy is highest (>90%) if there has been a previously affected fetus with intracranial haemorrhage.

DIFFERENTIAL DIAGNOSIS

The differential diagnosis for thrombocytopaenia includes the following:
▶ congenital infection (e.g., TORCH);
▶ sepsis or other causes of disseminated intravascular coagulation (DIC);
▶ placental insufficiency;
▶ perinatal asphyxia;
▶ thrombosis (e.g., renal vein);
▶ Kasabach-Merritt syndrome;
▶ hereditary thrombocytopaenia;
▶ aneuploidy;
▶ maternal autoimmune conditions (idiopathic thrombocytopaenic purpura, systemic lupus erythematosus); and
▶ marrow infiltration.

CONSEQUENCES

The consequences of FMAIT include:
▶ asymptomatic with a birth platelet count of $>50 \times 10^9$/L: common (60–80%) if appropriate antenatal treatment has been initiated;
▶ petechiae and bruising in 80–90%;
▶ intracranial haemorrhage occurs in 2–3% with antenatal treatment and 10–20% without antenatal treatment; the majority (50–75%) occur *in utero*;
▶ severe disability after intracranial haemorrhage occurs in about 20%; and
▶ death after intracranial haemorrhage occurs in about 10–30%.

MANAGEMENT—ANTENATAL

The mother should be under the care of a maternal fetal medicine specialist.

The treatment can be stratified according to severity of outcome in the previously affected fetus; if intracranial haemorrhage occurred, maternal therapy should be commenced as early as possible (e.g., from 12 weeks gestation). Treatments include:
▶ regular immunoglobulin infusion (typically 1 g/kg once or twice a week);
▶ oral glucocorticoids (typically prednisone 0.5 mg/kg/day);
▶ combination therapy (immunoglobulin and prednisone) is appropriate where there has been a previous severely affected fetus; and

▶ fetal blood sampling (with or without intrauterine platelet transfusion) may occasionally be necessary, but should be minimised due to the higher risk of associated morbidity/mortality in FMAIT (as compared with Rh disease).

The parents should also see a paediatric haematologist antenatally.

MANAGEMENT—LABOUR / DELIVERY

Delivery should be in a centre that has a neonatal intensive care unit.

It is difficult to predict the baby's platelet count at delivery (even with antenatal treatment), unless fetal blood sampling has been done. HPA-1a negative platelets should be available if possible.

Instrumental delivery should be avoided, as should fetal scalp monitoring. Delivery by elective caesarean section should be considered for selected cases.

NEONATAL MANAGEMENT

Cord blood will be taken for an urgent platelet count. If cord blood cannot be collected then blood will be taken from the baby as soon as possible after birth.

A platelet transfusion (10–20 mL/kg) will be given if the platelet count is $<30 \times 10^9$/L if baby is well, or $<50 \times 10^9$/L if the baby is unwell (e.g., low Apgar scores). **Platelet transfusion should not be delayed** while waiting for HPA-matched units; random donor platelets are suitable. Transfusion of maternal platelets is possible, but preparation is technically demanding, and may increase antibody exposure.

Other treatments to be considered include:
▶ intravenous immunoglobulin 1 g/kg daily for 2 days; and
▶ methylprednisolone 1 mg IV q8h for 2–3 days.

A head ultrasound will be done as soon as possible. This is important for management as the platelet count should be kept $>100 \times 10^9$/L if there is any intracranial haemorrhage. The presence of an intracranial haemorrhage is a prognostic indicator for subsequent pregnancies.

Baby will be admitted to the neonatal unit unless completely well with a platelet count $>50 \times 10^9$/L with no intracranial haemorrhage.

Platelet counts will be monitored regularly. The count often falls during the first week of life. Continued monitoring is necessary until the count has been normal off treatment (typically by 2–4 weeks of age).

RECURRENCE

If the father is homozygous for HPA-1a, and the mother is homozygous for HPA-1b, the risk of recurrence is 100%.

If the father is heterozygous (HPA-1a1b) the risk of recurrence is 50%. In these circumstances (or if the father is not available), fetal HPA genotyping is indicated (via amniocentesis or fetal blood sampling).

In most cases, if untreated, an HPA-incompatible fetus will be ***at least*** as severely affected as the previous affected sibling.

Further Reading

Arnold DM, Smith JW, Kelton JG. Diagnosis and management of neonatal alloimmune thrombocytopenia. *Transfus Med Rev.* 2008;22(4):255–267.

Bussel JB, Sola-Visner M. Current approaches to the evaluation and management of the fetus and neonate with immune thrombocytopenia. *Semin Perinatol.* 2009;33(1): 35–42.

Knight M, Pierce M, Allen D, et al. The incidence and outcomes of fetomaternal alloimmune thrombocytopenia: a UK national study using three data sources. *Br J Haematol.* 2011;152(4):460–468.

Vinograd CA, Bussel JB. Antenatal treatment of fetal alloimmune thrombocytopenia: a current perspective. *Haematologica.* 2010;95(11):1807–1811.

Section 8
Aneuploidy

CHAPTER 28
Down Syndrome

Judy Williams, Rachel Susman, Garry DT Inglis

Trisomy 21 is a form of aneuploidy (abnormal chromosome number) characterised by an extra copy of chromosome 21 in the cells of the body. Down syndrome is the clinical manifestation, or phenotype, caused by trisomy 21. It was named after Dr John Langdon Down, who first described the syndrome in 1866.

The ethics of antenatal screening for trisomy 21 have been debated for many years and can be a polarising topic. This chapter will not discuss the ethics of screening and assumes that the diagnosis either has already been made or is strongly suspected.

AETIOLOGY

In 95% of cases there is an extra complete copy of chromosome 21 in all cells of the body. This is commonly what is meant by "trisomy 21".

In 3–4% of cases the extra copy of chromosome 21 is attached (translocated) to another chromosome. This is sometimes called "translocation Down syndrome". This is usually a Robertsonian translocation—a translocation involving the loss of the p (short) arms of two acrocentric chromosomes and the fusion of the q (long) arms to form a single long chromosome. This most commonly involves chromosomes 21 and 14, but can also involve chromosomes 13, 15 or 22. Of the Down syndrome cases caused by a Robertsonian translocation, 75% arise *de novo*, while 25% are familial (i.e., carried by one of the parents).

In 1–2% of cases there is mosaicism; i.e., there are two cell lines, with one being normal and one having trisomy 21. This is known as "mosaic trisomy 21".

Figure 28.1 shows a karyotype with trisomy 21.

EPIDEMIOLOGY

Down syndrome occurs in approximately 1 in 800 live births and occurs equally in all ethnic groups. The incidence varies with maternal age:

- 25 years—1 : 1250;
- 30 years—1 : 1000;

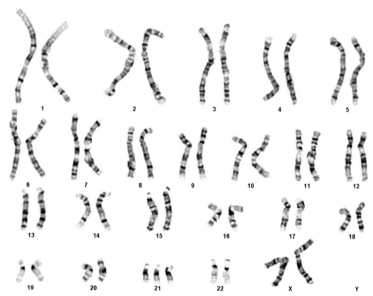

Figure 28.1 A karyotype showing trisomy 21.

- 35 years—1:400;
- 40 years—1:100; and
- 45 years—1:30.

PRENATAL TESTING
Screening
There is no screening test that either accurately detects all cases of trisomy 21 or excludes it completely. That is, there are false positive and false negative results with all forms of screening.

Five percent of screened fetuses will be identified as having an "increased risk" but the majority of these will not have trisomy 21. Screening tests have a very low positive predictive value.

First trimester screening, done from 11–13½ weeks, entails:
- a fetal ultrasound with nuchal translucency measurement which will identify 80% of fetuses with trisomy 21; and
- a maternal blood test measuring Pregnancy Associated Plasma Protein A (PAPP-A) and human chorionic gonadotrophin (hCG) which will identify 80–90% of fetuses with trisomy 21.

Second trimester screening, done from 14–20 weeks (ideally 15–17 weeks) can include either:

▶ the "quad test" (maternal blood levels of alpha fetoprotein, unconjugated oestriol, hCG and inhibin A) will detect about 80% of fetuses with trisomy 21; or

▶ the "triple test" (alpha-fetoprotein, unconjugated oestriol and human chorionic gonadotrophin).

If, after screening, a pregnancy is deemed to be at increased risk, the parents will require further counselling and should be offered a diagnostic test.

Diagnosis

Diagnostic testing requires a fetal karyotype, and has a false negative rate of less than 1%.

The specimen for karyotyping is obtained from the following:

▶ during the first trimester, a chorionic villus sampling (CVS); or

▶ during the second trimester, an amniocentesis.

FISH (fluorescence in situ hybridisation) testing for trisomy 21 may provide more rapid confirmation of the diagnosis.

DIFFERENTIAL DIAGNOSIS

If there is convincing clinical evidence of Down syndrome (see below) but the karyotype is normal, the baby should have blood sent for karyotype after delivery.

If the postnatal blood karyotype is normal, then consider trisomy 21 mosaicism. Mosaicism can be detected on a blood karyotype but this needs to be specifically requested. A skin karyotype can also be performed from a skin biopsy and this may be required for an accurate diagnosis.

Tell the parents that the karyotype takes several days to a couple of weeks to be reported.

Aside from the limitations of screening as mentioned above, it is uncommon for Down syndrome to be falsely diagnosed if the fetus or infant has convincing clinical features. The differential diagnosis includes other disorders that have some facial features similar to Down syndrome. These include other chromosomal disorders (such as chromosome 9q34 deletion) and Zellweger syndrome (a disorder of lipid metabolism).

ASSOCIATED FINDINGS

The characteristic dysmorphic features of Down syndrome include:

▶ facial features—a flat facial profile, depressed nasal bridge, epicanthic folds, upward slanting of palpebral fissures, Brushfield spots, small mouth, protruding tongue and small ears;

▶ excessive skin at the nape of the neck;

▶ microcephaly and brachycephaly, large fontanelles;

▶ a single transverse palmar crease;

▶ a short fifth finger (aplasia or hypoplasia of middle phalanx); and
▶ an increased space between first and second toes.

Cardiac anomalies occur in 40–50% of cases. The most common lesions are ventricular septal defects and atrio-ventricular septal defects.

Gastrointestinal atresia occurs in about 12% of cases, the most common being duodenal atresia.

There is an association with Hirschsprung disease, but this occurs in less than 1% of cases.

The parents should be warned that not all the associated congenital abnormalities can be detected antenatally.

CONSEQUENCES

There is a spontaneous loss-of-pregnancy rate of about 25% (miscarriage or intra-uterine fetal death).

With more aggressive management of the associated illnesses, life expectancy has improved but is still significantly shorter than in the general population. Overall life expectancy is currently 50–60 years with a median age at death of 49 years. Survival to 60 years is 44% (normal is 86%) and survival to 68 years is 14% (normal is 78%). Some of this excess mortality is due to cardiac defects and leukaemia, but not all. There is an increased morbidity and mortality from infectious diseases.

Neonatal pulmonary hypertension is more common, and may be more severe, in babies with Down syndrome than in others.

A leukaemoid reaction (also known as transient abnormal myelopoiesis or myeloproliferative syndrome) and polycythaemia occur in up to 10% of newborns. There is also an increased risk of leukaemia later in childhood, being 10–20 times more common in those with Down syndrome than in others. However, leukaemia still occurs in only 1% of children with Down syndrome.

Neurological findings include:
▶ intellectual impairment which is almost universal—usually mild (IQ 50–70) to moderate (IQ 30–50), although occasionally it can be severe;
▶ low muscle tone;
▶ hearing impairment (lifetime incidence of 75%);
▶ eye disease in 60%, including severe refractive errors (50%), strabismus (25–55%), nystagmus (20%) and cataracts (15%);
▶ psychiatric conditions, especially autism (7%);
▶ epilepsy;
▶ atlantoaxial joint instability (13%) and features of spinal cord compression (2%); and
▶ Alzheimer disease, which is becoming more common as life expectancy has increased, with the onset much earlier than in the general population.

Growth and development are affected. Feeding difficulties are common. Almost all have delayed achievement of milestones. For example, the average age at sitting is 11 months, crawling is 17 months, first word is 18 months and walking is 26 months.

Short stature and obesity are very common. Obstructive sleep apnoea is also common, with a lifetime incidence of 50–75%.

Virtually all adults with Down syndrome will need some level of day-to-day supervision.

Other recognised health problems include:

▶ otitis media (50–70%);
▶ thyroid disease (15%);
▶ diabetes mellitus (3 times more common than in the general population) (1–10%);
▶ coeliac disease (5–12%);
▶ acquired hip dislocation (6%); and
▶ arthropathy (almost 1%).

MANAGEMENT—ANTENATAL

The antenatal management will depend on the associated or anticipated problems. For example, with duodenal atresia there will likely be polyhydramnios, which may warrant amnioreduction.

Otherwise, the focus of antenatal management will be on providing information and counselling for the parents.

Some parents elect to terminate a pregnancy where the fetus is found to have trisomy 21.

OTHER CONSULTS REQUIRED

Refer to a geneticist for counselling. Arrange for a paediatric cardiologist to perform an antenatal echocardiogram. Other antenatal referrals will be dictated by the associated findings.

The parents may wish to consider seeking the help of a support group or Down syndrome association during the pregnancy.

MANAGEMENT—LABOUR AND DELIVERY

In the absence of specific abnormalities, such as congenital heart disease and duodenal atresia, the baby does not need be delivered in a tertiary centre. Delivery should be planned in a hospital that has a paediatric unit with a general paediatrician available.

There is no specific indication for operative delivery. Obstetric staff may request the presence of paediatric staff at the delivery, but this is not mandatory in all cases.

MANAGEMENT—POSTNATAL

Resuscitation should proceed as for any newborn. At delivery, or very soon after, the baby should be examined for evidence of pulmonary hypertension, cardiac lesions and gut atresias. In many neonatal units, the baby will be admitted to the special care nursery until these problems are excluded.

A thorough physical examination should confirm and note the presence of dysmorphic features of Down syndrome. Blood should be collected for a full blood count and film examination and a karyotype. The blood collection for a karyotype should be clean but does not need to be sterile in the manner of a blood culture (i.e., a venepuncture specimen or a sample from an arterial line is satisfactory, heel prick collection is not).

Babies with poor feeding may require tube feeds. A lactation consultant may be able to assist with establishment of breast feeding.

Thyroid function tests should be done on day 4 of life.

If not already done, the family should be referred to relevant support groups. A social worker can assist with accessing social services and carer allowances, etc.

Referral to a general or developmental paediatrician should be arranged. The paediatrician will play a significant role in the child's ongoing management and, along with the family doctor, is best placed to coordinate other relevant referrals, such as:

▶ early interventional developmental and educational services;
▶ diagnostic audiology; and
▶ an ophthalmologist.

Regular (6-monthly) health check-ups are recommended with the paediatrician or family doctor. Some advocate a X-ray of the cervical spine (for possible atlantoaxial joint instability), although there is debate over whether this is necessary unless the child becomes involved in sports.

All routine vaccinations are especially important.

If a translocation is found, arrange for the parents to have karyotyping to identify carrier status. If indicated (e.g., if one of the parents is a Robertsonian translocation carrier), refer the parents to a geneticist for reproductive counselling. Counselling regarding contraception may need to be arranged.

RECURRENCE

The recurrence risk is extremely variable, depending on the situation. This is summarised in Table 28.1.

ETHICS

Prospective parents faced with having a child with trisomy 21 will face numerous ethical dilemmas. For many, the decision of whether to terminate or continue with the pregnancy is very difficult.

For those who have a child with trisomy 21, some may choose to foster or adopt their child.

How aggressively to treat major morbidities, such as structural cardiac lesions and leukaemia, is also the subject of much debate. Aggressive management has become more common in recent years.

Table 28.1 Recurrence risk for trisomy 21 in various scenarios

For parents who have a child with trisomy 21		
Type of Trisomy	**Maternal Age**	**Recurrence Risk**
standard trisomy 21	<39 years	almost 1%
	39+ years	age-related
mosaic trisomy 21	<39 years	almost 1%
	39+ years	age-related
de novo Robertsonian translocation		<1%
mother carrier of Robertsonian translocation		10–15%
father carrier of Robertsonian translocation		1%
either parent carrier of 21:21 translocation		100%
For a person with trisomy 21		
Sex		**Recurrence Risk**
female with trisomy 21		50%
male with trisomy 21		rare case reports of fertility

Further Reading

American Academy of Pediatrics, Committee on Genetics. Health Supervision for Children With Down Syndrome. *Pediatrics*. 2001;107:442–449. Available at http://aappolicy.aappublications.org/cgi/content/full/pediatrics;107/2/442.

Barlow-Stewart K. Trisomy 21—Down syndrome [internet]. Centre for Genetic Education, NSW Health. 2007. Available at: http://www.genetics.edu.au/factsheet.

Firth HV, Hurst JA. *Oxford Desk Reference: Clinical Genetics*. Oxford: Oxford University Press. 2005.

Hunter AGW. Down Syndrome. In: Cassidy SB, Allanson JE, eds. *Management of Genetic Syndromes*. 3rd ed. Hoboken, NJ, USA: John Wiley & Sons, Inc; 2010.

McKinlay Gardner RJ, Sutherland GR, eds. *Chromosome Abnormalities and Genetic Counseling*. 3rd ed. Oxford: Oxford University Press Inc; 2003.

CHAPTER 29

Patau and Edwards Syndromes

Tammy Brinsmead, Julie Mcgaughran

With recent improvements in antenatal diagnosis, more pregnancies with these conditions are being identified before birth. As a result, they are seen less commonly in the neonatal period.

The diagnosis is usually made when a fetal karyotype is done following detection of anomalies on an ultrasound scan.

PATAU SYNDROME
Patau syndrome occurs when there is trisomy for all or a large part of chromosome 13.

Aetiology
Full trisomy or mosaicism occurs when there is abnormal chromosomal distribution during cell division. Partial trisomy 13 can occur when a portion of chromosome 13 has become attached to another chromosome (i.e., a translocation).

The prevalence is about 1 in 5000 births.

The differential diagnosis is broad given that the phenotype of trisomy 13 can vary considerably; a number of multiple congenital anomalies or chromosomal syndromes may need to be considered in the differential diagnosis. Chromosome analysis may identify a number of these. Referral to a clinical geneticist should also be considered.

Associated Abnormalities
A large variety of abnormalities may be present. These include:
- severe central nervous system anomalies—microcephaly, microphthalmia, holoprosencephaly (with severe mid-face abnormalities), neural tube defects;
- dysmorphic features—hand and foot abnormalities (polydactyly, flexed fingers, rocker-bottom feet);
- serious cardiac anomalies;
- cleft lip and/or palate; and
- omphalocele.

Consequences
About 80% of infants die within the first month of life; 95% die within the first six months. The most common causes of death are cardio-respiratory failure, congenital heart disease and infection.

Rare survivors with Patau syndrome consistently exhibit severe neurological and cognitive impairment with gross developmental delay. Seizures may occur. Failure to thrive is inevitable.

Management—Antenatal

If Patau syndrome is suspected then a fetal karyotype is recommended. If congenital anomalies were detected on a prenatal scan, a fetal karyotype and/or maternal fetal medicine specialist assessment may have already been done. However, there may be a concern about the possible diagnosis of trisomy 13 or Patau syndrome antenatally without confirmation of the diagnosis; sometimes the parents may not want a karyotype done.

In confirmed cases, the universally poor outcome will guide interventions if complications arise. Many parents will elect to terminate the pregnancy if diagnosis occurs at an appropriate gestation.

Operative interventions (e.g., caesarean section) are contraindicated for fetal indications.

Other consults required include clinical genetics and other specialties may be sought as determined by the specific congenital abnormalities identified.

Management—Postnatal

Active treatment, resuscitation and advanced life support are not considered appropriate. Comfort care should be provided. The parents should be informed that not all babies will die soon after birth.

Recurrence Risk

All families should be offered genetic counselling, with possible genetic testing of the parents for balanced translocations where indicated.

Recurrence in cases of full trisomy 13 is rare.

In cases of partial trisomy 13 (i.e., duplication of part of chromosome 13) a definite cause should be sought. There may be an unbalanced translocation therefore parental chromosomal analysis should be considered. The recurrence risk is dependent on the cause.

Recurrence in cases of mosaicism is rare.

EDWARDS SYNDROME

Edwards syndrome occurs when there is trisomy for all or a large part of chromosome 18.

Aetiology

Full trisomy or mosaicism occurs when there is abnormal chromosomal distribution during cell division. Partial trisomy 18 can occur with chromosomal breakage or translocation.

The prevalence is about 1 in 8000 births (it is the second most common syndrome with multiple malformations).

The differential diagnosis is extensive given the varied phenotype of trisomy 18; a number of syndromes with chromosomal abnormalities or other multiple congenital anomalies should be considered in the differential diagnosis. Chromosome analysis will identify a number of these. Referral to a clinical geneticist is recommended.

Associated Abnormalities

A large variety of abnormalities may be present (more than 130 abnormalities have been reported in the literature). These include:

▶ severe central nervous system anomalies—microcephaly, microphthalmia, cerebellar hypoplasia, neural tube defects;
▶ dysmorphic facial features—malformed ears, micrognathia or retrognathia, microstomia;
▶ severe congenital heart disease;
▶ renal tract malformations;
▶ clenched fingers; and
▶ gut abnormalities—oesophageal atresia, omphalocele, malrotation.

Consequences

About half the babies born with Edwards syndrome die within the first week of life; 90–95% die within the first year of life. Infants usually die from the cardiac and renal abnormalities, feeding difficulties, infection and apnoea caused by the central nervous system anomalies.

Survivors have severe physical and intellectual disability. They are usually unable to walk or use more than a few words.

Management—Antenatal

The approach when managing Edwards syndrome is similar to that for Patau syndrome; the universally poor outcome will guide obstetric and neonatal interventions. Many parents will elect to terminate the pregnancy if diagnosis occurs at an appropriate gestation.

Operative interventions (e.g., caesarean section) are contraindicated for fetal indications.

Other consults required include clinical genetics and other specialties may be sought as determined by the specific congenital abnormalities identified.

Management—Postnatal

Active treatment, resuscitation and advanced life support are not considered appropriate. Comfort care should be provided. The parents should be warned that not all babies will die soon after birth.

Recurrence Risk

All families should be offered genetic counselling, with possible genetic testing of the parents for balanced translocations where indicated.

Recurrence in cases of full trisomy 18 occurs in less than 1% of cases.

In cases of partial trisomy 18 (i.e., duplication of part of chromosome 18) a definite cause should be sought. There may be an unbalanced translocation therefore parental chromosomal analysis should be considered. The recurrence risk is dependent on the cause.

Recurrence in cases of mosaicism is rare.

ETHICS

The value of any interventions should be considered in the context of the condition's poor prognosis for both survival and quality of life.

Further Reading

Jones KL. *Smith's Recognizable Patterns of Human Malformation*. 6th ed. Saunders, Pennsylvania. Elsevier; 2006.

Weremowicz S. Cytogenetic abnormalities in the embryo, fetus, and infant. In: Lockwood C, Wilkins-Haug L, Firth H, et al, eds. *UpToDate*. 2010.

CHAPTER 30
Congenital Diaphragmatic Hernia

Alice E Stewart

A congenital diaphragmatic hernia (CDH) consists of a developmental defect of the diaphragm with herniation of abdominal contents into the chest. More than 95% are due to a defect in the posterolateral diaphragm (at the posterior foramen of Bochdalek) and 80% of these are left-sided. Less commonly, defects occur in the anterior midline (at the foramen of Morgagni) or in the crural diaphragm (i.e., paraoesophageal). Complete diaphragmatic agenesis is rare.

AETIOLOGY/PATHOPHYSIOLOGY/EMBRYOLOGY
Isolated congenital diaphragmatic hernia is a largely sporadic condition.

The diaphragmatic defect is thought to arise from failure of pleuroperitoneal canal closure at 8–10 weeks gestational age. Herniation of the abdominal contents into the thorax causes compression of the developing lungs which leads to disruption of bronchial and pulmonary artery branching (i.e., pulmonary hypoplasia) The ipsilateral lung is more severely affected than the contralateral lung.

Animal models of congenital diaphragmatic hernia suggest that pulmonary hypoplasia may initially occur independently of the diaphragmatic defect but this mechanism is not fully understood.

The primary pathological process in congenital diaphragmatic hernia arises from both pulmonary and pulmonary vascular hypoplasia. The combination of fewer generations of airways, fewer alveoli and abnormal pulmonary vasculature results in reduced surface area for gas exchange, severe restriction to pulmonary blood flow due to fixed high vascular resistance, and ventilation-perfusion mismatch. Surgical repair of the diaphragm will not correct this.

PREVALENCE
Congenital diaphragmatic hernia is reported in 1 in 2500–3000 births. The male to female ratio is estimated at 1.5 : 1.

DIFFERENTIAL DIAGNOSIS

Antenatal differential diagnoses include:
- congenital cystic adenomatoid malformation;
- bronchopulmonary sequestration;
- congenital lobar emphysema;
- bronchogenic cysts;
- pulmonary agenesis; and
- diaphragmatic eventration.

Congenital diaphragmatic hernia is differentiated from these conditions by the intra-thoracic location of abdominal organs.

ASSOCIATED ABNORMALITIES

Additional congenital anomalies occur in 10–40% of affected fetuses. These may involve the cardiac, renal, gastrointestinal and central nervous systems.

An underlying syndrome or chromosomal anomaly should be considered when there are one or more additional congenital anomalies.

Genetic syndromes in which congenital diaphragmatic hernia is a cardinal feature include Fryns syndrome and Donnai-Barrow syndrome. Others associated with congenital diaphragmatic hernia include Beckwith-Wiedemann, Simpson-Golabi-Behmel and Brachmann-de Lange syndromes.

No single chromosome has been implicated. There is an association with aneuploidy; e.g., trisomies 13, 18 and 21 and Turner syndrome (45,X).

CONSEQUENCES

Mortality

The survival rate is very much dependent on the population studied. Data from the population-based study of Colvin et al[1] are shown in Table 30.1. These data demonstrate the differences in mortality depending on the population studied. They also provide useful ball-park figures to use when counselling parents.

Tertiary paediatric surgical centres have reported survival rates of up to 90% but these figures reflect case selection bias.

Population-based studies which include *in utero* death, prenatal termination or death before transfer to a tertiary centre show static mortality rates in the range of 60–70%. This is despite the introduction of new treatments for pulmonary hypertension.

One year survival in live-born infants with prenatally diagnosed congenital diaphragmatic hernia has been reported as low as 30%.

Morbidity

Survivors have a high risk of significant morbidity, both early and late. Early on, the baby will be critically ill and will require a prolonged time on respiratory support and many weeks in hospital. Late morbidity impacts on quality of life.

Table 30.1 Outcomes from the population based study of Colvin et al[1]

Outcomes of Cases of CDH in Western Australia, 1991–2002

| | | n (%) | |
Outcomes	All Cases (N = 116)	Prenatal Diagnosis (N = 61)	Postnatal Diagnosis (N = 55)
Live-born	71 (61)	30 (49)	41 (74)
Elective termination	38 (33)	30 (49)	8 (15)
Spontaneous abortion	4 (3)	0 (0)	4 (7)
Stillborn	3 (3)	1 (2)	2 (4)
Survived to surgical centre	46 (40)	13 (21)	33 (60)
Survived to surgery	40 (34)	12 (21)	28 (51)
Survived > 1 y	37 (32)	10 (16)	27 (49)
Died at < 7 d	31 (27)	18 (30)	13 (24)
Died at 7–28 d	2 (2)	1 (2)	1 (2)
Died at 29 d to 1 y	1 (1)	1 (2)	0 (0)

Persistent pulmonary hypoplasia can lead to chronic lung disease and long-term oxygen requirement. Bronchodilator-responsive obstructive airways disease and recurrent respiratory tract infections are common.

Pulmonary hypertension carries significant morbidity and may persist beyond the neonatal period despite improvement in respiratory function.

Neurodevelopmental sequelae including cognitive and motor impairment, developmental delay and sensorineural hearing impairment are common in survivors. Only a minority of survivors will be free of neurodevelopmental deficits.[2–4]

Musculoskeletal deformities such as chest wall asymmetry, pectus deformity and scoliosis are common.

Gastrointestinal complications include gastro-oesophageal reflux disease which occurs in up to 50% of survivors and may contribute to respiratory morbidity. Gastrostomy feeds may be required for failure to thrive due to the increased metabolic demands of chronic lung disease.

Hernia recurrence is well documented.

MANAGEMENT—ANTENATAL

Detailed evaluation is indicated to confirm the diagnosis, to assess the severity of the defect and to detect the presence of other congenital anomalies. This includes detailed ultrasound imaging, fetal magnetic resonance imaging (MRI), echocardiography and fetal karyotyping.

There are no effective fetal interventions for congenital diaphragmatic hernia. *In utero* patch closure of the diaphragmatic defect has been shown to confer no survival benefit. Trials of fetal tracheal occlusion for treatment of pulmonary hypoplasia have been inconclusive.

Accurate prognostic information is essential for non-directive antenatal counselling. The presence of an additional major congenital anomaly carries a very poor prognosis. Other prognostic indicators include liver herniation and contralateral lung area to head circumference ratio. In cases where the liver is above the diaphragm, the mortality has been reported between 50% and 65%. Although the lung area to head circumference ratio correlates with severity of congenital diaphragmatic hernia, its value as an independent predictive indicator is diminished by observer-dependence.

Parents should be fully informed of the severity of this condition, and of the expected outcome. This includes a discussion of both mortality risk and of the significant cardiorespiratory, neurological and gastrointestinal morbidity.

MANAGEMENT—LABOUR / DELIVERY / IMMEDIATE POSTNATAL MANAGEMENT

Delivery should occur at a tertiary referral centre that has an intensive care nursery with paediatric surgeons and paediatric cardiological support available.

There is no evidence that delivery mode influences outcome.

Minimise gaseous distension of the herniated bowel by intubating and ventilating immediately; i.e., avoid non-invasive positive pressure ventilation (e.g., bag and mask). A large bore gastric tube should be used to decompress the stomach.

Umbilical arterial and venous catheters should be inserted. Get a chest X-ray (see Figure 30.1).

A lung protective ventilatory strategy is recommended. This is achieved by using an adequate positive end expiratory pressure to optimise lung recruitment, allowing permissive hypercapnia, targeting pre-ductal saturations of $\geq 85\%$ (and not targeting hyperoxia), and avoidance of peak inspiratory and mean airway pressures that over-distend the lung. The use of high frequency oscillatory ventilation (HFOV).

Serial echocardiography should be performed to assess the degree of pulmonary hypertension and ductus arteriosus patency and shunt direction. Right-to-left ductal shunting can help to preserve right ventricular function in severe pulmonary hypertension, and a prostaglandin (PGE_1) infusion is sometimes used to maintain duct patency. Inhaled nitric oxide is sometimes used but there is no evidence of benefit in congenital diaphragmatic hernia.

Where available, extracorporeal membrane oxygenation (ECMO) may be considered for infants with hypoxic respiratory failure which has not responded to conventional management. However, it has proven difficult

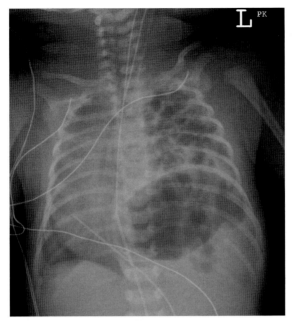

Figure 30.1 Chest X-ray on the first day of life showing stomach and bowel in the left chest with gross displacement of the heart to the right.

to identify those infants who are most likely to benefit without incurring significant morbidity.[5]

Surgery is delayed until cardiorespiratory stability is achieved. The herniated abdominal contents are reduced and the diaphragmatic defect is repaired either through primary closure or the use of a prosthetic patch. The parents should know that surgery will not improve baby's condition; only time and lung growth will do that.

Chromosomal analysis should be performed if there are additional congenital anomalies.

OTHER CONSULTS REQUIRED

Paediatric surgical consultation will be required. Genetics counselling may be indicated depending on the presence of additional congenital anomalies, a positive family history and abnormal fetal or infant karyotype.

MANAGEMENT—POSTNATAL

Follow-up of growth and development and surveillance for known neurological, respiratory, gastrointestinal and musculoskeletal complications should be undertaken by a general paediatrician, with sub-specialty involvement as indicated.

Surveillance may include chest X-rays to detect hernia recurrence, respiratory function testing and echocardiographic screening for pulmonary hypertension.

Surgical follow-up includes monitoring and intervention for hernia recurrence, chest wall deformities and scoliosis.

RECURRENCE

The recurrence risk is 2% for isolated congenital diaphragmatic hernia in the absence of a positive family history.

Where there is a positive family history, a specific syndromal diagnosis or chromosomal abnormality, the recurrence risk may be as high as 50%, warranting detailed genetic counselling.

ETHICS

Given that there are no effective fetal interventions for congenital diaphragmatic hernia and that this condition carries a very high risk of mortality and morbidity, it is important that thorough antenatal evaluation is followed by non-directive counselling that allows for fully informed decision making by parents.

REFERENCES

1. Colvin J, Bower C, Dickinson J, Sokol J. Outcomes of congenital diaphragmatic hernia: a population-based study in Western Australia. *Pediatrics*. 2005;116: e356–e362.
2. Bagolan P, Morini F. Long-term follow up of infants with congenital diaphragmatic hernia. *Seminars in Pediatric Surgery*. 2007;16:134–144.
3. Benjamin JR, Bizzarro MJ, Cotton CM. Congenital diaphragmatic hernia: updates and outcomes. *Neoreviews*. 2011;12:e439–e452.
4. Chiu P, Hedrick H. Postnatal management and long-term outcome for survivors with congenital diaphragmatic hernia. *Prenatal Diagnosis*. 2008;28:592–603.
5. Harrington K, Goldman A. The role of extracorporeal membrane oxygenation in congenital diaphragmatic hernia. *Seminars in Pediatric Surgery*. 2005;14:72–76.

Further Reading

Hedrick H. Management of prenatally diagnosed congenital diaphragmatic hernia. *Seminars in Fetal & Neonatal Medicine*. 2009;15:21–27.
Kitano Y. Prenatal intervention for congenital diaphragmatic hernia. *Seminars in Pediatric Surgery*. 2007;16:101–108.
Robinson P, Fitzgerald D. Congenital diaphragmatic hernia. *Paediatric Respiratory Reviews*. 2007;8:323–335.
Stege G, Fenton A, Jaffray B. Nihilism in the 1990s: the true mortality of congenital diaphragmatic hernia. *Pediatrics*. 2003;112(3 Pt 1):532–535.

CHAPTER 31

Congenital Cystic Adenomatoid Malformation

David Hou

Congenital cystic adenomatoid malformations (CCAM) are congenital cystic lung malformations characterised by cystic, dilated terminal bronchioles lined with epithelial cells. They have a normal vascular supply and communicate in a normal way with the bronchial tree. Congenital pulmonary airway malformation (CPAM) is a more recent and more accurate term as not all cystic adenomatoid malformations contains cysts and it is difficult to differentiate them from other congenital cystic lung malformations.

AETIOLOGY

One hypothesised pathogenesis is that bronchial maturation ceases during the pseudoglandular phase of lung development (before 16 weeks gestation) with overgrowth of mesenchymal elements.

The pathological classification was originally proposed then adapted by Stocker (2009)[1] and it is shown in Table 31.1. The classification is based on the presumed site of development of the malformation (from proximal to distal in the respiratory tree).

The antenatal ultrasound classification was proposed by Adzick et al:[2]

▶ type 1—macrocystic, with cysts >5 mm, has a good prognosis; and
▶ type 2—microcystic, with cysts <5 mm, has a solid appearance and has a poor prognosis.

While antenatal ultrasound scanning is extremely sensitive, it has poor correlation with histology and it is difficult to estimate prognosis for antenatal counselling.

PREVALENCE

Congenital cystic adenomatoid malformation is the most common congenital cystic lung malformation, but is overall quite uncommon. Historically, the incidence has been quoted as 1 in 10,000–1 in 35,000. The prevalence is about 9 in 100,000 live births.[3] More recent reports suggest an increase in the detection of congenital lung lesions, perhaps due to the increased sensitivity of antenatal ultrasound scanning.

DIFFERENTIAL DIAGNOSIS

The differential diagnoses include:

▶ congenital cystic lung malformations:
  • pulmonary sequestration,
  • hybrid lesions (elements of both CCAM and sequestration),

Table 31.1 Pathological classification of congenital cystic malformations based on the presumed site of development.[1]

Type	Original CCAM Type	Pathology	Percent of All Cystic Adenomatoid Malformations (%)
0		acinar dysplasia	<2
1	I	single or multiple cysts >2 cm in size	60–70
2	II	single or multiple cysts <2 cm in size	15–20
3	III	mainly solid with cysts <0.5 cm	5–10
4		large air filled cysts (often single)	<10

- congenital lobar emphysema,
- bronchogenic cysts;
▶ congenital high airway obstruction syndrome;
▶ congenital diaphragmatic hernia;
▶ tumours:
  - pleuropulmonary blastomas,
  - bronchopulmonary alveolar carcinomas, and
  - fetal lung interstitial tumours.

ASSOCIATED ABNORMALITIES

Poor prognostic signs include bilateral cystic adenomatoid malformations, hydrops fetalis and hypoplastic lungs (lung-to-thorax ratio of <0.25). Polyhydramnios and mediastinal shift are not associated with a poor prognosis.

Cloutier et al[4] reported that 18% of patients had associated anomalies such as renal agenesis, cardiac anomalies and pectus excavatum. With increased detection of even smaller lesions, this proportion may now be significantly decreased.

CONSEQUENCES

Respiratory insufficiency can occur if there is associated pulmonary hypoplasia or pleural effusions. Babies with congenital cystic adenomatoid malformations have an increased risk of pneumothorax.

Part of the justification for the early resection of cystic adenomatoid malformations is that some may undergo malignant change. In infants and young children, pleuropulmonary blastomas occur and in older children and adults bronchopulmonary alveolar carcinomas dominate. Pleuropulmonary blastomas are difficult to differentiate clinically, radiographically and pathologically from type 4 cystic adenomatoid malformations. This adds further to the argument that all cystic adenomatoid malformations should be resected (see below). As pleuropulmonary blastomas progress from large cysts to more solid tumours, the prognosis deteriorates.

Cystic adenomatoid malformations can become infected and present as lung abscesses, recurrent pneumonia or empyema. The most common presentation outside the neonatal period is infection.

MANAGEMENT—ANTENATAL

Regular antenatal ultrasound scans should be performed to monitor the size of the lesions and, if large, to monitor for hydrops fetalis. The natural course is for continued growth until 28 weeks and then regression with decreasing size.

Fetal echocardiography could be considered to look for cardiac abnormalities and cardiac function (hydrops fetalis). Magnetic resonance imaging (MRI) could be considered for further differentiation of the lesion.

Ten percent of cystic adenomatoid malformations need fetal intervention. Polyhydramnios may be improved by a simple amniotic fluid reduction or a thoraco-amniotic shunt. The development of hydrops fetalis may signal the need to consider premature delivery at 30–32 weeks with postnatal resection of the adenomatoid lesion. Antenatal corticosteroids have been shown to resolve hydrops and improve both fetal and postnatal survival without decreasing the size of the lesion.

Larger lesions or lesions with other associated abnormalities should be delivered in a tertiary centre. Smaller lesions can be delivered in the referring centre. If the cystic adenomatoid malformation is uncomplicated, there is no indication for delivery by caesarean section.

Antenatal consultation with a paediatric surgeon should be considered, particularly if the lesion is large or does not regress.

MANAGEMENT—POSTNATAL

The immediate postnatal management depends on the degree of respiratory distress after birth. Respiratory compromise may require intubation and mechanical ventilation. Any respiratory compromise requires immediate referral to a paediatric surgeon for investigation and management.

A chest X-ray (CXR) is the usual first-line investigation. An example is shown in Figure 31.1. However, a normal chest X-ray is not evidence the lesion has resolved. Over half of those whose antenatal ultrasound and postnatal chest X-ray appeared to show resolution of the lesion had a cystic adenomatoid malformation detectable on computed tomography (CT) scan or required surgery. The CT scan of the lesion shown in Figure 31.1 is shown in Figure 31.2.

If there is no respiratory compromise, the baby can be referred for outpatient follow-up. A CT scan of the chest would usually occur at one month of age. This confirms the diagnosis and delineates the vasculature for surgery.

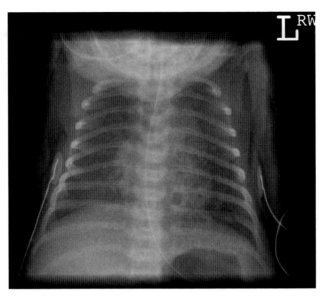

Figure 31.1 Chest X-ray of a term newborn baby with a left lower lobe cystic adenomatoid malformation.

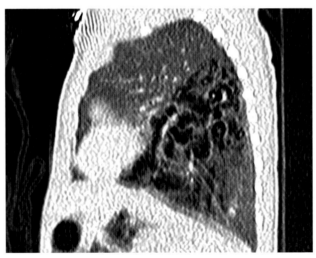

Figure 31.2 A coronal slice of the chest CT scan of a term newborn baby with a left lower lobe cystic adenomatoid malformation.

There is consensus that all symptomatic cystic adenomatoid malformations should be resected. The management of asymptomatic lesions remains controversial. Some continue to manage conservatively with regular outpatient CT scans (which carries the unwanted effect of radiation exposure). Expectant management may be appropriate in those with small lesions (either <3 cm or <25% of ipsilateral lung volume). Others would resect by 6–12 months of age because of the risk of infection and malignant change as well as the chance of compensatory lung growth following resection. Resection when asymptomatic may result in fewer complications and shorter hospital stay.

REFERENCES

1. Stocker JT. Cystic lung disease in infants and children. *Fetal and Pediatric Pathology.* 2009;28:155–184.
2. Adzick NS, Harrison MR, Glick PL, et al. Fetal cystic adenomatoid malformation: prenatal diagnosis and natural history. *J Pediatr Surg.* 1985;20:483–488.
3. Stanton M, Davenport M. Management of congenital lung lesions. *Early Hum Dev.* 2006;82:289–295.
4. Cloutier MM, Schaeffer DA, Hight D. Congenital cystic adenomatoid malformation. *Chest.* 1993;103:761–764.

Further Reading

Laberge J-M, Puliganda P, Flageole H. Asymptomatic congenital lung malformations. *Seminars in Pediatric Surgery.* 2005;14:16–33.

Lakhoo K. Management of congenital cystic adenomatous malformations of the lung. *ADCFN.* 2009;94:F73–F76.

Peranteau WH, Wilson RD, Liechty KW, et al. Effect of maternal betamethasone on prenatal congenital cystic adenomatoid malformation growth and fetal survival. *Fetal Diagn Ther.* 2007;22:365–371.

Priest JR, Williams GM, Hill DA, et al. Pulmonary cysts in early childhood and the risk of malignancy. *Ped Pulm.* 2009;44:14–30.

CHAPTER 32

Congenital Heart Disease in the Fetus

Pieter J Koorts

Congenital heart disease affects about 1% of live born infants. It is the most common congenital anomaly.

Khoo et al[1] found an incidence of congenital heart disease of 10.7 in 1000 births in South Australia.

The increased availability of antenatal ultrasound has made prenatal diagnosis of congenital heart disease widely available.

Some structural lesions are difficult to pick up *in utero*. A normal ultrasound early in gestation does not rule out any congenital heart disease at birth. Some lesions, especially left-sided lesions, can get more severe with increasing gestation.

There is increasing evidence that prenatal diagnosis improves postnatal outcome, especially with duct-dependent lesions, as this ensures prompt appropriate medical care, such as maintaining an open ductus arteriosus to avoid severe cyanosis.

A prenatal diagnosis of congenital heart disease is associated with increased parental understanding at discharge.

Congenital heart disease encompasses a wide range of lesions, ranging from lesions that do not require treatment, to lesions that require cardiac surgery, to lesions that may need palliation, such as hypoplastic left-heart syndrome.

AETIOLOGY

The aetiology is multifactorial, with mostly a combination of genetic predisposition and environmental factors.

ASSOCIATED ABNORMALITIES

Eight per cent of patients with congenital heart disease have a specific syndrome, such as trisomy 13, 18 and 21, Turner syndrome or DiGeorge syndrome with q22 deletion. Increased nuchal translucency, measured on a fetal ultrasound at around 12 weeks gestational age, is an early marker of aneuploidy.

Much of the mortality and morbidity associated with congenital heart disease is attributable to the extra cardiac malformations.

Two per cent of patients with congenital heart disease have known environmental factors, such as rubella, maternal alcohol use (drugs such as anticonvulsants, lithium and amphetamines), maternal diabetes and systemic lupus erythematosus (SLE).

COUNSELLING—ANTENATAL

A multidisciplinary approach is advised. Depending on the presumed diagnosis, obstetricians, maternal fetal medicine specialists, neonatologists, cardiologists, cardiac surgeons, geneticists and nursing staff will need to be involved.

The details of the counselling will depend on the diagnosis (see Box 32.1), how certain the diagnosis is, if there are any non-cardiac associations, the natural course of the lesion *in utero* (severity may increase with gestation) and *ex utero*, and the treatment options (and their outcomes).

Box 32.1 EXAMPLES OF CONGENITAL HEART DISEASE DETECTED ANTENATALLY: LISTED FROM MOST COMMON TO LESS COMMON.[1]

Ventricular septal defect (VSD)
Tetralogy of Fallot
Transposition of the great arteries (TGA)
Atrio-ventricular septal defect (AVSD)
Coarctation of the aorta
Total anomalous pulmonary venous return (TAPVR)
Ebstein's anomaly
Truncus arteriosus
Tetralogy of Fallot with pulmonary atresia
Pulmonary atresia with intact ventricular septum
Severe aortic stenosis
Double outlet right ventricle
Complex TGA
Complex corrected TGA
Tricuspid atresia, double inlet right ventricle
Hypoplastic left-heart syndrome
TAPVR with obstruction

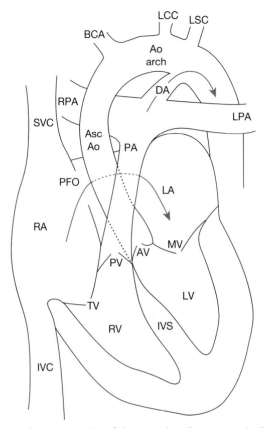

Figure 32.1 A schematic drawing of the normal cardiac anatomy in the fetus. Key: Ao arch—aortic arch, Asc Ao—ascending aorta, AV—aortic valve, BCA—brachiocephalic artery, DA—ductus arteriosus, Dsc Ao—descending aorta, IVC—inferior vena cava, IVS—interventricular septum, LA—left atrium, LCC—left common carotid artery, LPA—left pulmonary artery, LSC—left subclavian artery, LV—left ventricle, MV—mitral valve, PA—pulmonary artery, PFO—patent foramen ovale, PV—pulmonary valve, RA—right atrium, RPA—right pulmonary artery, RV—right ventricle, SVC—superior vena cava, TV—tricuspid valve.

Available locally and elsewhere. The parents should be made aware that any diagnoses made antenatally carry a degree of uncertainty and that postnatal tests are always required to provide a more definitive diagnosis. A diagram of the normal cardiac anatomy can be a useful adjunct when explaining congenital heart defects (see Figures 32.1 and 32.2).

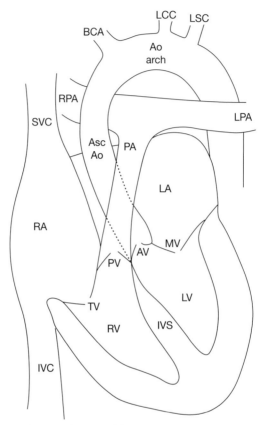

Figure 32.2 A schematic drawing of the normal cardiac anatomy after birth. Key: Ao arch—aortic arch, Asc Ao—ascending aorta, AV—aortic valve, BCA— brachiocephalic artery, Dsc Ao—descending aorta, IVC—inferior vena cava, IVS—interventricular septum, LA—left atrium, LCC—left common carotid artery, LPA—left pulmonary artery, LSC—left subclavian artery, LV—left ventricle, MV—mitral valve, PA—pulmonary artery, PV—pulmonary valve, RA—right atrium, RPA—right pulmonary artery, RV—right ventricle, SVC—superior vena cava, TV—tricuspid valve.

The following chapters provide more specific details on right and left ventricular outflow tract obstructions, hypoplastic left-heart syndrome, transposition of the great arteries and dysrhythmias.

Management options may include termination of pregnancy or transferring care to a more appropriate tertiary perinatal centre that deals with cardiac babies.

MANAGEMENT—POSTNATAL

The postnatal management will depend on the diagnosis. Please refer to the following chapters for diagnosis-specific management (Chapters 33, 34, 35, 36 and 37).

Some complex lesions will not fit any particular simple diagnosis. Nevertheless, each infant with the antenatally diagnosed congenital heart disease should have a detailed plan documented for management in the immediate postnatal period.

REFERENCE

1. Khoo N, Van Essen P, Richardson M, et al. Effectiveness of prenatal diagnosis of congenital heart defects in South Australia: A population analysis 1999–2003. *Australian and New Zealand Journal of Obstetrics and Gynaecology.* 2008;48:559–563.

Further Reading

Allan L, Huggon I. Counselling following a diagnosis of congenital heart disease. *Prenat Diagn.* 2004;24:1136–1142.

Cohen MS. Fetal Diagnosis and management of congenital heart disease. *Clin Perinatol.* 2001 March;28:(1):11–29.

Williams I, Shaw R, Kleinman C, et al. Parental understanding of neonatal congenital heart disease. *Pediatric Cardiology.* 2008;29:1059–1065.

CHAPTER 33

Right Ventricular Outflow Tract (RVOT) Abnormalities

Tim Colen, Alice Stewart

Abnormalities of the right ventricular outflow tract (RVOT) include numerous obstructive lesions such as tetralogy of Fallot, hypoplastic right heart and pulmonary atresia.

CONDITIONS

The tetralogy of Fallot (TOF) consists of the following abnormalities (see Figure 33.1):

▶ pulmonary stenosis;
▶ perimembranous ventriculoseptal defect (VSD);
▶ right ventricular (RV) hypertrophy; and
▶ an aorta that over-rides the ventriculoseptal defect.

An example of the anatomy in tetralogy of Fallot is shown in Figure 33.1.

Variants of the classical tetralogy include pulmonary atresia with a ventriculoseptal defect with or without major aorto-pulmonary collateral arteries (MAPCAs).

Pulmonary atresia with an intact ventricular septum is a different pathology, compared with pulmonary atresia with a ventriculoseptal defect, and it is associated with a small (hypoplastic) right ventricle and a small tricuspid valve.

Right ventricular outflow tract lesions are diagnosed using screening ultrasound. The abnormalities seen include an abnormal outflow tract (stenosis or atresia), a large ventriculoseptal defect as part of a tetralogy of Fallot, or a hypoplastic right ventricle or tricuspid valve in cases of pulmonary atresia with an intact ventricular septum.

If an abnormality is suspected then fetal echocardiography should be done by a paediatric cardiologist to delineate the cardiac anatomy and pathology and to allow in-depth counselling.

AETIOLOGY / PATHOPHYSIOLOGY / EMBRYOLOGY

The exact cause of these abnormalities is largely unknown. The majority of cases occur sporadically.

Right ventricular outflow tract abnormalities are associated with following conditions:

▶ 22q11 deletion;
▶ aneuploidy (trisomy 13, 18 or 21);

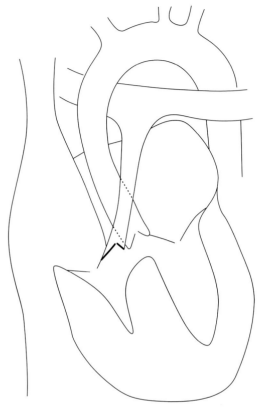

Figure 33.1 A schematic diagram of the heart showing the anatomy of the tetralogy of Fallot (compare with Figures 32.1 and 32.2 in Chapter 32)—there is pulmonary valve stenosis and narrowing of the pulmonary artery, a ventriculoseptal defect with an overriding aorta, and right ventricular hypertrophy.

- Alagille syndrome;
- Holt-Oram syndrome; and
- fetal rubella exposure.

PREVALENCE

Right ventricular outflow tract obstruction is one of the most common causes of cyanotic heart disease (along with transposition of the great arteries). It occurs in 1 in 3500 live births, accounting for around 3.5% of congenital heart disease.[1]

DIFFERENTIAL DIAGNOSIS

The differential diagnosis includes tetralogy of Fallot, pulmonary atresia with a ventriculoseptal defect, pulmonary atresia with an intact ventricular septum and truncus arteriosus.

CONSEQUENCES

Almost all patients require surgery at some stage.

Infants with tetralogy of Fallot will require surgery within the first 6–9 months of age. They may also need further surgery later in life for ongoing stenosis or regurgitation. The one-year survival rate is about 97% and the 30-year survival rate is greater than 90%. The risk of problems in late childhood and adulthood relates predominantly to rhythm disturbance and sudden cardiac death (3–6% of patients).

Infants with pulmonary atresia with a ventriculoseptal defect have a higher mortality rate at all stages and higher re-intervention rates.

For infants with pulmonary atresia with an intact ventricular septum there are two potential surgical strategies (biventricular or univentricular) dependent on the size of the tricuspid valve and the right ventricle, and the coronary artery anatomy. Mortality rates are about 15–20% in first year, with 80% survival up to 15 years.[1] Long-term survival rates with current management strategies are not well known.

MANAGEMENT—ANTENATAL

There are no specific antenatal treatments. There is currently limited experience with fetal pulmonary valvuloplasty aiming to promote right ventricular growth and neonatal biventricular circulation. The experience is mainly in fetuses with critical pulmonary stenosis or pulmonary atresia with an intact ventricular septum, however there is no clear benefit. The mortality rate for similar interventions for aortic stenosis is 15%.[2]

MANAGEMENT—LABOUR / DELIVERY / IMMEDIATE POSTNATAL

Affected babies should be delivered at a tertiary neonatal unit with 24-hour paediatric cardiology support.

Babies who are likely to have ductal-dependent pulmonary circulation (e.g., pulmonary atresia with a ventriculoseptal defect or an intact ventricular septum), require initiation of prostaglandin E_1 (Alprostadil, PGE_1) and early postnatal echocardiogram by a paediatric cardiologist. PGE_1 may cause apnoeas at high doses requiring medical management (caffeine) or invasive respiratory support.

Baby will remain in hospital until early surgery is done (systemic-pulmonary shunt i.e., modified Blalock-Taussig shunt), or until saturations are deemed adequate without surgery (e.g., in the presence of MAPCAs). The admission duration tends to be 2–4 weeks.

Babies with tetralogy of Fallot require saturation monitoring and review by a paediatric cardiologist and an echocardiogram on the first day of life.

The majority of patients remain adequately saturated and are discharged home in the first week of life. Significant neonatal desaturations (<75%) may require early surgery, either a modified Blalock-Taussig shunt or repair, prior to discharge. The parents of patients discharged without repair or shunt need counselling regarding hypercyanotic spells (i.e., presenting symptoms and management at home).

OTHER CONSULTS REQUIRED
Genetic counselling and general paediatric review for babies with associated conditions.

MANAGEMENT—POSTNATAL
Infants with tetralogy of Fallot require regular clinical follow-up by a paediatric cardiologist until the time of complete repair. The timing of repair is determined by oxygen saturations or the occurrence of hypercyanotic spells—early repair or a modified Blalock-Taussig shunt if saturations are less than 70–75%; otherwise complete repair between 3 and 9 months of age if saturations are stable (>75%). The exact timing varies between institutions. Repair involves ventriculoseptal defect closure and relief of pulmonary stenosis. The long-term management involves regular clinical review with assessment of right ventricle function, pulmonary valve stenosis or incompetence and monitoring for arrhythmia (ventricular). Further surgery may be required for significant pulmonary incompetence causing a dilated and/or dysfunctional right ventricle or for significant pulmonary stenosis.

Infants with pulmonary atresia with a ventriculoseptal defect require follow-up as above. Surgical repair is dependent on the size of the pulmonary arteries as determined by echocardiography and/or cardiac catheterisation. Repair includes closure of the ventriculoseptal defect and placement of a conduit (allograft, xenograft or artificial) from the right ventricle to the pulmonary arteries. Ongoing follow-up by a paediatric cardiologist is required with monitoring for obstruction to the conduit. The conduit will need replacement as the child grows (every 3–10 years in childhood and about every 10 years in adults).

Infants with pulmonary atresia with an intact ventricular septum require follow-up as above. Specific management depends on which pathway is chosen—either biventricular or univentricular.

With the biventricular pathway, the pulmonary valve is opened (with either surgery or via a catheter) with or without a Blalock-Taussig shunt in the first month of life. Further surgery may be required for ongoing pulmonary stenosis and to close the shunt if the right ventricle is growing appropriately.

With the univentricular pathway, the baby has a Blalock-Taussig shunt initially, followed by the Glenn operation and likely eventual Fontan procedure (single ventricle palliation).

RECURRENCE

Recurrence risks for tetralogy of Fallot have been reported as less than 3% in siblings, similar to other congenital heart lesions. If more than one first degree relative is affected the risk is doubled.[3]

REFERENCES

1. Shinebourne EA, Rigby ML, Carvalho JS. Pulmonary atresia with intact ventricular septum: from fetus to adult: Congenital heart disease. *Heart*. 2008;94;1350–1357.
2. Sekar P, Hornberger L. The role of fetal echocardiography in fetal intervention: a symbiotic relationship. *Clinics in Perinatology*. 2009;36:301–327.
3. Nora JJ, McGill CW, McNamara DG. Empiric recurrence risks in common and uncommon congenital heart lesions. *Teratology*. 1970;3:325–330.

Further Reading

Keane JK, Lock JE, Fyler DC. *Nadas' Pediatric Cardiology*. 2nd ed. Saunders Elsevier; 2006.

Shinebourne EA, Babu-Narayan SV, Carvalho JS. Tetralogy of Fallot: from fetus to adult. *Heart*. 2006;92;1353–1359.

CHAPTER 34
Transposition of the Great Arteries

Paul G Woodgate

Transposition of the great arteries (TGA) is a form of congenital heart disease where the aorta arises from the right ventricle and the pulmonary artery from the left ventricle (see Figure 34.1). This leads to the oxygenated blood returning to the left side of the heart and recirculating through the lungs, whilst the desaturated blood returning from the body leaves the right side of the heart and returns to the body via the aorta. Some mixing is provided by the foramen ovale and ductus arteriosus. The aorta is anterior and to the right of the pulmonary artery, which leads to the term *d-TGA*, the *d* indicating a dextropositioned aorta.

INCIDENCE
Congenital heart disease occurs in 0.5–1% of live births. Transposition of the great arteries accounts for approximately 5% of all congenital heart disease. It has been reported to occur in 0.26 in 1000 births.[1]

ASSOCIATED ANOMALIES
A ventricular septal defect (VSD) is also present in about 50% of cases of transposition of the great arteries. Some form of left ventricular outflow tract obstruction is also common. More complex congenital cardiac defects can also have transposition of the great arteries as part of the overall abnormality.

AETIOLOGY
The cause of most congenital heart disease is not known. Transposition of the great arteries is more common in infants of diabetic mothers. The male:female ratio is 3:1. It can be associated with a deletion of chromosome 22q11 (CATCH 22 or DiGeorge syndrome).

CONSEQUENCES
Transition to extrauterine life, and survival beyond the immediate newborn period, requires adequate delivery of oxygenated blood to the brain and body. In the presence of transposition of the great arteries, this depends upon some mixing of the two circulations via the foramen ovale and ductus arteriosus. Once the ductus begins to close following birth, the mixing of systemic and pulmonary blood is severely restricted. The newborn presents with cyanosis, tachypnoea and severe hypoxaemia within hours of birth. Adequate mixing, and therefore systemic oxygenation, may occur if there is a non-restrictive ventricular septal defect.

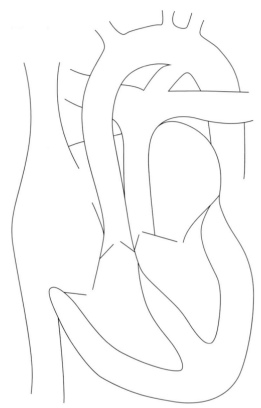

Figure 34.1 A schematic diagram of the heart showing the anatomy of transposition of the great arteries (compare with Figures 32.1 and 32.2 in Chapter 32)—the aorta arises from the right ventricle and the pulmonary artery from the left ventricle.

MANAGEMENT—ANTENATAL

If transposition of the great arteries is identified, or suspected, on antenatal ultrasound scan, referral for a tertiary level scan and counselling by a paediatric cardiologist is recommended.

Delivery of babies with known or suspected transposition should be planned to occur in a centre with an intensive care nursery and specialist cardiological and cardiac surgical services. The ideal gestational age for delivery is 39–40 completed weeks of gestation.[2]

MANAGEMENT—POSTNATAL

Immediately following birth, an infusion of prostaglandin E_1 should commence to maintain ductal patency. Initially this is best given through an umbilical venous catheter.

The cardiological service should be immediately alerted so that a detailed echocardiogram can be done to confirm the cardiac anatomy, and to determine the need for an atrial septostomy.

Significant haemodynamic compromise may result if there is an intact ventricular septum and a restrictive atrial septum.[3] If significant hypoxaemia persists despite the prostaglandin infusion, a balloon atrial septostomy may be required. Acidosis may require treatment and hypoglycaemia will require prompt correction. Apnoea due to the prostaglandin infusion may necessitate intubation and mechanical ventilation.

The arterial switch procedure is the definitive surgical treatment for transposition of the great arteries. This is usually performed within the first two weeks of life, and has a survival rate of better than 95%. Most babies will go home after 1–2 weeks.

Further surgery is required in about 5% of cases. Infrequently, the cardiac anatomy is not suitable for arterial switch and some form of atrial switch is required.

Long-term outcomes have not been well studied. Some cohorts of patients that have had the arterial switch operation have mean motor and cognitive scores within the normal range.[4] Bellinger et al[5] followed a cohort of children to 8 years of age after arterial switch surgery—3% had general intelligence quotient scores below 70; other abnormalities on neurological examination (neurocognitive, motor function, gait) were more common (around two-thirds) but were generally mild.

RECURRENCE

There is a 2–6% risk for transposition of the great arteries in a subsequent pregnancy. The risk of recurrence is also increased if there is an affected parent. The recurrence risk may be increased to 20–30% if there are two affected first-degree relatives.

REFERENCES

1. Brenner JI. Prevalence of congenital heart disease. In: Kleinman CS, Seri I, Polin RA, eds. *Hemodynamics and Cardiology: Neonatology Questions and Controversies.* Philadelphia: Saunders Elsevier; 2008:269–274.
2. Costello JM, Polito A, Brown DW, et al. Birth before 39 weeks' gestation is associated with worse outcomes in neonates with heart disease. *Pediatrics.* 2010;126(2): e277–e284.
3. Johnson BA, Ades A. Delivery room and early postnatal management of neonates who have prenatally diagnosed congenital heart disease. *Clin Perinatol.* 2005;32:921–946.
4. Snookes SH, Gunn JK, Eldridge BJ, et al. A systematic review of motor and cognitive outcomes after early surgery for congenital heart disease. *Pediatrics.* 2010;125: e818–e827.

5. Bellinger DC, Wypij D, duPlessis AJ, et al. Neurodevelopmental status at eight years in children with dextro-transposition of the great arteries: The Boston Circulatory Arrest Trial. *J Thorac Cardiovasc Surg.* 2003;126:1385–1396.

Further Reading

Bernstein D. Epidemiology and genetic basis of congenital heart disease. In: Kliegman RM, Stanton BMD, St. Geme J, et al, eds. *Nelsons Textbook of Pediatrics.* 19th ed. Philadelphia: Saunders; 2011:1362–1363.

Menahem S, Grimwade J. Pre-natal counselling—helping couples make decisions following the diagnosis of severe heart disease. *Early Human Development.* 2005;81(7):601–607.

Khoo N, Van Essen P, Richardson M, et al. Effectiveness of prenatal diagnosis of congenital heart defects in South Australia: A population analysis 1999–2003. *Australian and New Zealand Journal of Obstetrics and Gynaecology.* 2008;48:559–563.

Martins P, Castela E. Transposition of the great arteries. *Orphanet Journal Of Rare Diseases.* 2008;3:27.

Skinner J, Hornung T, Rumball E. Transposition of the great arteries: from fetus to adult. *Heart.* 2008;94(9):1227–1235.

CHAPTER 35

Hypoplastic Left-Heart Syndrome

Adam B Hoellering, Pieter J Koorts

Hypoplastic left-heart syndrome represents a spectrum of cardiac malformations characterised by varying degrees of hypoplasia of left-sided cardiac structures: mitral valve, left ventricle, aortic valve and aorta (see Figure 35.1). This results in a left ventricle that is unable to maintain an adequate systemic circulation after delivery.

INCIDENCE
Hypoplastic left heart syndrome is an uncommon condition, affecting approximately 1 in 5000 newborn infants. It occurs more frequently in males than females with a 2:1 male predominance.

DIFFERENTIAL DIAGNOSIS
The differential diagnosis includes any left-sided obstructive lesions where the systemic circulation is dependent on ductal flow; e.g., critical aortic stenosis, coarctation of the aorta, interrupted aortic arch.

Postnatally, non-structural cardiac conditions such as myocarditis can present the same way (with cardiogenic shock). Neonatal infection and inborn errors of metabolism can also cause shock and mimic hypoplastic left-heart syndrome.

AETIOLOGY
Like other congenital structural heart conditions, hypoplastic left-heart syndrome is thought to have multiple interacting underlying causes.

Although specific genes are yet to be identified, genetic abnormalities are believed to be particularly important. The incidence is increased in Turner syndrome, Noonan syndrome, Smith-Lemli-Opitz syndrome and Holt-Oram syndrome. Extracardiac anomalies can be found in 28% of cases of hypoplastic left-heart syndrome.[1]

ASSOCIATED FINDINGS
In addition to the associated genetic abnormalities detailed above, babies with hypoplastic left-heart syndrome are more likely to be low birth weight.

There is also an increased risk of abnormal brain findings, including periventricular leukomalacia (about 15% of complex cardiac lesions before surgery, and around half after surgery) and microcephaly.

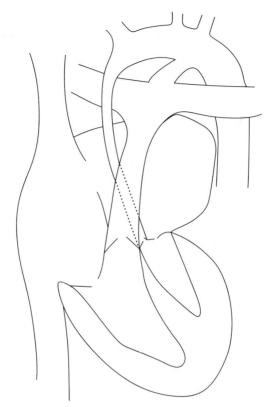

Figure 35.1 A schematic diagram of the heart showing the anatomy of hypoplastic left heart syndrome (compare with Figures 32.1 and 32.2 in Chapter 32)—the left ventricle and aorta are small and the systemic circulation is dependent on the patent ductus arteriosus.

PATHOPHYSIOLOGY

Hypoplastic left-heart syndrome is not clinically significant *in utero*, with fetal compromise being very rare.

The systemic circulation is maintained via flow from the pulmonary artery across the widely patent ductus arteriosus. Perfusion to the coronary and carotid arteries is via retrograde flow from the blood crossing the ductus arteriosus. Blood returning from the fetal lungs drains into the left atrium and has to shunt across a patent foramen ovale as normal passage to the left ventricular outflow tract is obstructed.

Because the cerebral circulation is supplied by retrograde flow from blood flowing right-to-left across the patent ductus arteriosus, there is a risk of inadequate blood supply to the developing fetal brain. This may in part explain the poor neurodevelopmental outcome seen in children with hypoplastic left-heart syndrome.

After birth, the right ventricle is responsible for maintaining the blood flow to both the lungs and the systemic circulation. Infants are often asymptomatic initially, until the onset of constriction of the ductus arteriosus (day 2–3) which results in markedly reduced systemic perfusion. This leads them to become hypoxaemic, shocked and acidotic. Due to mixing of the systemic and pulmonary venous return in the left atrium, the newborn is often mildly cyanosed from birth.

PROGNOSIS

Without surgical intervention, hypoplastic left-heart syndrome is lethal, usually within two weeks of delivery.

For low-risk patients who have had the staged surgery for hypoplastic left-heart syndrome, survival to school age is around 80–85%.

Risk factors for poor outcome include:

- prematurity;
- associated chromosomal or genetic abnormalities;
- other extracardiac abnormalities;
- an abnormal tricuspid valve with severe regurgitation; and
- an intact atrial septum.

In those who survive surgical treatment for hypoplastic left-heart syndrome, there is an increased risk of a variety of problems.[2] These include neurodevelopmental problems such as:

- motor delay;
- learning disabilities;
- behavioural problems (up to 70% have attention deficit hyperactivity disorder); and
- cognitive impairment (18%).

Exercise limitation, an increased risk of thrombosis, atrial arrhythmias and protein-losing enteropathy are also common.

RECURRENCE RISK

Hinton et al[3] report a recurrence risk of around 8%.

TREATMENT OPTIONS

Antenatal diagnosis may result in termination of up to half of pregnancies with hypoplastic left-heart syndrome.

Where the parents have opted to continue the pregnancy, delivery should be planned in a specialist centre that has an intensive care nursery with on-site paediatric cardiology services and cardiac surgery.

The initial care, including any necessary resuscitation, should proceed as for any newborn infant.

An intravenous infusion of prostaglandin E_1 to maintain ductal patency should be started as soon as possible after birth. Usually an umbilical venous catheter is inserted initially for intravenous access. The baby should be referred to a paediatric cardiologist soon after birth.

Tibballs and Cantwell-Bartl[4] report that, in a cohort of babies admitted to a children's hospital, most families with an antenatal diagnosis opted for surgical intervention; if the diagnosis is not made until after delivery half of the parents chose to not proceed with surgery.

Surgery consists of a series of major procedures which are undertaken at only a small number of specialist cardiac centres (only in Melbourne and Sydney in Australia). The first stage (the Norwood procedure) involves major restructuring of the circulation so that the right ventricle is connected to the aorta; it is done in the first week or two life. Most babies will go home after 2–4 weeks.

The aim of the second stage (at 4–6 months) and third stage (at 18 months–3 years) is to separate the pulmonary and systemic circulations. The process is technically challenging and complications are common.

The parents should know that the process is not curative. The aim is to create a circulation that can sustain life until a donor heart becomes available for transplantation.

There is considerable concern that those patients who survive surgical treatment for hypoplastic left-heart syndrome are at significantly increased risk of poor neurodevelopmental outcome.

Some families elect not to undertake the surgical option, because of the poor quality of life in survivors. In this case it is perfectly acceptable to redirect care towards comfort, compassion and maintenance of dignity. The infant may appear well at delivery, but will gradually become shocked and acidotic as the duct closes. The process of dying may take several days during which time the family are encouraged to hold and comfort their baby. Medications can be prescribed to minimise any distress in the infant. Early involvement of a palliative care team should be considered.

ETHICS

The key issue facing the parents in this condition is whether or not to embark on a long, difficult and uncertain surgical course of palliation or to elect comfort care following delivery. Complete, accurate, up-to-date data presented clearly and honestly to the family is imperative.

ASPECTS OF COUNSELLING

In addition to a neonatologist, early involvement of a paediatric cardiologist is essential as they are best qualified to answer questions regarding the technical aspects of the Norwood procedure and its complications and outcomes.

It may also be appropriate to involve a clinical geneticist.

REFERENCES

1. Natowicz M, Chatten J, Clancy R, et al. Genetic disorders and major extra-cardiac anomalies associated with the hypoplastic left heart syndrome. *Pediatrics.* 1988;82: 698–706.
2. Rychik J. Hypoplastic left heart syndrome: From in-utero diagnosis to school age. *Seminars in Fetal & Neonatal Medicine.* 2005;10:553–566.
3. Hinton RB, Martin LJ, Tabangin ME, et al. Hypoplastic left heart syndrome is heritable. *Journal of the American College of Cardiology.* 2007;50:1590–1595.
4. Tibballs J, Cantwell-Bartl A. Outcomes of management decisions by parents for their infants with hypoplastic left heart syndrome with and without a prenatal diagnosis. *J Paediatr Child Health.* 2008;44:321–324.

Further Reading

Fyler DC. Report of the New England Regional Infant Cardiac Program. *Pediatrics.* 1980;65(2 part 2):375–461.

Mahle WT, Clancy RR, McGaurn SP, et al. Impact of prenatal diagnosis on survival and early neurologic morbidity in neonates with hypoplastic left heart syndrome. *Pediatrics.* 2001;107:1277–1282.

Rychik J, Szwast A, Natarajan S, et al. Perinatal and early surgical outcome for the fetus with hypoplastic left heart syndrome: a 5-year single institutional experience. *Ultrasound Obstet Gynecol.* 2010;36:465–470.

Tabbutt S, Nord AS, Jarvik GP, et al. Neurodevelopmental outcomes after staged palliation for hypoplastic left heart syndrome. *Pediatrics.* 2008;121(3):476–483.

CHAPTER 36

Other Left Ventricular Outflow Tract (LVOT) Abnormalities

Ben Reeves, Pieter Koorts

Apart from hypoplastic left-heart syndrome, abnormalities of the left ventricular outflow tract (LVOT) include numerous obstructive lesions such as aortic stenosis, coarctation of the aorta and an interrupted aortic arch. Examples of the anatomy are shown in Figure 36.1.

Signs suggestive of left-sided obstruction on a fetal ultrasound include:
- asymmetry of ventricle size (i.e., right ventricle bigger than the left) or discrepant outflow tracts (pulmonary artery bigger than the aorta);
- the ductal diameter larger than the aortic isthmus in coarctation;
- flow reversal in the arterial duct or transverse arch;
- a left-to-right atrial shunt;
- abnormal colour Doppler through the mitral or aortic valves;
- interrupted colour flow in the aortic arch; and
- endocardial fibroelastosis seen as a bright endocardial border.

Coarctation of the aorta can be considered a spectrum of abnormalities with variable degrees and sites of obstruction, with the extreme end of the spectrum being interruption of the aorta.

The normal values for the diameter of the aortic annulus (average range) are:
- 18–20 weeks gestational age—3–4 mm;
- 28 weeks gestational age—4–6 mm;
- 36 weeks gestational age—7–10 mm.

INCIDENCE

Aortic stenosis occurs in 1 in 2500 live births. A bicuspid aortic valve is much more common occurring in 1–2% of live births.

Coarctation of the aorta occurs in 1 in 12,000 live births and is slightly increased in males. It is found in up to 10% of children with Turner syndrome.

An interrupted aortic arch is uncommon but it makes up 1% of all "critical cardiac disease". Interruption type B is strongly associated with 22q11 deletion (two-thirds of cases with type B interruption have 22q11 deletion).

AETIOLOGY / PATHOPHYSIOLOGY / EMBRYOLOGY

Arterial valves are first seen at around week 7 of embryonic development. The trifoliate arrangement of aortic and pulmonary valves develops from

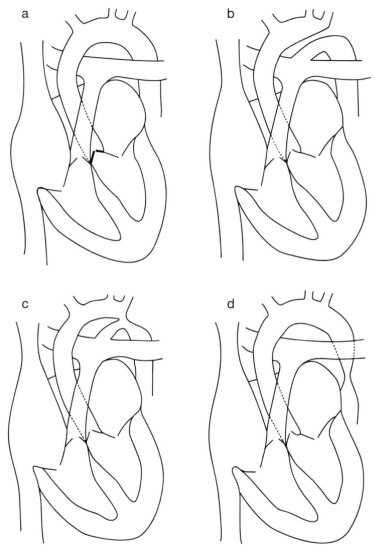

Figure 36.1 A schematic diagram of the heart showing the anatomy of four examples of LVOT obstruction (compare with Figures 32.1 and 32.2 in Chapter 32)—a) aortic valve stenosis, b) interrupted aortic arch, c) peri-ductal coarctation of the aorta, and d) post-ductal coarctation of the aorta.

cavitation of outflow cushions which are critical in the formation of the outflow tracts. Disruption of this process leads to valve stenosis or, in extreme cases, atresia.

Interrupted aortic arch has a multifactorial inheritance. Neural crest cells populate the aortic arches, hence its association with 22q11 deletion, another disorder of neural crest migration.

The morphogenesis of aortic arch abnormalities, including coarctation, is thought to be related to abnormal arch embryogenesis (from the fourth branchial arch), abnormal development of the arterial duct, and *in utero* changes in the ratio of flow between pulmonary and systemic arterial pathways (for example subarterial ventricular septal defect redirecting fetal flow away from the aorta).

DIFFERENTIAL DIAGNOSIS

Severe left-sided arch obstruction may be associated with varying degrees of left ventricular hypoplasia and can be part of the spectrum of hypoplastic left-heart syndrome. It can therefore be difficult in equivocal cases to counsel parents on the likelihood of a biventricular repair, or need for univentricular palliation with all the attendant increased morbidity and mortality.

Examination for other sites of left-heart obstruction should be made; e.g., "Shone syndrome"—parachute mitral valve, supravalvar left atrial ring, subaortic stenosis and aortic coarctation.

ASSOCIATED ABNORMALITIES

There is a recognised association between interruption of the aortic arch and patent ductus arteriosus (PDA), ventricular septal defect (VSD) (seen in 75% of patients with interruption) and inter-atrial communication. The associated ventricular septal defect is often described as a "malalignment-type" VSD, which tends to reduce flow through the systemic pathway in fetal life.

Interruption of the arch may be associated with an aorto-pulmonary window rather than a ventricular septal defect in some cases. Rarely, an interruption may exist in isolation.

Coarctation of the aorta frequently coexists with other left-sided obstructive lesions, especially bicuspid aortic valve.

Interruption or coarctation may also be associated with anomalies of the subclavian artery (the commonest is a right subclavian artery arising from the aorta distal to the arterial duct).

CONSEQUENCES

Aortic stenosis or a bicuspid aortic valve tends to reduce aortic flow during fetal life and may predispose to aortic arch abnormalities or hypoplasia of the left ventricle with the attendant risk of development of the hypoplastic left-heart syndrome.

The clinical condition depends on severity of left-sided obstruction and the presence or absence of associated lesions.

MANAGEMENT—ANTENATAL

In utero aortic valve dilation, with the aim of averting the natural trend of severe aortic stenosis progressing to hypoplastic left-heart syndrome, has been attempted with some limited success since 1991.

Counselling on likely surgical options and decisions for optimal delivery can be made following antenatal diagnosis. This should be done by a paediatric cardiologist.

Prenatal diagnosis of coarctation of the aorta is known to improve survival and pre-operative clinical condition, but a recent review suggests postnatal diagnosis is more frequent.[1]

MANAGEMENT—LABOUR / DELIVERY / IMMEDIATE POSTNATAL

Delivery should be in a tertiary neonatal centre for those with severe lesions. Operative delivery is not necessary unless required for maternal factors.

Each infant with an antenatally diagnosed left ventricular outflow tract abnormality should have a detailed plan documented for management in the immediate postnatal period.

A postnatal echocardiogram to confirm the anatomical diagnosis, with full clinical assessment, should be done to determine the requirement for prostaglandin infusion to maintain ductal patency (to augment systemic perfusion). An umbilical venous catheter should be inserted initially if prostaglandin infusion is required.

In all cases, surgical repair of the arch should follow resuscitation and stabilisation of the infant to optimise outcome.

MANAGEMENT—POSTNATAL

An end-to-end repair is recommended as the treatment of choice for severe coarctation or aortic interruption, with management of associated abnormalities as required.

Hypertension following coarctation repair is seen in older children presenting with coarctation, occasionally requiring medical therapy, and may exist without any residual coarctation.

Aortic balloon valvuloplasty is the treatment of choice for critical or severe aortic stenosis, but operative intervention may be required if this technique is unsuccessful, or obstruction worsens despite an initial good result.

Echocardiographic surveillance for re-coarctation is required. Balloon dilation of residual coarctation with or without insertion of a stent can frequently delay or avoid the need for further surgical intervention.

Berry aneurysm is a significant cause of late mortality after coarctation and relates to vascular wall abnormalities at sites distal to the coarcted segment. There seems also to be a predisposition to aortic dissection or rupture as a result.

Balloon dilation of the aortic valve is associated with an appreciable risk of aortic regurgitation, which can rarely be severe enough to require urgent surgical repair. Recurrence of stenosis following balloon dilation is a risk and further balloon dilation or eventual surgical repair or valve replacement may be required. Infants with aortic stenosis not requiring early intervention will require regular review every 2–3 months, as obstruction can progress rapidly.

Specialist referral may be required for children with 22q11 deletion or other syndromes; disorders of parathyroid function and immune deficiency are of concern.

ETHICS

Considerable debate exists about fetal intervention for severe left-sided obstructive lesions, with attendant high mortality rates from intervention *versus* long-term morbidity and mortality with single-ventricle palliation (see Chapter 35). No large scale randomised control trials exist to provide guidance on this topic.

REFERENCE

1. Gardiner HM. The case for fetal cardiac intervention. *Heart.* 2009;95:1648–1652.

Further Reading

Anderson RH, Baker EJ, Redington A, et al, eds. *Paediatric Cardiology.* 3rd ed. Philadelphia USA: Churchill Livingstone; 2010.

Chew C, Halliday JL, Riley MM, et al. Population-based study of antenatal detection of congenital heart disease by ultrasound examination. *Ultrasound Obstet Gynecol.* 2007;29:619–624.

Franklin O, Burch M, Manning N, et al. Prenatal diagnosis of coarctation of the aorta improves survival and reduces morbidity. *Heart.* 2002;87:67–69.

Fyler DC, Buckley DC, Hellenbrand WC, et al. Report of the New England Regional Infant Cardiac Program. *Pediatrics.* 1980;65:375–461.

Maxwell D, Allan L, Tynan MJ. Balloon dilatation of the aortic valve in the foetus: a report of two cases. *British Heart Journal.* 1991;65:256–258.

Shone JD, Sellers RD, Anderson RC, et al. The development complex of "parachute mitral valve," supravalvar ring of left atrium, subaortic stenosis and coarctation of the aorta. *Am J Cardiol.* 1963;11:714–725.

Wilkins-Haug LE, Benson CB, Tworetzky W, et al. In-utero intervention for hypoplastic left heart syndrome—a perinatologist's perspective. *Ultrasound in Obstetrics and Gynecology.* 2005;26:281–486.

CHAPTER 37

Fetal Arrhythmias

Ben Anderson, Luke A Jardine

Disorders of fetal cardiac rate and rhythm are broadly classified into either bradycardia or tachycardia. Approximately 1–3% of pregnancies are affected by some form of dysrhythmia; around 40% of these are brady arrhythmias and 60% are tachyarrhythmias.[1,2] In 10% of affected pregnancies, the arrhythmia (tachy or brady) may be life threatening.[2]

BRADYCARDIA

Bradycardia is defined as a fetal heart rate of <100 beats per minute. There are three main groups:[1,3]

1. **Sinus bradycardia**—there is a slowing of the atrial and ventricular rates with normal 1:1 conduction. Brief and clinically irrelevant decelerations are often observed in the first and second trimester ultrasound scans.[3]
2. **Blocked atrial beats**—these occur when the atrial rate is faster than the ventricular rate. Premature atrial beats (often atrial bigeminy) are sufficiently early to arrive at the atrio-ventricular node during the refractory period, and are therefore not conducted. Ventricular rates are typically 70–80 bpm.[1]
3. Second and third degree **atrio-ventricular (AV) block** (including complete AV block)—complete AV block occurs when there is a normal atrial rate with regular dissociated ventricular bradycardia. Half of these are related to structural heart disease with abnormal placement of the conducting bundle and consequent interruption of this pathway.

Of fetuses with persistent bradycardia, sinus bradycardia accounts for around 12%, atrial bigeminy 20% and complete AV block 60%.[1,3] Complete AV block is rare and occurs in 1 in 15,000–1in 22,000 live births.[4]

Aetiology

Sinus bradycardia can occur in the following settings:
- if the sinus bradycardia is of early onset and persistent then up to 17% are associated with inherited channelopathies (e.g., long QT syndrome)— particularly if accompanied by runs of ventricular tachycardia and 2:1 AV block;[2]
- structural heart disease (e.g., heterotaxy syndromes, sinus node dysfunction);

▶ central nervous system disorders; and
▶ metabolic derangement, including fetal hypoxia, acidosis and inadvertent poisoning.
  Blocked atrial beats usually have no significant associations, although AV block will need to be excluded.

  AV block is associated with:
▶ Structural heart disease is found in 50% of cases (commonly left atrial isomerism and congenitally corrected transposition of the great arteries).[5,6]
▶ Maternal collagen vascular diseases are present in most of those with structurally normal hearts; e.g., systemic lupus erythematosus (SLE), rheumatoid arthritis, dermatomyositis, Sjögren's syndrome. These disorders may be asymptomatic in the mother. They can cause an inflammatory myocarditis in the fetus which leads to disruption of the developing conduction system between 18 and 32 weeks gestation. Auto-antibodies are present in 2% of pregnant women with 1–2% of exposed fetuses developing complete AV block.[7]

Consequences
In sinus bradycardia and blocked atrial beats, the fetus usually compensates for the decreased heart rate by increasing its stroke volume.

Complete AV block may be complicated by fetal hydrops, endocardial fibroelastosis and fetal death.

Management
In general there are three options for the management of fetal bradycardia, depending upon the cause and the effects on the fetus. These options are:

1. observation without treatment;
2. drug therapy (either trans-placental via the maternal circulation or direct fetal administration); or
3. delivery and postnatal management (preferably ≥37 weeks gestation).[7]

Antenatal Management
Pregnancies with an antenatal diagnosis of sustained fetal bradycardia should be referred to a fetal cardiologist for further assessment, including detailed fetal echocardiography.

In cases of sinus bradycardia, the family history should be checked for possible long QT syndrome (e.g., family history of syncope, seizures, congenital sensorineural deafness, sudden infant death syndrome (SIDS) and sudden unexplained death). Also investigate for causes of underlying systemic disease in the mother and look for possible causes of fetal hypoxia.

There is generally no treatment required for fetuses with blocked atrial beats. Follow-up antenatal scans are advised as there is a small risk of the fetus developing tachyarrhythmia.[4]

In fetuses with AV block, there is no universal consensus on management. The mother should be checked for anti-Ro/La antibodies. Consider weekly echocardiographic assessment from 20–24 weeks gestation.

Specific management for fetal AV block may include:

▶ Maternal steroids if there is first or second degree AV block and endocardial fibroelastosis—this may resolve incomplete block, although endocardial fibroelastosis is often already present and tends to progress rapidly.[3]

▶ Maternal dexamethasone in high doses (4–8 mg/day and weaning[1,7]) from diagnosis to delivery may improve fetal AV block, improve the hydrops and myocardial dysfunction and improve survival to 93%,[3] although some report no change in outcome.[6] This therapy remains the subject of further research. The amniotic fluid volumes should be monitored.

▶ If the fetal heart rate is <55 bpm then consider treating the mother with a beta-sympathomimetic (e.g., salbutamol 10 mg three times a day orally) as this increases the fetal heart rate by 5–10 bpm,[1,5] although this may not improve survival.[7]

▶ Maternal immunoglobulin therapy (70 g every 2–3 days) if the fetus has endocardial fibroelastosis, cardiac dysfunction or incomplete block.[7]

▶ Some have recommended elective delivery at 37 weeks gestation if the AV block is uncomplicated; however, there is no evidence to suggest this improves outcome.[7] Delivering the baby preterm for immediate pacing is not advised as this may place the infant at greater risk of other complications.[6,7]

Babies with a diagnosis of fetal bradycardia should be delivered in a hospital with an intensive care nursery with on-site availability of paediatric cardiologists.

Post Delivery

Babies should be resuscitated as for any other newborn infant; those with hydrops and cardiac failure causing respiratory compromise may require intubation and mechanical ventilation. The baby should be referred to a paediatric cardiologist.

Fetuses with sinus bradycardia usually do not require any specific treatment after birth. An electrocardiogram (ECG) should be done, as well as a 24-hour halter monitor ECG. The family history should be checked for possible long QT syndrome (e.g., family history of syncope, seizures, congenital sensorineural deafness, SIDS and sudden unexplained death). Any underlying disorders (e.g., structural heart disease, central nervous system pathology, poisoning, metabolic abnormalities) should be managed appropriately. If the bradycardia is severe or symptomatic the baby may need treatment with isoprenaline, atropine or adrenaline. Temporary external pacing can be used where there is cardiac arrest.

Blocked atrial beats do not usually require any specific treatment after birth. An ECG should be done and continuous rhythm monitoring started to ensure the cardiac rhythm normalises post-delivery.

Babies with AV Block do not often require pacing. Pacing may be considered if the heart rate is <55 bpm, if there are signs of hydrops or heart failure or if there is metabolic acidosis or other significant symptoms.[2,6] If the bradycardia is severe or symptomatic the baby may need treatment with isoprenaline, atropine or adrenaline. Immunoglobulin therapy (2 g/kg IV as a single dose) is considered if the fetus has endocardial fibroelastosis, cardiac dysfunction or incomplete block.[7] A pacemaker is inserted if:[2]

- the ventricular rate is <50 bpm (if there is no structural heart disease) or <70 bpm (if there is structural disease);
- there is a wide complex QRS (>80 ms);
- there are complex ventricular arrhythmias; or
- there is significant ventricular dysfunction or hydrops.

These babies require long-term follow-up with a paediatric cardiologist.

Outcomes

Babies with sinus bradycardia very occasionally develop progressive sinus node dysfunction. Infants with persistent sinus bradycardia without explanation should be referred for cardiology assessment.

In babies with blocked atrial beats, the rhythm usually resolves spontaneously without treatment by the time of or soon after delivery. If it does not then these infants should be referred for cardiology assessment.

AV block has a number of risk factors for poor prognosis including:[4]

- fetal hydrops;
- endocardial fibroelastosis;
- premature delivery;
- heart rate <55 bpm;
- complete AV block in association with congenital heart disease (<20% survival[1]); and
- complete AV block associated with left atrial isomerism—it is almost universally fatal.[3]

Untreated isolated complete AV block has a perinatal mortality of 18–43%.[4,7] Treated complete AV block has a live birth rate of 95% and a 95% one-year survival (86% if the heart rate is <55 bpm.[3,7] Late cardiomyopathy and ventricular dysfunction are still a risk long term.

Recurrence

The risk of complete AV block in fetuses of mothers with known antibodies increases by up to 10 times in subsequent pregnancies.[8] The recurrence risk is likely to be between 10% and 20%.[4]

Maternal intravenous immunoglobulin has been used in subsequent high risk pregnancies, although recurrences were observed.[8]

TACHYCARDIA

Tachycardia is defined as a fetal heart rate of >180 beats per minute (bpm). There are four main groups:[1,2,4]

1. **Sinus tachycardia** accounts for 6% of cases—this occurs when the atrial rate is 180–200 bpm with 1 : 1 AV conduction and some variability of the heart rate. There are a number of fetal and maternal causes (e.g., maternal thyrotoxicosis, beta adrenergic drugs, congenital heart disease, early fetal hypoxia).

2. **Ectopic beats** causing irregular fetal heart rhythm. Ectopic beats are common and may be found in up to 1.7% of fetuses between 36 and 41 weeks.[9] This is the most frequent diagnosis in fetuses referred for assessment of tachycardia (up to 43% of all referrals[10]). Ectopic beats are due to premature contractions and are more commonly atrial in origin rather than ventricular.

3. **Supra-ventricular tachycardia** (SVT) accounts for 40–90% of cases—this is characterised by a persistent tachycardia with little rate variation; often between 210 and 320 bpm. It is often related to a re-entrant pathway. Supra-ventricular tachycardia usually presents between 28 and 30 weeks gestation; however, it may be seen as early as 18 weeks.[2]

4. **Atrial flutter** (AF) accounts for 10–30% of cases—this results from an intra-atrial macro-re-entrant circuit. The atrial rate is between 300 and 550 bpm with a resulting irregular ventricular rate between 150 and 250 bpm due to variable AV block. Atrial flutter often has onset later in the pregnancy or during labour and is usually persistent once present.

Associations

An associated abnormality may be detected in up to one-third of early presentations; these include:

- an accessory AV conducting pathway in 70%;[2]
- structural cardiac defects in 14%[11] (e.g., Ebstein anomaly, coarctation of the aorta, cardiac tumours[4]);
- chromosomal anomalies;
- fetal distress;
- anaemia;
- infection;
- maternal beta-stimulation; and
- fetal thyrotoxicosis.[1]

Consequences

Sustained tachyarrhythmia compromises the cardiac output and function as the high rates increase cardiac metabolic demand in the face of inadequate filling times. Severely compromised cardiac output leads to the development of hydrops fetalis. Fetuses with supra-ventricular tachycardia with a heart rate of >230 bpm for more than 12 hours will often develop hydrops fetalis.[2]

Supra-ventricular tachycardia has an antenatal mortality of 2–38% if associated with hydrops compared with 0–4% without hydrops.[1,2,4,11] Prenatal control of the heart rate is achievable in up to 92% of non-hydropic fetuses and 63% of hydropic fetuses.[12] If untreated postnatally, half will have recurrence with more resolving by one year of age.[2] If episodes of supra-ventricular tachycardia persist beyond one year of age, resolution is unlikely. Of those who are treated over the first 6 months, 40% have no recurrence. About one-third of all cases will have a recurrence of their supra-ventricular tachycardia in the teenage years. Long-term neurological outcome is good, even following hydrops, with normal cognitive function reported in 73% of survivors.[13]

Atrial flutter has an antenatal mortality of 6–30%;[2] this is lower if the onset is near term. Recurrence after cardioversion is uncommon.[1,12] Long-term prophylactic treatment is usually not required.[1]

Antenatal Management

In general the options for the management of antenatal tachycardia are the same as for fetal bradycardia:

1. observation without treatment;
2. anti-arrhythmic drug therapy (maternal or fetal); or
3. delivery and postnatal management, particularly if tachycardia occurs at or after 36 weeks.[11]

All babies with fetal tachycardia should be assessed by a fetal cardiologist and have an echocardiographic assessment.

For babies with sinus tachycardia, treatment is aimed at the underlying cause.

For babies with isolated ectopics, spontaneous resolution is often the rule with most not requiring treatment.[4] Isolated ectopics are not an indication for delivery as there is only a small risk of them ever triggering a tachyarrhythmia (<5%).[4] The fetus should be reviewed every 2–4 weeks with fetal heart rate and rhythm assessment.

Mothers of fetuses with supra-ventricular tachycardia should be admitted to hospital for assessment and monitoring of the fetal heart rate. Transplacental drug therapy via the mother should be considered; the choice of medication varies between centres (e.g., digoxin, sotalol, flecainide, amiodarone).[1,2,5,12] Cardioversion *in utero* will occur in 65–95% after 6–10 days of therapy.[4] If near term, the baby can be delivered and managed *ex utero*.

Mothers of fetuses with atrial flutter may require admission to hospital for assessment and monitoring of the fetal heart rate. Maternal drug therapy may be considered. Sotalol appears to be more effective than digoxin.[1]

If there is fetal compromise or ongoing arrhythmia, delivery should occur in a tertiary hospital with an intensive care nursery and access to paediatric cardiology and other paediatric sub-specialty services. If there is no *in utero* cardioversion and the hydrops doesn't resolve within 2 weeks then delivery and postnatal treatment is recommended.

Postnatal Management

Babies should be resuscitated as for any other newborn infant; those with hydrops and cardiac failure causing respiratory compromise may require intubation and mechanical ventilation. The baby should be referred to a paediatric cardiologist. An ECG should be performed on all babies with an *in utero* diagnosis of tachycardia.

Babies with sinus tachycardia need to have the underlying metabolic or structural disease treated (e.g., thyroid dysfunction).

Babies who have supra-ventricular tachycardia may require the following treatments: vagal manoeuvres (including a cold pack on the forehead, massage of a single carotid sinus); intravenous adenosine, beta-blockers and/ or DC cardioversion. Ablation of aberrant conduction pathways may be required when the baby is older or larger (usually >15 kg).

Babies who have atrial flutter often require similar treatment to supra-ventricular tachycardia. They may need to be cardioverted following delivery and can be pre-treated with digoxin for control of the heart rate.[2] Sotalol therapy (effective in 80%) appears to be more effective than amiodarone (effective in 30%).[2]

Recurrence

In general, the risk of recurrence in future pregnancies is very low unless there is associated congenital heart disease. If associated with congenital heart disease, then chromosomal causes that may have increased risk of recurrence must be considered (e.g., 22q11 deletion, Down syndrome, etc). There are some reported familial cases of supra-ventricular tachycardia but these are very rare. There are currently no recommendations to screen siblings for tachyarrhythmia.

ETHICS

The maternal risks of trans-placental therapy for fetuses with any form of arrhythmia must be weighed against the potential fetal benefits, particularly in areas where the risk:benefit ratio is still being investigated.

REFERENCES

1. Jaeggi E, Nii M. Fetal brady- and tachyarrhythmias: New and accepted diagnostic and treatment methods. *Seminars in Fetal and Neonatal Medicine.* 2005;10:504–514.
2. Strasberger J, Cheulkar B, Wichman H. Perinatal Arrhythmias: Diagnosis and Management. *Clinics in Perinatology.* 2007;34:627–652.
3. Jaeggi E, Friedberg M. Diagnosis and Management of Fetal Bradyarrhythmias. *Pace.* 2008;31:S50–S53.
4. Api O, Carvalho J. Fetal Dysrhythmias. *Best Practice and Research Clinical Obstetrics and Gynaecology.* 2008;22:31–48.

5. Maeno Y, Hirose A, Kanbe T, et al. Fetal arrhythmia: Prenatal diagnosis and perinatal management. *Journal of Obstetrics and Gynaecology*. 2009;35(4):623–629.

6. Wren C. Cardiac arrhythmias in the fetus and newborn. *Seminars in Fetal and Neonatal Medicine*. 2006;11:182–190.

7. Weber R, Golding F, Jaeggi E. Managing the fetus with atrioventricular block. *Heart Rhythm*. 2008;5:1347–1349.

8. Brucato A. Prevention of congenital heart block in children of SSA-positive mothers. *Rheumatology*. 2008;47:iii35–iii37.

9. Southall DP, Richards J, Hardwick RA, et al. Prospective study of fetal heart rate and rhythm patterns. *Archives of Disease in Childhood*. 1980;55:506–511.

10. Copel JA, Liang RI, Demasio K, et al. The clinical significance of the irregular fetal heart rhythm. *American Journal of Obstetrics and Gynaecology*. 2000;182:813–817.

11. Jurjevic R, Podnar T, Vesel S. Diagnosis, clinical features, management and post-natal follow-up of fetal tachycardias. *Cardiology in the Young*. 2009;19:486–493.

12. Kothari D, Skinner J. Neonatal tachycardias: an update. *Archives of Disease in Childhood, Fetal and Neonatal Edition*. 2006;91:F136–F144.

13. Oudijk MA, Gooskens RH, Stoutenbeek P, et al. Neurological outcome of children who were treated for fetal tachycardia complicated by hydrops. *Ultrasound in Obstetrics and Gynaecology*. 2004;24:154–158.

Section 11
Gut Problems

CHAPTER 38
Gastroschisis

Mark W Davies

Gastroschisis is a congenital anterior abdominal wall defect with the uncovered abdominal contents (usually small and large bowel) protruding through the defect. Why it develops is not definitively known.

Gastroschisis occurs in about 5 in 10,000 live births. It has been associated with mothers who are young, smoke and use other recreational drugs; as well as poor socioeconomic status and education.

ANTENATAL DIAGNOSIS

The overwhelming majority of babies with gastroschisis will have their condition diagnosed antenatally. The diagnosis is usually made on ultrasound scan in the second or third trimester. See Figures 38.1 and 38.2.

Gastroschisis is not usually associated with other congenital abnormalities other than gut atresia and vascularly compromised gut. There is an increased risk of intra-uterine growth restriction.

The main differential diagnosis is omphalocele/exomphalos, especially if ruptured.

Because the risk of chromosomal abnormality is extremely low, fetal karyotyping is not usually offered.

The parents should also see a paediatric surgeon antenatally.

DELIVERY

The baby should be delivered in a centre that has paediatric surgeons available and a neonatal intensive care unit. There is no advantage to either vaginal or caesarean birth. There is no reason to deliver early in the absence of general fetal compromise.

PROBLEMS EXPECTED AT BIRTH

There is an increased risk of being born preterm (up to 60%) and small for gestational age (up to 70%).

The major risks to the infant with gastroschisis are compromised circulation to the gut, gut obstruction, loss of heat and water from the exposed bowel and infection.

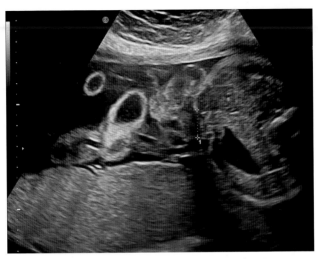

Figure 38.1 Fetal ultrasound at 30 weeks gestational age showing a transverse section of the abdomen on the right and bowel outside the abdomen on the left. The callipers span the abdominal wall defect.

Call a paediatric surgeon prior to delivery if the diagnosis was made antenatally, or as soon as the baby is stabilised.

EARLY NEONATAL MANAGEMENT

Upon delivery, the baby is resuscitated as for any baby.

Any respiratory problems will be managed as for babies without gastroschisis. Keep in mind that some surgeons would prefer that nasal continuous positive airway pressure (CPAP) is not used to avoid the gut filling with gas.

The baby will not be fed and a nasogastric tube will be inserted and left on free drainage and aspirated frequently.

The bowel will need to be supported so that the external bowel is not on the stretch and checked to make sure that it is not twisted on itself. See Figure 38.3.

The bowel will be covered usually by covering the whole abdomen or lower body using either clear polyethylene film ("kitchen wrap" or "cling wrap") or a "bowel bag".

Intravenous antibiotics (metronidazole, gentamicin, penicillin) will be started.

Maintenance intravenous fluids will be given.

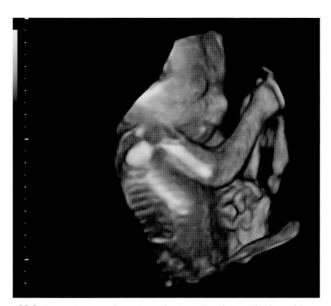

Figure 38.2 A 3D ultrasound at 19 weeks gestational age. The bowel is seen just below the fetus's right arm.

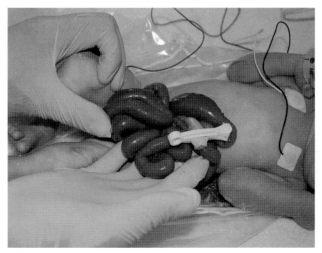

Figure 38.3 Term baby with gastroschisis an hour after birth.

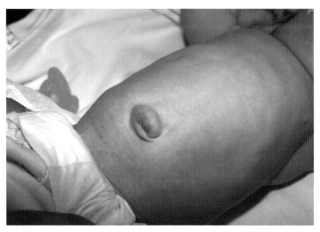

Figure 38.4 The appearance of the umbilicus 4 weeks after gastroschisis reduction—the reduction was done in the neonatal unit, without general anaesthesia, in the first few hours of life.

SUBSEQUENT MANAGEMENT

A paediatric surgeon should be involved early (preferably present at delivery). After the baby has been admitted to the neonatal unit and the above treatment started, then early, safe return of the external abdominal contents to the abdominal cavity is the aim. See Figure 38.4.

This is either done in the neonatal unit without general anaesthesia or in the operating theatre. Primary reduction and closure is the preferred option but this depends on whether there is enough space in the abdominal cavity (as judged by the surgeon during initial attempts at reduction). If there is not, then a staged closure will be necessary, with the external abdominal contents placed in a silo attached to the defect with subsequent slow reduction of the contents over days. The baby may require multiple operations.

Abdominal compartment syndrome occurs when the venous return and circulation to the lower body (including the kidneys) is compromised because of increased pressure in the abdomen. It can occur if too much is pushed back into the abdomen and an excessively tight abdominal wall results. This can prolong the post-operative ileus and further damage the gut.

Any gut with compromised circulation may need to be excised and this can result in short gut syndrome.

THE PARENTS ALSO NEED TO KNOW

The overall mortality is around 10%, usually from infection, dead gut or short gut.

Even if all goes well, feeds take a long time to start and establish with full enteral feeds usually reached at about 4–5 weeks old. Some babies will take up to 10 weeks.

Late morbidity is often due to infection and/or short gut.

Babies usually require 4–5 weeks of total parenteral nutrition, with some needing up to 10 weeks.

As for any baby requiring prolonged hospital admission, the parents may require psychosocial support and the involvement of a social worker.

The long-term outlook is very good for the majority. Some children continue to grow poorly. There is a risk of gut adhesions with or without obstruction, and functional gut problems.

RECURRENCE

The recurrence risk for gastroschisis is very low.

Further Reading

David AL, Tan A, Curry J. Gastroschisis: sonographic diagnosis, associations, management and outcome. *Prenat Diagn.* 2008;28:633–644.

Holland AJ, Walker K, Badawi N. Gastroschisis: an update. *Pediatric Surgery International.* 2010;26(9):871–878.

CHAPTER 39

Omphalocoele

Melissa Lai

Omphalocoele is a midline defect in the anterior abdominal wall that results in the herniation of abdominal contents into a membrane-covered sac. The sac is contiguous with the umbilical cord. The terms omphalocoele and exomphalos are used interchangeably. The contents of the sac include the intestines, but can also contain liver and/or stomach.

The defect can be confirmed as early as 12–14 weeks gestational age (see Figure 39.1). Before 12 weeks gestational age, the abdominal wall is not complete and there is normal physiological midgut herniation. After 12 weeks, bowel loops in the umbilical cord are no longer physiological. Protrusion of the liver and/or stomach is abnormal at any gestation.

CLASSIFICATION
Omphalocoele can be classified as either:
- small—containing either bowel and/or stomach;
- giant—containing bowel, stomach and liver; or
- ruptured.

AETIOLOGY/PATHOPHYSIOLOGY/EMBRYOLOGY
The prevailing theory is that omphalocoele results from a failure of gut loops to return to the body cavity after their normal physiological herniation into the umbilical cord from the 6th–10th week of development. The underlying reasons for this failure are poorly understood.

PREVALENCE
Omphalocoele occurs in about 2.5 in 10,000 live births. The incidence has remained stable, or actually decreased in terms of cases per live births due to a high rate of pregnancy termination with large defects.

DIFFERENTIAL DIAGNOSIS
Most abdominal wall defects are accurately diagnosed using antenatal ultrasound. However, the differential diagnoses include:
- gastroschisis (prenatally ruptured omphalocoeles may be difficult to distinguish from gastroschisis if there is no liver involved);
- bladder exstrophy;
- body stalk anomaly; and
- urachal abnormalities.

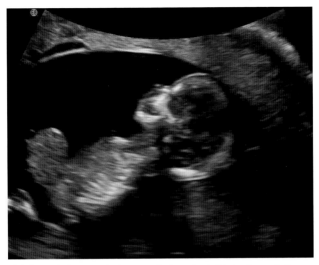

Figure 39.1 Fetal ultrasound of an omphalocoele at 14 weeks gestation.

ASSOCIATED ABNORMALITIES

Omphalocoeles may be isolated defects or associated with syndromes and chromosomal abnormalities:

▶ up to 70% are associated with other malformations, chromosomal abnormalities or genetic syndromes;

▶ up to 50% of fetuses have cardiac defects including ventricular septal defects, atrial septal defects or coarctation of the aorta;

▶ Beckwith-Wiedemann is the most common syndrome of which omphalocoele is a common feature and is marked by macroglossia, organomegaly and hypoglycaemia secondary to hyperinsulinism;

▶ omphalocoele is also associated with Pentalogy of Cantrell and the OEIS (omphalocoeles, exstrophy, imperforate anus and spinal defects) complex; and

▶ associated chromosomal disorders include trisomy 13, 18, 21, Turner's syndrome and triploidy.

CONSEQUENCES

In cases of isolated omphalocoele, survival rates are between 75% and 95%.

Survival is much lower in those with associated chromosomal and syndromic abnormalities. Of the survivors, the majority have significant impairment. Parental counselling is essential and parents may consider termination of pregnancy.

In cases of large omphalocoele, early respiratory distress or pulmonary insufficiency from pulmonary hypoplasia is a strong predictor of poor outcome.

MANAGEMENT—ANTENATAL
An amniocentesis is advised for fetal karyotype.

Serial assessment of fetal growth and amniotic fluid volume is done, as there is increased risk of fetal growth restriction, polyhydramnios and intrauterine death. An estimate of lung size is useful just before delivery.

MANAGEMENT—LABOUR/DELIVERY/IMMEDIATE POSTNATAL MANAGEMENT
Delivery should occur in a centre that has paediatric surgeons available and a neonatal intensive care unit. Most should be delivered vaginally as it is considered safer for the mother. Those with a giant omphalocoele should undergo caesarean delivery to avoid injury to abdominal viscera.

Rupture of the sac increases the risk of infection and can lead to intestinal or hepatic trauma and can limit options for delayed closure. Antibiotics will be started immediately if the sac is ruptured.

There is a high likelihood that the baby will need immediate intubation and ventilation at delivery. An oro- or nasogastric tube will be inserted immediately.

With large omphalocoeles, the sac is loosely covered with gauze and another mildly compressive gauze wrap is placed around the abdomen to minimise fluid and heat loss and to stabilise the sac. Some prefer to wrap in clear polyethylene film ("kitchen wrap" or "cling wrap")—check with your local paediatric surgeons.

Baby will have a peripheral intravenous cannula inserted and a drip started upon admission to the nursery. Do not attempt to use the umbilical vessels for access.

Most will have prophylactic antibiotics started on day 1.

Communication is crucial—the obstetric staff must give the nursery and surgical staff adequate warning of the baby's pending delivery. Urgent surgical review is required after the baby is born.

OTHER CONSULTS REQUIRED
Other specialists that should be consulted include:
▶ maternal fetal medicine specialist;
▶ paediatric surgeon; and
▶ geneticist.

MANAGEMENT—POSTNATAL
Surgical repair of the omphalocoele is usually not urgent. The baby should be stabilised and associated abnormalities identified. Use of oscillator

ventilation, nitric oxide or even ECMO may be required in those with severe lung problems. This may further delay the surgical repair.

An early echocardiogram is recommended due to the high incidence of associated cardiac anomalies.

The baby will require vigilant monitoring of blood sugar levels—those with Beckwith-Wiedemann syndrome are at risk of profound or prolonged hypoglycaemia.

Consider karyotyping if it has not been done prenatally. Confirmation of trisomy 13 or 18 will alter the clinical strategy.

Complications include feeding difficulties, gut dysmotility, necrotising enterocolitis and wound failure.

RECURRENCE

Omphalocoele is typically a sporadic congenital anomaly and recurrence risks are generally considered negligible; however in familial cases which involve autosomal dominant or vertical transmission, recurrence may be as high as 50%.

ETHICS

Significant ethical considerations arise with cases that involve life-limiting chromosomal abnormalities and other associated anomalies (see Chapters 28 and 29).

Further Reading

Islam S. Clinical care outcomes in abdominal wall defects. *Current Opinion in Pediatrics.* 2008;20:305–310.

Mann S, Blindman TA, Wilson RD. Prenatal and postnatal management of omphalocele. *Prenatal Diagnosis.* 2008; 28:626–632.

Pryde PG, Greb A, Isada NB, et al. Familial omphalocele: considerations in genetic counselling. *American Journal of Medical Genetics.* 1992 Nov 15;44(5):624–627.

Sadler TW. The embryologic origin of ventral body wall defects. *Seminars in Paediatric Surgery.* 2010;19:209–214.

CHAPTER 40

Oesophageal Atresia and Tracheo-Oesophageal Fistula

Kelly M Dixon

Oesophageal atresia is a congenital, anatomical interruption of the oesophagus resulting in a lack of direct communication from the pharynx to the stomach. It is the most common congenital anomaly affecting the oesophagus. More than 90% have an associated tracheo-oesophageal fistula. In the most common form, the upper oesophagus ends as a blind pouch and a fistula connects the trachea to the distal oesophagus, as shown in Figure 40.1.

EMBRYOLOGY
In normal development, the respiratory and digestive tubes originate from a diverticulum of the primitive foregut. This separates to form the oesophagus and trachea. Atresia occurs when this process fails.

PREVALENCE
Oesophageal atresia occurs in 1 in 3000–4500 live births. The incidence is higher in twins than in singletons (relative risk is about 2.5). There is a slight male predominance.

ASSOCIATED ANOMALIES
Overall, about 50% have associated anomalies. Associated anomalies are more common in those with antenatally diagnosed oesophageal atresia (about 80%) than in those who are diagnosed postnatally.

The most common associated anomalies (occurring in 30–40%) are skeletal (vertebral or limb) and cardiac (e.g., ventricular septal defect, tetralogy of Fallot).

Other associated findings include:
- renal anomalies, including the Potter deformation sequence (oligohydramnios, renal anomalies, pulmonary hypoplasia);
- aneuploidy (trisomies 18, 21, 13);
- 22q11 deletions;
- Feingold syndrome (microcephaly, limb anomalies, oesophageal atresia, duodenal atresia, developmental delay);
- other atresias of the gastrointestinal tract;

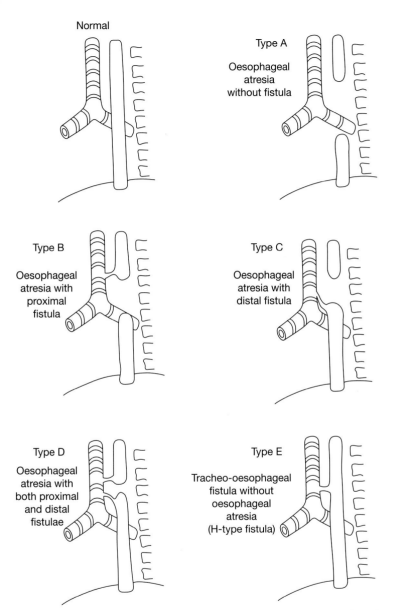

Figure 40.1 Anatomical variants of oesophageal atresia and tracheo-oesophageal fistula (posterior view). Type C is the most common anomaly, representing 85–90% of cases. Type A occurs in about 5–8%. Type E occurs in about 4%. Types B and D are rare, representing about 1% each. Note that in Type E there is no oesophageal atresia.

▶ VATER/VACTERL association (vertebral anomalies, anal atresia, cardiovascular anomalies, tracheo-oesophageal fistula, oesophageal atresia, renal and/or radial anomalies, limb defects); and
▶ CHARGE syndrome (coloboma, central nervous system abnormalities, congenital heart defects, choanal atresia, growth restriction, neurodevelopmental delay, genital and/or urinary tract abnormalities, ear and/or hearing defects).

There is also increased risk of preterm delivery and low birth weight.

The parents should be warned that there may be associated anomalies that are not able to be detected antenatally.

CONSEQUENCES

The prognosis is related to any co-morbidities or associated anomalies. A birth weight of <1500 g and congenital cardiac disease are independent predictors of morbidity and mortality. Infants born weighing >1500 g with no cardiac abnormality have >95% survival. Infants with either a cardiac abnormality or a birth weight of <1500 g have a 60–80% survival. Infants born weighing <1500 g with a cardiac anomaly have a 22–50% survival. Overall, those diagnosed antenatally have much higher mortality rates than those presenting postnatally.

MANAGEMENT—ANTENATAL

The antenatal diagnosis is based on the combined ultrasound findings of polyhydramnios and a small or absent stomach pouch/bubble. However, there are many false positives and false negatives. Fetal magnetic resonance imaging may be helpful to diagnose the associated anomalies, but generally does not help to confirm or exclude the oesophageal atresia. A H-type, or type E, fistula is very difficult to diagnose antenatally.

The antenatal management is basically that of polyhydramnios (see Chapter 12) and any associated anomalies. There is no specific treatment of the oesophageal atresia antenatally.

Delivery should occur in a maternity centre with a neonatal intensive care nursery that has full paediatric surgical support.

OTHER CONSULTS REQUIRED

Antenatal consultation with a paediatric cardiologist and a paediatric surgeon should be arranged. The cardiologist can perform a fetal echocardiogram, the results of which may dictate further management. Other consultations are arranged according to the other associated findings (e.g., nephrologist, geneticist).

MANAGEMENT—IMMEDIATE POSTNATAL

Delivery will be attended by a paediatric registrar and neonatal nurse. At delivery a large (8–10 FG) "orogastric" tube should be inserted. If an oesophageal atresia is present, resistance will be met at about 10 cm from the mouth. Smaller gauge tubes easily coil in the oesophageal pouch and should therefore be avoided.

The need for resuscitation and ventilation will be determined as for any baby; however if the baby requires mechanical ventilation, this should be done as gently as possible to minimise the chance of gastric over-distension (air readily gets into the stomach via any fistula). In general, intubation and ventilation should be avoided if possible.

The baby will be admitted to the intensive care nursery.

A chest and abdominal X-ray is done to confirm the placement of the tube. The presence of gas in the stomach confirms a distal tracheo-oesophageal fistula. Associated spinal skeletal anomalies may be evident on these films.

If oesophageal atresia is confirmed, the orogastric tube is removed and a Replogle tube placed in the upper oesophagus to permit continuous suction of saliva and secretions.

A peripheral intravenous cannula is inserted and maintenance fluids started. The paediatric surgical team should see the baby and begin planning for a repair. Some paediatric surgeons request an urgent echocardiogram to exclude associated cardiac defects and right-sided aortic arch prior to surgery. If surgery is going to be delayed, monitor electrolytes and fluid balance, although the fluid losses are not usually enough to cause significant electrolyte disturbance.

MANAGEMENT—POSTNATAL

Surgery is usually performed on day 1 or 2 of life, once the baby is stabilised. The likelihood of aspiration is increased if surgery is delayed.

In more than 80% of cases, primary anastomosis of the oesophagus and ligation of the fistula is achieved. Some may need a staged procedure involving the creation of a gastrostomy for feeding and waiting several weeks for the oesophagus to grow. Occasionally a neo-oesophagus is formed using segments of stomach, jejunum or colon. The latter situations are most likely to occur with a long gap atresia (>3–4 cm)—most likely to be seen in type A atresia (atresia without fistula).

The usual surgical approach is to make the incision in the right side of the chest and to leave a trans-anastomotic nasogastric tube in place for at least 5 days. Also, warn the parents that the baby may return from the surgery with a chest drain in place.

Most babies are successfully extubated within 24 hours of surgery if there are no associated morbidities. About 10% develop a pneumothorax post-operatively.

Broad spectrum antibiotics will usually be given for a few days, as directed by the surgical team.

Encourage the mother to begin expressing milk as soon after delivery as practical. The time to tube-feeding is determined by the surgical team but is generally within several days. An oesophageal contrast study may be performed about 5 days after surgery to check the integrity of the anastomosis, before suck feeds are started. The median length of stay in hospital is about 3 weeks.

Significant long-term complications are common—at least 50% in the first year. Almost all patients have a degree of gastro-oesophageal reflux. Other complications include:

▶ oesophageal dysmotility and dysphagia (40–50%);
▶ anastomotic strictures (30–50%);
▶ the need for tube feeding beyond three months of age (20%);
▶ scoliosis and chest wall deformity (20%; higher in those with skeletal abnormalities);
▶ anastomotic leaks (15–20%);
▶ tracheomalacia and/or bronchomalacia (10–20%); and
▶ recurrent fistula (10%).

RECURRENCE
While the recurrence rate of 1% is considered low, this is much higher than in the general population.

Further Reading

Achildi O, Grewal H. Congenital anomalies of the esophagus. *Otolaryngologic Clincs of North America.* 2007;40:219–244.

Castilloux J, Noble AJ, Faure C. Risk factors for short- and long-term morbidity in children with esophageal atresia. *The Journal of Pediatrics.* 2010;156:755–760.

de Jong EM, de Haan MAM, Gischler SJ, et al. Pre- and postnatal diagnosis and outcome of fetuses and neonates with esophageal atresia and tracheoesophageal fistula. *Prenatal Diagnosis.* 2010;30:274–279.

de Jong EM, Felix JF, de Klein A, et al. Etiology of esophageal atresia and tracheoesophageal fistula: "Mind the gap". *Curr Gastroenterol Rep.* 2010;12:215–222.

Holland AJA, Fitzgerald DA. Oesophageal atresia and tracheo-oesophageal fistula: current management strategies and complications. *Paediatric Respiratory Reviews.* 2010;11:100–107.

Kinottenbelt G, Skinner A, Seefelder C. Tracheo-oesophageal fistula (TOF) and oesophageal atresia (OA). *Best Practice and Research. Clinical Anaesthesiology.* 2010;24:387–401.

CHAPTER 41

Other Gut Atresias

Kelly M Dixon

A complete congenital occlusion of the bowel lumen is known as an atresia. Atresia of the gut can occur at any point along its length. Oesophageal atresia is discussed in Chapter 40.

Evidence of gut atresias can be seen on fetal ultrasound scans with dilation of the stomach or bowel (see Figure 41.1), or they may present with polyhydramnios.

Intestinal atresia is the most common cause of bowel obstruction in neonates. The ileum is the most commonly affected site.

Gut atresias are classified into four types:

▶ type 1—the lumen is obstructed by a diaphragm or membrane of mucosa and submucosa, there is no gap in bowel continuity;
▶ type 2—there is a gap in bowel continuity with the proximal and distal segments connected by short fibrous band;
▶ type 3—
  • 3A—there is a gap in bowel continuity without a connecting band, there is an associated gap in the mesentery,
  • 3B—there is a proximal small bowel atresia, with absence of the mid-small bowel that is normally supplied by the distal superior mesenteric artery, and a large gap in the small bowel mesentery (the small bowel distal to the atresia is shortened and coiled; it receives its blood supply from the ileocolic, right colic or inferior mesenteric artery); and
▶ type 4—multiple type 2 and type 3A atresias.

Anal atresia can occur in isolation or as part of more significant ano-rectal malformations. These may involve the genito-urinary tract.

EMBRYOLOGY

The foregut forms the mouth, pharynx, oesophagus, stomach and first third of the duodenum. The midgut forms the second two-thirds of the duodenum, small intestine, ascending colon and two-thirds of the transverse colon. The hindgut forms the distal third of the transverse colon, descending colon, rectum and anus.

In normal development, during weeks 6 and 7 of gestation, parts of the intestinal tract become occluded as the endodermal epithelium proliferates. Then during weeks eight to ten recanalisation of the gut lumen occurs.

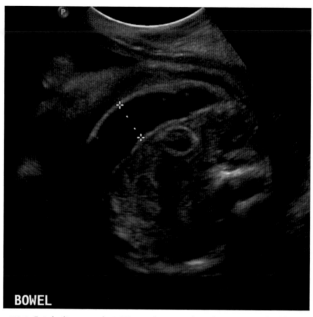

Figure 41.1 Fetal ultrasound at 32 weeks gestation shows a single dilated loop of bowel—the baby had a jejunal atresia.

Duodenal atresia results from failure of the normal recanalisation.

Jejunal and ileal atresia are acquired lesions thought to result from vascular disruption leading to ischaemic necrosis of the fetal intestine. Necrotic tissue is resorbed, leaving blind proximal and distal ends, often with a gap in the mesentery. The causes include segmental or midgut volvulus, intussusception, internal hernia and interruption of the segmental mesenteric blood supply. The risk is increased with maternal smoking and the use of vasoconstrictive drugs that interrupt mesenteric blood flow in the first trimester, including methylenedioxymethamphetamine, pseudoephedrine and ephedrine.

Type 3B may result from a volvulus of all or part of the midgut. Much of the gut supplied by the superior mesenteric artery disappears, leaving a high jejunal or distal duodenal atresia. The distal ileum winds around a thin vascular stalk, which usually consists of the left branch of the ileocolic artery. A large gap in the mesentery is present along with intestinal malrotation and a microcolon.

INCIDENCE
Ileal and jejunal atresia occurs in 1 in 1500–5000 births. Duodenal atresia occurs in 1 in 20,000–40,000 births. Atresia of the colon occurs in 1 in 40,000 births. Anorectal malformations occur in about 1 in 4000 births.

ASSOCIATED ABNORMALITIES
An atresia in any part of the gut increases the likelihood of an atresia in another part of the gut. Other associations include:
‣ about half of the cases of duodenal atresia have some other abnormality (e.g., heart, genitourinary tract, ano-rectal);
‣ Down syndrome—almost one-third (30%) of infants with duodenal atresia have Down syndrome;
‣ gastroschisis is often complicated by intestinal atresia;
‣ about half of the cases of anorectal malformation have some other abnormality (e.g., genitourinary tract (including fistulae), intestinal atresia, vertebral anomalies, central nervous system anomalies, VATER/VACTERL association);
‣ Hirschsprung disease; and
‣ inherited thrombophilia.

ANTENATAL PRESENTATION
The fetal ultrasound may show polyhydramnios, dilated stomach and/or bowel (a classic double bubble is seen in duodenal atresia, see Figure 41.2) or echogenic bowel wall. The more distal the obstruction, the later any dilated bowel is likely to be seen on ultrasound. The fetal abdomen can be distended and active peristalsis may be observed. If bowel perforation occurs, evidence of meconium peritonitis, including ascites, may be seen.

Proximal atresias are more likely than distal lesions to be detected prenatally. The more proximal the obstruction, the more likely the development of polyhydramnios. Polyhydramnios occurs in >50% of patients with duodenal atresia. Overall, 15–20% of cases of polyhydramnios are associated with fetal intestinal obstruction.

Lesions in the proximal jejunum result in more severe dilation of the proximal bowel due to continuing fetal swallowing of amniotic fluid which outpaces intestinal absorption.

Anal atresia can be diagnosed on fetal ultrasound, especially in the presence of a dilated rectum or distal colon. Cases of anal atresia without other significant abnormalities may not be diagnosed before birth.

The mother should be referred for a tertiary fetal ultrasound to look for other gut abnormalities, other structural anomalies and evidence of aneuploidy.

Testing for a fetal karyotype should be considered.

OTHER CONSULTS REQUIRED
Other specialists to be consulted are a paediatric surgeon and a paediatric cardiologist for fetal echocardiogram and counselling.

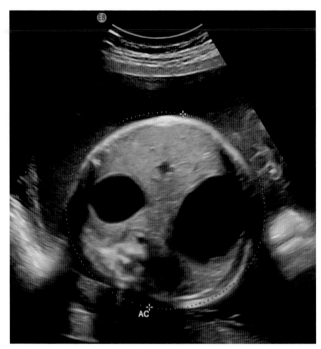

Figure 41.2 Fetal ultrasound at 34 weeks gestation shows the classic double bubble (dilated stomach and proximal duodenum) seen in duodenal atresia.

MANAGEMENT—POSTNATAL

The baby may require active resuscitation if there is significant abdominal distension and respiratory compromise. This may be complicated by large amounts of fluid from the stomach (this will be bile stained with any obstruction distal to the opening of the bile duct).

Any baby who has had evidence of gut obstruction on fetal ultrasounds should be treated as though they have a gut obstruction until it can be excluded. Initially the baby should not be fed, a nasogastric tube should be inserted and intravenous fluids started. The baby should be referred to a paediatric surgeon.

A physical examination should look for evidence of other congenital abnormalities, especially anal atresia and Down syndrome. The following investigations should be done:

▶ a plain abdominal X-ray;
▶ upper and/or lower gastrointestinal tract contrast study—depending on whether the obstruction is likely to be proximal or distal;

- echocardiogram;
- renal ultrasound scan;
- rectal biopsy to exclude Hirschsprung disease (this needs excluding in any case of a distal gut obstruction);
- cystic fibrosis gene testing and sweat test if there is an associated meconium ileus; and
- ultrasound and X-ray of the spine in cases of anal atresia.
    Surgical correction of the atresia will be necessary.

MANAGEMENT—SURGICAL
The nature of the surgery will depend on the specific site of the atresia. In most cases a simple end-to-end or end-to-back anastomosis can be done. The possibility of a second or multiple atresias should be excluded either by inspection at the time of surgery or with a subsequent gastrointestinal tract contrast study. If there are multiple atresias with short bowel segments between them it may be preferable to resect the entire section of involved bowel rather than perform multiple anastomoses.

After any small bowel resection, the length of remaining small bowel should be estimated. The absolute minimum length required is 30 cm of jejunum and ileum if the ileocaecal valve is intact. At least 75 cm remaining is preferred.

In small bowel atresia with gastroschisis a primary repair can be performed at the time of reduction of the bowel and closure of the abdominal wall, or surgical correction can be delayed until several weeks after repair of the gastroschisis. Alternatively, a stoma can be made at the time of abdominal wall repair and reanastomosed later.

In cases of colonic atresia, primary repair is possible, or exteriorise the proximal colon as a colostomy and defer anastomosis until the child is several months of age.

The extent of the surgery required for anal atresia will vary with the severity of the ano-rectal malformation. Low lesions may only require straightforward incision and anal dilatation. If there is a fistula then this will need excision and the anus repaired. High lesions will usually require a colostomy as soon as practicable after birth with more definitive surgery after a few months.

POSTOPERATIVE CARE
Intravenous fluids and a nasogastric tube will be required until bowel function returns. Total parenteral nutrition (TPN) is started once electrolyte balance is normalised and continued until full enteral feeding is established. A percutaneously inserted central venous line will be required for the parenteral nutrition. Most infants recover uneventfully following repair of intestinal atresia.

COMPLICATIONS
In some case the bowel proximal to the atresia will take a long time to recover. Sometimes a severely dilated segment does not recover. This may cause delayed emptying. Further surgery may be required.

Other complications include:

‣ short bowel syndrome;
‣ infection (if there is prolonged gut dysfunction and/or prolonged parenteral nutrition); and
‣ recurrent obstruction from anastomotic dysfunction, stricture and adhesions (these are likely to occur in complex atresias).

Anastomotic dysfunction complicates the recovery of infants with type 3B atresia who require prolonged parenteral nutrition.

PROGNOSIS

The prognosis in cases of atresia without other abnormalities is very good. Most mortality occurs in infants with medical conditions such as prematurity (especially with respiratory distress syndrome), associated anomalies or complications such as short gut syndrome.

The prognosis of complex atresias depends upon the length and function of the remaining bowel. The bowel function determines the required duration of parenteral nutrition with its associated risks of sepsis and cholestasis.

Patients at especially high risk for short bowel syndrome include those with type 4 atresias and gastroschisis.

Babies with a low anal atresia, with or without a fistula, have a good prognosis with minimal incontinence and/or constipation. High anal atresia has a worse prognosis; most children will have severe constipation and/or faecal incontinence.

RECURRENCE

Most cases of intestinal atresia are sporadic. Some familial cases of type 3B atresia have been reported. Multiple atresias also have been reported to recur in families.

Further Reading

1. Bales C, Liacouras C. Intestinal atresia, stenosis, and malrotation. In: Kliegman RM, Stanton BF, St Geme III JW, et al, eds. *Nelson Textbook of Pediatrics*. 19th ed. Philadelphia: Saunders Elsevier; 2011:322.
2. Brantberg A, Blaas HG, Haugen SE, et al. Imperforate anus: A relatively common anomaly rarely diagnosed prenatally. *Ultrasound in Obstetrics & Gynecology*. 2006; 28(7):904–910.
3. Hutson MH, O'Brien M, Woodward AA, et al, eds. Anorectal anomalies. In: *Jones' clinical paediatric surgery*. 6th ed. Carlton: Blackwell Publishing; 2008:61–65.
4. Vijayaraghavan SB, Prema AS, Suganyadevi P. Sonographic depiction of the fetal anus and its utility in the diagnosis of anorectal malformations. *Journal of Ultrasound in Medicine*. 2011;30(1):37–45.
5. Wesson DE. Intestinal atresia; 2011. Up To Date [web]. Accessed 5 August 2011. Available at <http://www.uptodate.com/contents/intestinal-atresia?source=search_result &selectedTitle=1%7E19>.

CHAPTER 42

Echogenic Bowel

Greg Duncombe, Peter G Davis

Echogenic (hyperechogenic) bowel is one of a number of so-called "soft markers" observed on ultrasounds during the second trimester (ultrasounds which are of progressively higher resolution). It falls into a group of findings that are associated with an increased risk of fetal abnormality, although most fetuses with these findings are normal. The most commonly accepted definition for echogenic bowel is an ultrasound appearance where the bowel is as bright as, or brighter than, the surrounding bone.

PREVALENCE
Echogenic bowel is reported to occur in about 1% of fetuses.

PATHOPHYSIOLOGY
The exact cause for the increased echogenicity of the bowel wall is unknown. It is thought to be due to an activation or stimulation of the fetal bowel lining and wall by irritants. Factors thought to lead to this hyperechogenicity include swallowed blood, fetal bowel obstruction or a reduction in gut motility, abnormal meconium, vasculitis or a viraemia-induced endocolitis. There may be an associated accumulation of meconium in the small bowel.

ASSOCIATED FINDINGS
The appearance of echogenic bowel may represent a normal variant. In the majority of cases isolated echogenic bowel is seen in an otherwise normal fetus. However, it is known to be associated with a number of important serious abnormalities and these are outlined below:

▶ chromosomal abnormalities:
  • most commonly trisomy 21 but trisomies 13 and 18, and sex chromosome abnormalities have been observed,
  • 1–2% of fetuses with echogenic bowel have trisomy 21—trisomy 21 is more likely if other structural abnormalities/significant markers are also seen (e.g., short femur/humerus, cardiac abnormalities, ventriculomegaly);

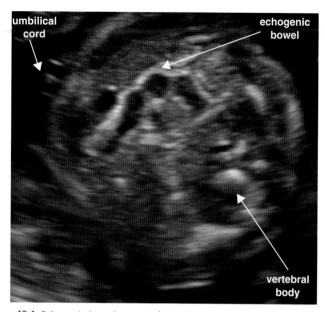

Figure 42.1 Echogenic bowel seen on fetal ultrasound at 20 weeks gestational age—the image shows a transverse section of the fetal abdomen.

▶ cystic fibrosis:
  • the risk varies with the population base (i.e., higher in northern Europeans);
▶ infection:
  • cytomegalovirus and toxoplasmosis are the most common (herpes zoster and parvovirus have also been reported),
  • 1–2% of infants with echogenic bowel have an *in utero* infection—other ultrasound signs should be looked for (e.g., microcephaly and periventricular calcification);
▶ gastrointestinal disorders:
  • the most common pathology is meconium ileus usually secondary to cystic fibrosis,
  • other primary bowel pathologies are usually accompanied by dilated bowel loops, polyhydramnios and/or fetal ascites; and
▶ fetal growth restriction:
  • 18% of fetuses with echogenic bowel develop *in utero* growth restriction,
  • growth restriction may accompany or follow the appearance of echogenic bowel.

MANAGEMENT—ANTENATAL

Antenatal management focuses on detecting or excluding known associated abnormalities. The following tests should therefore be considered:

▶ a detailed fetal ultrasound scan to assess for structural anomalies and fetal biometry;
▶ amniocentesis for fetal karyotype (with a sample kept for parallel assessment for cystic fibrosis after parental genotype/carrier status has been assessed);
▶ cystic fibrosis screening for the presence of the most common gene mutations;
▶ maternal serology for cytomegalovirus and toxoplasmosis; and
▶ serial fetal ultrasounds to assess growth and fetal well being (including Doppler analysis) and to check for the development of any other anatomical abnormalities (e.g., bowel obstruction).

If these tests are normal, newborn infants should be cared for in the usual manner. In these cases (i.e., the majority with echogenic bowel), parents should be reassured that there is no evidence of any serious long-term bowel or other pathology associated with this finding.

Further Reading

Hill LM, Fries J, Hecker J, et al. Second-trimester echogenic small bowel: an increased risk for adverse perinatal outcome. *Prenat Diagn.* 1994;14:845–850.

Patel Y, Boyd PA, Chamberlain P, et al. Follow-up of children with isolated fetal echogenic bowel with particular reference to bowel-related symptoms. *Prenat Diagn.* 2004;24:35–37.

Penna L, Bower S. Hyperechogenic bowel in the second trimester fetus: a review. *Prenat Diagn.* 2000;20:909–913.

Ruiza MJ, Thatcha KA, Fishera JC, et al. Neonatal outcomes associated with intestinal abnormalities diagnosed by fetal ultrasound. *J Pediatr Surg.* 2009;44:71–75.

CHAPTER 43

Developmental Kidney Disorders

Steven McTaggart, Dirk Bassler

Developmental malformations of the kidney can involve gross and/or microscopic anatomical abnormalities in renal structure that may be associated with abnormal renal function and urinary flow.

Antenatal diagnosis of these abnormalities usually relies on routine fetal ultrasound scans.

EPIDEMIOLOGY

Renal and urinary tract malformations occur in up to 2% of newborns, making up one of the largest groups of congenital anomalies. Lower urinary tract abnormalities represent about half of these conditions.

EMBRYOLOGY

Kidney development commences with the process of induction which involves an outgrowth of the mesonephric duct (the ureteric bud) invading the metanephric blastema. The ureteric bud forms the collecting duct, calyces, renal pelvis and ureter while the metanephric blastema forms the glomerulus, proximal and distal convoluted tubule and the loop of Henle.

The embryonic kidney has a lobulated appearance and ascends from its initial pelvic location to the lumbar region during the 6th–9th week. Fetal urine is produced from the 10th week and after 15 weeks approximately two-thirds of the amniotic fluid is produced by fetal urination and one third by the lungs.

An adequate volume of urine allows free movement of the fetus and is important for lung and skeletal development, although some reports suggest that abnormal lung dysplasia may precede the advent of oligohydramnios in fetuses with intrinsic defects of renal parenchymal development.[1]

Nephrogenesis finishes at 34 weeks gestation, signalling the end of kidney development.

The glomerular filtration rate is very low *in utero* but increases rapidly after birth. Serum creatinine within the first 48 hours of life reflects maternal rather than neonatal kidney function.

PATHOPHYSIOLOGY AND CONSEQUENCES
Disorders of Induction

1. Renal agenesis

   Unilateral renal agenesis occurs in 1 in 500–1000 newborns and has a generally excellent long-term prognosis. There may be associated congenital urinary tract abnormalities and ultrasound examination is therefore warranted.

   There are no specific recommendations for diet or restriction of activity throughout childhood. A blood pressure check and dipstick urinalysis is recommended every 1–2 years in adulthood.

   Bilateral renal agenesis (1 in 5000–10,000 newborns) is not compatible with life.

2. Duplex kidney

   Duplex kidneys are relatively common, occurring in about 1% of people.[2] Females are twice as likely as males to have a duplex kidney. They are bilateral in about 20%. It arises due to the development of two ureteric buds, and may result in a bifid ureter or complete duplication.

   Complex duplex systems may have vesicoureteric reflux into the lower moiety. The upper moiety is prone to obstruction, particularly if associated with an ureterocoele.

   For those with a simple duplex kidney (i.e., where there is no dilatation of either moiety and no evidence of obstruction or reflux), observation only is required.

3. Dysplasia/hypoplasia

   Dysplastic kidneys consist of areas of abnormal, malformed nephrons, often with coexistent cystic change (cystic dysplasia). Hypoplasia refers to a small kidney that has fewer nephrons than normal. Hypoplastic kidneys may have associated areas of dysplasia (hypodysplasia).

   Unilateral dysplasia is usually asymptomatic unless associated with other structural abnormalities such as vesicoureteric reflux or a duplex system.

   Bilateral renal dysplasia may also be asymptomatic but in severe cases may progress to kidney failure.

4. Multicystic dysplastic kidney (MCDK)

   Multicystic dysplastic kidney occurs in about 1 in 5000 newborns. It is a developmental anomaly in which the kidney is completely replaced by large fluid-filled cysts with no excretory function, and attached to an atretic or absent ureter.

   Vesicoureteric reflux commonly occurs in the contralateral kidney (about 20% of cases) but is often low grade and therefore a routine micturating cystourethrogram is not recommended. Pelviureteric junction obstruction has also been described in the contralateral kidney (7–15%) and should be looked for in infants with significant pelvicalyceal dilatation.

   Routine nephrectomy is not recommended as the majority of multicystic dysplastic kidneys undergo involution over about

9 months–10 years. The risk of hypertension is no higher than that of the general population and rates of malignant transformation of multicystic dysplastic kidneys are equivalent to or less than the risk in the general population.

Disorders of ascent

1. Ectopic kidney

   Kidneys that fail to ascend are most commonly located in the pelvis. Less commonly, kidneys may lie on the contralateral side (crossed ectopia) and may fuse with the normally located kidney (crossed fused ectopia).

   A number of urological abnormalities have been associated with renal ectopia, with vesicoureteric reflux the most common (seen in 20–30%). Ectopic kidneys may also be associated with dysplasia. Therefore an annual blood pressure check and dipstick urinalysis is recommended.

2. Horseshoe kidney

   Horseshoe kidney is relatively common (the incidence is 1 in 500) and occurs when there is fusion of lower poles of both kidneys during development. It is associated with Turner syndrome.

   In the majority, horseshoe kidney is asymptomatic but complications may include urinary tract infections, vesicoureteric reflux, renal calculi, haematuria and an increased risk of Wilms' tumour (in children) and transitional cell carcinoma (in adults).

Bladder abnormalities

1. Obstructive uropathy

   Obstructive uropathy is characterised by bladder distension and may be accompanied by a decrease in amniotic fluid volume. The obstruction can be complete or partial.

   In males it involves a spectrum of abnormalities from complete urethral atresia to a partially obstructing membrane in the membranous/prostatic urethra (posterior urethral valves).

   In females it indicates a complex urogenital malformation commonly grouped under the term "cloacal abnormality".

ASSOCIATED ABNORMALITIES

Up to 35% of patients with dysplastic kidneys may have extra-renal anomalies, especially of the heart, spine and extremities. Thirty to fifty per cent of kidneys contralateral to dysplastic kidneys are either structurally abnormal or affected by vesicoureteric reflux.

There are more than 100 syndromes described that are associated with renal and urinary tract malformations. Examples include:

▶ Turner syndrome (especially horseshoe kidneys);
▶ Potter syndrome;

▶ VATER/VACTERL association (vertebral anomalies, anal atresia, cardiovascular anomalies, tracheo-oesophageal fistula, oesophageal atresia, renal and/or radial anomalies, limb defects); and

▶ CHARGE syndrome (colobomata, heart defects, choanal atresia, retarded growth and/or development, genital hypoplasia, ear malformations).

In cases of bilateral renal disease or obstruction with decreased fetal urine output, oligohydramnios will result. With very low liquor volumes, or anhydramnios, pulmonary hypoplasia is a serious life-threatening consequence.

MANAGEMENT—ANTENATAL

In the majority of structural malformations, no specific antenatal management is required.

Following detection of antenatal renal tract dilatation, around 50% of postnatal scans will subsequently be normal.

Fetuses with ultrasound findings suggestive of obstructive uropathy and oligo-/anhydramnios can be considered for vesicoamniotic shunting. Although early intervention might prevent progressive renal deterioration or improve long-term renal outcomes,[3] vesicoamniotic shunting is also associated with a significant morbidity, perinatal mortality and shunt complications.[4]

An assessment of fetal kidney function is performed prior to shunting by examination of fetal urine obtained by aspiration of the fetal bladder. Favourable urinary parameters may be associated with reasonable long-term outcomes but their utility in accurately predicting kidney outcomes is generally low.

There is currently no evidence that preterm delivery leads to a better prognosis in cases of obstructive uropathy and renal dysplasia. Therefore, in the absence of other factors, preterm delivery should not be done to benefit the baby.

MANAGEMENT—LABOUR / DELIVERY / IMMEDIATE POSTNATAL MANAGEMENT

Where there is significant oligohydramnios or anhydramnios, delivery should be planned in a hospital that has an intensive care nursery and paediatric renal services. There are no specific requirements during labour and delivery.

If there is pulmonary hypoplasia, the baby will almost always require intubation and mechanical ventilation. They will need to be admitted to the intensive care nursery and require vascular access (usually umbilical lines). The mortality of pulmonary hypoplasia is high (>50%). Pneumothoraces are a common complication. The baby will usually require a prolonged duration of respiratory support.

If the lungs have developed normally, then intubation and mechanical ventilation will not usually be needed and resuscitation and immediate postnatal care should proceed as for any other baby.

For bilateral kidney abnormalities:

⏵ perform a renal ultrasound at about 48 hours of age;
⏵ check serum electrolytes, including creatinine, at 72 hours of age (note that severe kidney failure is rare in the neonatal period due to the physiological increase in glomerular filtration rate that occurs in the first few postnatal weeks).

For unilateral abnormalities, perform a renal ultrasound at 4–5 days of age.

Prophylactic antibiotics could be considered for significant structural abnormalities of the urinary tract although supportive evidence is currently lacking.

OTHER CONSULTS REQUIRED

Where there are complex structural abnormalities, refer to a paediatric nephrologist and, if surgical intervention is likely to be needed, a paediatric surgeon or urologist.

RECURRENCE

There is a 2–3% risk of recurrence of dysplasia unless it is associated with a genetically inherited syndrome. In siblings, consider a detailed antenatal morphology scan and/or postnatal ultrasound.

ETHICS

In babies with no recoverable renal function and pulmonary hypoplasia, it is often considered inappropriate to initiate life-sustaining measures, particularly in the presence of additional congenital abnormalities. The option of not providing these measures, if the infant is severely affected, should be discussed with the parents before delivery.

In those with life-threatening renal failure where there is little or no prospect of recovery, the place of dialysis (and renal transplantation) is often raised. Haemofiltration and haemodialysis are technically difficult and have a high risk of complications. Peritoneal dialysis is likewise technically difficult in small infants but may be feasible in some infants without other significant comorbidities. In many cases, dialysis is not considered a feasible option and the family may need to be counselled accordingly.

REFERENCES

1. Smith NP, Losty PD, Connell MG, et al. Abnormal lung development precedes oligohydramnios in a transgenic murine model of renal dysgenesis. *The Journal of Urology*. 2006;175:783–786.
2. Whitten SM, McHoney M, Wilcox DT, et al. Accuracy of antenatal fetal ultrasound in the diagnosis of duplex kidneys. *Ultrasound in Obstetrics and Gynecology*. 2003; 21:342–346.

3. Chevalier RL, Kim A, Thornhill BA, et al. Recovery following relief of unilateral ureteral obstruction in the neonatal rat. *Kidney International.* 1999;55(3):793–807.
4. Coplen DE. Prenatal intervention for hydronephrosis. *Journal of Urology.* 1997;157:2270–2277.

Further Reading

Rosenblum ND, Salomon R. Disorders of Kidney Formation. In: Geary DF, Schaefer F, eds. *Comprehensive Pediatric Nephrology.* Philadelphia: Elsevier; 2008:131–141.
Wiesel A, Queisser-Luft A, Clementi M, et al. EUROSCAN Study Group. Prenatal detection of congenital renal malformations by fetal ultrasonographic examination: an analysis of 709,030 births in 12 European countries. *European Journal of Medical Genetics.* 2005;48:131–144.

CHAPTER 44

Dilated Renal Pelvis

Garry DT Inglis

Dilatation of the fetal renal pelvis is detected on ultrasound at the time of a routine antenatal scan or when a scan is done at any other time for any reason. The kidneys are examined on antenatal ultrasound to detect those fetuses who may need postnatal treatment (including surgery) in order to minimise the risk of complications and to preserve or restore as much kidney function as possible.

DEFINITION
When the kidneys are examined routinely on antenatal ultrasound, the width of the renal pelvis is measured. The standard measurement is the anteroposterior diameter. Pelvicalyceal dilatation is present at the following thresholds:
- second trimester >6 mm;
- third trimester >10 mm; and
- postnatal >10 mm.

PREVALENCE
Pelvicalyceal dilatation is found in 1–5% of fetuses. Predominantly males are affected (male-to-female ratio is 2 : 1–3 : 1).

DIFFERENTIAL DIAGNOSIS
Given that the diagnosis of pelvicalyceal dilatation is based on a measurement, there is usually no doubt about the diagnosis—either it is dilated or it isn't. On the other hand, there are numerous possible underlying causes and these should be looked for, although in the vast majority it is an isolated finding. The likelihood of associated or underlying renal tract pathology is roughly proportional to the anteroposterior diameter.

The most common underlying pathology is obstruction to urine flow—usually pelvi-ureteric junction obstruction; occasionally urethral or bladder outlet obstruction (see Chapters 43 and 45).

Non-obstructive renal pathologies (see Chapter 43) include:
- vesico-ureteric reflux (the correlation with vesico-ureteric reflux is poor);
- renal duplication;
- renal agenesis; and
- dysplastic kidneys.

ASSOCIATED ABNORMALITIES

Associated anomalies are seen in about 10% of cases. These include hydrops, omphalocele, ventriculomegaly, cardiac anomalies and aneuploidy.

INVESTIGATIONS

If not already done, a thorough morphology scan should be done to check for the above associated abnormalities. Serial antenatal ultrasound scans to monitor progress may be warranted. If there is a suggestion of associated structural or obstructive pathology, then further imaging (e.g., MRI) may be arranged.

CONSEQUENCES

In the majority, it is an incidental finding (normal variant) which resolves spontaneously. A normal postnatal scan occurs in 75%. About 5% will require surgery; almost all of those requiring surgery will have a renal pelvis diameter of >15 mm.

Renal function is not related to degree of dilatation; loss of renal function is rare.

MANAGEMENT—ANTENATAL

Look for other evidence of renal tract dilatation, oligohydramnios or other anomalies.

If there is no evidence of obstruction or other significant pathology, then a suggested approach is:

▶ if dilated at <28 weeks, repeat the scan in the third trimester;
▶ if normal in the third trimester, no further investigation is needed; and
▶ if dilated in the third trimester, assess post-natally with a renal tract ultrasound.

MANAGEMENT—LABOUR / DELIVERY / IMMEDIATE POSTNATAL MANAGEMENT

There are no special precautions for labour and delivery. After delivery, the baby should have the following:

▶ physical examination on day 1 to check for grossly enlarged kidneys;
▶ observe for normal passage of urine (direct observation or wet nappies); and
▶ renal tract ultrasound—
  • day 1, if there was evidence of obstruction on the antenatal ultrasound,
  • day 3–7, if there was no evidence of obstruction.
  Antibiotic prophylaxis is controversial and falling out of favour.

If the postnatal scan is normal, and the renal pelvis anteroposterior diameter measures <10 mm, then no further investigation or treatment is required. If the postnatal scan is abnormal, refer to general paediatrician, renal physician and/or paediatric surgeon (depending on the specific findings) for ongoing management.

OTHER CONSULTS REQUIRED

If there is evidence of a problem that is likely to need surgery, then refer to a paediatric urologist antenatally for counselling. Genetic counselling is advised if there is evidence of aneuploidy or other abnormalities.

RECURRENCE

Most cases are sporadic; therefore, the risk of recurrence is very low.

Further Reading

Acton C, Pahuja M, Opie G, et al. A 5-year audit of 778 neonatal renal scans (Part 1): Perplexing pyelectasis and suggested protocol for investigation. *Australas Radiol.* 2003;47:349–353.

Chitty LS, Altman DG. Charts of fetal size: kidney and renal pelvis measurements. *Prenat Diagn.* 2003;23:891–897.

Cohen-Overbeek TE, Wijngaard-Boom P, Ursem NTC, et al. Mild renal pyelectasis in the second trimester: determination of cut-off levels for postnatal referral. *Ultrasound Obstet Gynecol.* 2005;25:378–383.

Gramellini D, Fieni S, Caforio E, et al. Diagnostic accuracy of fetal renal pelvis anteroposterior diameter as a predictor of significant postnatal nephrouropathy: Second versus third trimester of pregnancy. *Am J Obstet Gynecol.* 2006;194:167–173.

Ozcan Z, Anderson PJ, Gordon I. Prenatally diagnosed unilateral renal pelvic dilatation: a dynamic condition on ultrasound and diuretic renography. *J Urol.* 2004;172:1456–1459.

Wollenberg A, Neuhaus TJ, Willi UV, et al. Outcome of fetal renal pelvic dilatation diagnosed during the third trimester. *Ultrasound Obstet Gynecol.* 2005;25:483–488.

CHAPTER 45

Dilated Bladder

Lindsay Mildenhall, Roy Kimble

A dilated bladder can be seen on fetal ultrasound either as an isolated finding or in conjunction with dilatation of other parts of the renal collecting system.

DEFINITION OF DILATED BLADDER
In the first trimester, the bladder is considered dilated if the longitudinal diameter is >6 mm. If it is, there is an increased risk of chromosomal anomalies. A longitudinal diameter of >15 mm is associated with a poor prognosis.

In the second trimester, the bladder is considered dilated if there is a large bladder which fails to empty over 45 minutes.

EPIDEMIOLOGY
A dilated bladder is found in approximately 1 in 1831 pregnancies. About half of these cases resolve spontaneously.

DIFFERENTIAL DIAGNOSIS
The differential diagnosis includes:
▶ posterior urethral valves (PUV);
▶ urethral atresia/stenosis;
▶ prune belly syndrome (collecting system dilation, cryptorchidism and abnormal abdominal musculature);
▶ plunging ureterocele;
▶ megacystis-megaureter association (with vesico-ureteric reflux); and
▶ megacystis-microcolon syndrome.

The sex of the fetus should be determined and chromosome analysis done to exclude aneuploidy. The following should also be assessed at the time of fetal ultrasound:
▶ liquor volume (oligohydramnios);
▶ posterior urethral dilation (keyhole sign on ultrasound);
▶ thickness of bladder wall;
▶ patent urachus;
▶ ureteral dilation; and
▶ renal pelvic diameter.

SIGNIFICANCE
Posterior Urethral Valves
Posterior urethral valves occur in 1 in 5000–8000 male births. They are responsible for 25% of megacystis detected antenatally, although scans before 24 weeks gestational age may miss up to 92% of posterior urethral valves. The classic ultrasound sign is the keyhole sign caused by the appearance of a dilated posterior urethra. The overall mortality is 25–50% but this increases to >90% if there is oligohydramnios.

Urethral atresia or stenosis is the most common diagnosis when severe megacystis is seen in the first trimester. Of all the causes of megacystis urethral atresia has the worst prognosis.

Prune Belly Syndrome
Prune belly syndrome occurs in 1 in 30–50,000 live births. It occurs almost exclusively in males. In addition to the dilated bladder, bilateral hydroureters and hydronephrosis are seen. Prune belly syndrome is differentiated from posterior urethral valves on ultrasound because the **entire** urethra is dilated in prune belly syndrome.

Other
Ureteroceles usually cause upper collecting system dilation but they can plunge into the posterior urethra causing bladder outlet obstruction.

Megacystis-megaureter association occurs in the context of a dilated urinary tract, with high grade bilateral vesico-ureteric reflux and no obvious bladder neck or urethral obstruction.

Megacystis-microcolon syndrome is more common in females (F:M ratio of 4:1). There is a grossly dilated bladder and chronic intestinal obstruction. Incomplete intestinal rotation with microcolon is seen on contrast enema. Ultrasound evidence of megacystis and hydronephrosis helps distinguish microcolon from Hirschsprung disease. Megacystis-microcolon syndrome is very rare (only 70 cases have been described) and is generally fatal.

MANAGEMENT
A paediatric surgeon or urologist should be involved antenatally from the time of diagnosis.

Posterior Urethral Valves
Fetal karyotype is suggested. There is a worse prognosis with aneuploidy. If amniotic fluid index remains normal then no intervention is needed.

If >32 weeks gestational age and worsening oligohydramnios, consider delivery, urethral catheterisation and subsequent valve ablation.

If <32 weeks gestational age and there is worsening oligohydramnios then two approaches can be taken. The first is a non-operative expectant approach. The other approach is to assess renal function by serial bladder aspiration and urine analysis (hypotonic urine normal for fetus; isotonic urine and increased β2 microglobin levels are signs of poor renal function and poor prognosis). In the good prognostic group, vesico-amniotic shunting under ultrasound control can allow drainage of the fetal bladder and increase the amniotic fluid volume. Percutaneous fetal cystoscopy with direct visualisation and ablation of the posterior urethral valves has also been successfully performed in several centres. Both operative approaches are still considered experimental carrying a high incidence of fetal complications and morbidity in survivors. Results of current randomised controlled trials are awaited before these techniques can be recommended.

Long-term outcomes are dependent on renal function and continence. Continence is usually preserved by age 20 but up to 50% develop chronic renal failure.

Prune Belly Syndrome

Monitoring during pregnancy should focus on the degree of dilatation and amniotic fluid volume. A vesico-ureteric shunt may improve amniotic fluid status (see above).

Immediate postnatal assessment and management focuses initially on the respiratory status—intubation and mechanical ventilation are frequently required. Cardiac anomalies occur in 10% of cases; cardiology assessment and echocardiography is recommended. Ultrasound of the kidneys, ureters and bladder should be done. Orchidopexy and abdominoplasty will need to be considered. Urinary tract reconstruction including urethroplasty and ureteric re-implantations may be required. Chronic renal failure develops eventually in approximately 30% of cases.

LABOUR AND DELIVERY

Assuming that the baby will receive active resuscitation and treatment, the baby should be delivered in a centre with newborn intensive care and paediatric surgical care provided. Access to renal services is also required.

POSTNATAL CARE

Resuscitation with intubation and mechanical ventilation is often required, especially if there is oligohydramnios. The need for ongoing respiratory support is also common. Umbilical catheters will be required if the baby is unwell.

Once baby is stable, the investigations detailed above can be done to establish the cause of the dilated bladder. Any diagnosis made antenatally should be confirmed by postnatal investigation.

The paediatric surgeon or urologist should be notified as soon as the baby is born, if not before.

RECURRENCE

Posterior urethral valves have sporadic recurrence.

In the case of prune belly syndrome, polygenic or X-linked mechanisms have been postulated to explain the occurrence in siblings and the male predominance. However, it is generally accepted that the occurrence of prune belly syndrome is a sporadic event with low recurrence.

Further Reading

Lissauer D, Morris RK, Kilby MD. Fetal lower urinary tract obstruction. *Seminars In Fetal & Neonatal Medicine*. 2007 Dec;12(6):464–470.

Morris R, Malin G, Khan K, Kilby M. Systematic review of the effectiveness of antenatal intervention for the treatment of congenital lower urinary tract obstruction. *BJOG* 2010;117:382–390.

Woodward PJ, Kennedy A, Sohaey R, et al. *Diagnostic Imaging: Obstetrics*. Amirys; 2005.

Yiee J, Wilcox D. Abnormalities of the fetal bladder. *Seminars In Fetal & Neonatal Medicine*. 2008 Jun;13(3):164–170.

CHAPTER 46
Dandy-Walker Complex

Luke A Jardine

The Dandy-Walker complex refers to a spectrum of developmental anomalies of the brain that result from cystic dilatation of the fourth ventricle. It is often associated with dysgenesis or complete agenesis of the cerebellar vermis.

The most severe form is the Dandy-Walker malformation which is characterised by the presence of large posterior fossa cysts and severe atresia, or absence, of the cerebellar vermis. There may also be an elevated tentorium and dilatation of the third and lateral ventricles.

The Dandy-Walker variant is believed to be a less severe anomaly with mild hypoplasia of the cerebellar vermis, a small cystic cavity and normal sized posterior fossa (see Figure 46.1). Mega-cisterna magna is at the mildest end of the spectrum and consists of a large cisterna magna without cerebellar abnormalities.

PREVALENCE
The incidence of Dandy-Walker malformation is 1 in 30,000 births.[1]

DIFFERENTIAL DIAGNOSIS
The final development of the cerebellar vermis occurs somewhere between 16 and 29 weeks post-menstrual age. Care must therefore be taken to avoid a false early diagnosis of Dandy-Walker malformation.

Differentiation between the Dandy-Walker complex and an arachnoid cyst of the posterior fossa depends upon demonstration of a connection between the cyst with the fourth ventricle. Arachnoid cysts do not communicate with the fourth ventricle.

Joubert syndrome can normally be excluded by the absence of the "molar tooth" sign (a specific appearance of the cerebellar peduncles and vermis on magnetic resonance imaging).[2]

ASSOCIATED ABNORMALITIES
Hydrocephalus is frequently associated with Dandy-Walker malformation (55–96%); up to half of these cases may require shunting.

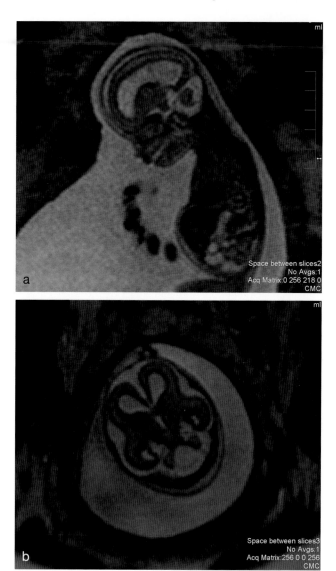

Figure 46.1 Fetal magnetic resonance imaging of the fetal brain with Dandy-Walker variant—a—sagittal view, b—transverse/coronal view.

Associated neurological disorders were seen in one-third of patients in one case series and included seizure disorders, cerebral palsy, hypotonia, progressive encephalopathy, autism, microcephaly and cortical blindness.[3] In the same series, 42% of patients had an associated cardiac abnormality, including patent ductus arteriosus, ventricular septal defect, atrial septal defect, hypoplastic right heart, transposition of the great vessels and mild pulmonary artery stenosis. Gastrointestinal anomalies were also observed in 21% of patients including congenital diaphragmatic hernia, malrotation of the gut, omphalocele, tracheo-oesophageal fistula and gastro-oesophageal reflux disease.

Numerous other associated abnormalities include:

▶ anal atresia;
▶ craniofacial anomalies (cleft palate, cleft lip, hypertelorism and Pierre Robin sequence with mandibular and maxillary hypoplasia);
▶ renal abnormalities (polycystic kidneys [Goldstrom syndrome] and renal agenesis);
▶ hypoplasia of the spleen;
▶ haemangioma;
▶ limb abnormalities; and
▶ syndactyly.

The following syndromes have also been associated with the Dandy-Walker complex:

▶ Pierre Robin sequence;
▶ Smith-Lemli-Opitz syndrome;
▶ Senior-Loken syndrome;
▶ Meknes syndrome;
▶ Coffin-Siris syndrome;
▶ Ehlers–Danlos syndrome; and
▶ neurocutaneous melanosis.

INVESTIGATIONS

It is essential that a tertiary level antenatal ultrasound scan be done to identify any other abnormalities. Fetal magnetic resonance imaging should also be considered to clarify the extent of the Dandy-Walker complex.

A fetal karyotype is recommended. Up to two-thirds of cases of Dandy-Walker malformation may have an associated chromosomal abnormality. Many different chromosomal abnormalities have been reported and including trisomy 13 and 18.

Rubella is a possible aetiological factor.

PROGNOSIS

Long-term outcome varies from normal to severe neurodevelopmental disability. The prognosis largely depends upon the degree of hydrocephalus and the presence of any associated abnormalities.

For mega cisterna magna with no associated abnormality, the outcome is essentially normal. Dror et al[4] reported a case series in which children with a large cisterna magna seen antenatally all had developmental scores in the normal range but had a significantly lower developmental quotient compared with non-affected patients.

Kolble et al[5] report that developmental delay was seen in half the patients in one case series with Dandy-Walker variant; half of those were severely affected.

Poor developmental outcome is reported in 55–100% of patients with Dandy-Walker malformation, depending upon the series. Approximately one-third of patients with Dandy-Walker malformation will have severe developmental delay.

Both fetal death and early childhood death have been reported.

MANAGEMENT—ANTENATAL

Given the severity of some cases, the option of providing comfort care following delivery should be discussed with the parents. Some parents may decide that advanced life support is not appropriate. Whatever course of action is decided upon, the plan for immediate postnatal management should be documented and known by staff attending the delivery. It may be appropriate to provide advanced life support whilst a definitive diagnosis is sought.

Delivery by caesarean section may be required where there is significant hydrocephalus and an enlarged head.

If significant abnormalities have been identified and active resuscitation and treatment is planned, delivery should be undertaken at a hospital that has an intensive care nursery.

For those cases with hydrocephalus, baby should be delivered at a hospital that has an intensive care nursery with paediatric neurosurgical services available.

POST DELIVERY

The baby should be examined carefully for other abnormalities. A cranial ultrasound scan should be arranged to check for the presence and degree of hydrocephalus and, if required, neurosurgical review should be arranged. If a shunt is required it will normally be done in the first few days of life.

A magnetic resonance imaging scan is recommended as it may identify other central nervous system abnormalities not previously identified.

Chromosomal studies should be undertaken if not already done antenatally. If a syndrome has been identified consider parental chromosomes looking for balanced translocation or mosaicism.

An ophthalmology assessment and auditory assessment should be undertaken prior to hospital discharge.

Long-term neurodevelopmental follow up will be required.

ETHICS

For severe cases, the options of termination of pregnancy or postnatal palliative care should be discussed with the parents, particularly if significant associated abnormalities have been identified.

RECURRENCE

Referral should be made to a genetic service to appropriately counsel parents about risk in subsequent pregnancies. Recurrence rate will depend upon the family history, environmental history, presence of chromosomal abnormalities and co-existing syndromes.

REFERENCES

1. Osenbach RK, Menezes AH. Diagnosis and management of the Dandy-Walker malformation: 30 years of experience. *Pediatric Neurosurgery.* 1992;18:179.
2. Maria BL, Bozorgmanesh A, Kimmel KN, et al. Quantitative assessment of brainstem development in Joubert syndrome and Dandy-Walker syndrome. *Journal of Child Neurology* 2001;16(10):751–758.
3. Sasaki-Adams D, Ababa SK, Jewells V, et al. The Dandy-Walker variant: a case series of 24 Pediatric patients and evaluation of associated anomalies, incidence of hydrocephalus, and developmental outcomes. *J Neurosurgery Pediatrics.* 2008; 2:194–199.
4. Dror R, Malinger G, Ben-Sira L, et al. Developmental outcome of children with enlargement of the cisterna magna identified *in utero*. *Journal of Child Neurology.* 2009;24(12):1486–1492.
5. Kolble N, Wisser J, Kurmanavicius J, et al. Dandy-Walker malformation: prenatal diagnosis and outcome. *Prenatal Diagnosis.* 2000;20:318–327.

Further Reading

Imataka G, Yamanouchi H, Arisaka O. Dandy–Walker syndrome and chromosomal abnormalities. *Congenital Anomalies.* 2007;47:113–118.

CHAPTER 47

Agenesis of the Corpus Callosum

Linda Mellick, Chris Burke, Pieter Koorts

Agenesis of the corpus callosum is a developmental cerebral anomaly in which the major commissure that joins the two cerebral hemispheres is partially or completely absent. Agenesis of the corpus callosum can occur as an isolated finding, in combination with other cerebral malformations or as part of a syndrome. The neurological sequelae are dependent upon the underlying aetiology and the presence of associated malformations.

PATHOGENESIS

The corpus callosum is the largest interhemispheric commissure, which forms between the 10th and 20th weeks of gestation. The corpus callosum develops in a rostral to caudal direction. Failure of the commissural axons to either develop or cross the midline accounts for the callosal defect. Agenesis of the corpus callosum can range in severity from complete to partial agenesis. In partial agenesis, the anterior portion of the corpus callosum (posterior genu and anterior body) is formed, but the posterior portion (posterior body and splenium) is not. The rostrum and the anterior/inferior genu are also not formed. Neuromediators, working with chemo-attractants and repellent proteins, guide the commissural axons and deficiencies can result in a failure of axonal guidance.

AETIOLOGY

The aetiology of agenesis of the corpus callosum is heterogenous. Agenesis can occur as an isolated condition or in combination with other cerebral abnormalities, often forming part of complex malformations. Associated malformations include the Arnold-Chiari malformation, Dandy-Walker syndrome, schizencephaly (clefts or deep divisions in the brain) and holoprosencephaly (failure of the forebrain to divide into lobes). Midline cysts or corpus callosum lipomas can also occur with agenesis of the corpus callosum.

Genetic causes of agenesis of the corpus callosum include chromosomal aneuploidy, Aicardi syndrome and the X-linked hydrocephalus spectrum. Aicardi syndrome is an X-linked dominant condition (lethal in males unless they have Klinefelter syndrome) which is characterised by the triad of infantile spasms, chorioretinal lacunae and agenesis of the corpus callosum. Aicardi syndrome is also associated with mental retardation, midline facial defects and a seizure disorder.

X-linked hydrocephalus, X-linked agenesis of the corpus callosum, MASA syndrome (mental retardation, aphasia, shuffling gait and adducted thumbs) and spastic paraparesis type 1 are all associated with mutations in the L1CAM gene (neural cell adhesion molecule L1) and are autosomal recessive in inheritance. X-linked lissencephaly with absent corpus callosum and ambiguous genitalia are caused by mutations in the ARX gene.

Other rare genetic causes include Andermann syndrome (autosomal recessive motorsensory neuropathy associated with developmental delay and mental retardation) and Mowat-Wilson syndrome (an autosomal dominant disorder caused by mutations in the zinc finger homeobox 1B [ZFHX1B] gene and characterised by agenesis of the corpus callosum, mental retardation, seizures, congenital heart disease, genitourinary anomalies and, although not a diagnostic criterion, Hirschsprung's disease).

Inborn errors of metabolism, including pyruvate dehydrogenase deficiency, nonketotic hyperglycinaemia, and maternal phenylketonuria have been reported to be associated with corpus callosum abnormalities. Other rare causes of agenesis of the corpus callosum include fetal alcohol syndrome and maternal drug ingestion.

No gene has as yet been identified for isolated agenesis of the corpus callosum.

PREVALENCE

A Californian study[1] reported that the combined prevalence of complete and partial agenesis of the corpus callosum was 1.8 in 10,000 live births from the period 1983–2003. However, other research has estimated a prevalence of 3–7 in 1000 in the general population. These figures correlate with the prevalence of agenesis of the corpus callosum on prenatal ultrasound at around 0.5–1.0 in 100.

Risk factors for agenesis of the corpus callosum noted in the Californian study include:

▶ male sex (52% of cases are male);
▶ prematurity (a four-fold increase); and
▶ advanced maternal age (≥40 years) especially associated with agenesis of the corpus callosum in the context of a chromosomal disorder.

Clinical associations with agenesis of the corpus callosum include other central nervous system malformations (50%), chromosomal abnormalities (17%), musculoskeletal defects (34%) and cardiac malformations (28%). There was no association with paternal age.

PROGNOSIS OF AGENESIS OF THE CORPUS CALLOSUM

The prognosis depends on the extent and severity of the callosal agenesis and any associated malformations. The reported neurodevelopmental outcome of patients who have isolated agenesis of the corpus callosum is that 55% develop normally, 25% have a moderate disability and 20% have a severe disability.

A prenatal diagnosis of isolated agenesis of the corpus callosum may not warrant a recommendation for termination of pregnancy, due to the variability in clinical presentation. Children with agenesis of the corpus callosum can be of average intelligence, but neuropsychological testing may reveal subtle differences in higher cortical function compared to individuals of the same age and education without agenesis of the corpus callosum. If associated with other cerebral malformations or a syndrome, many patients will have developmental delay, intellectual disability, neurological deficits and a seizure disorder.

MANAGEMENT—ANTENATAL
Antenatal ultrasound is reliable for the diagnosis of agenesis of the corpus callosum after the 20th week of gestation. The posterior horn of the lateral ventricle appears dilated, giving the ventricle a "tear drop" appearance.

A prenatal cerebral fetal magnetic resonance imaging (MRI) scan may be helpful in detecting other cerebral malformations.

Fetal karyotype and genetic testing should be considered.

In isolated agenesis of the corpus callosum, parental counselling is based on the prognosis (i.e., 55% normal, 25% moderate disability and 20% severe disability).

MANAGEMENT—LABOUR / DELIVERY / IMMEDIATE POSTNATAL
Babies with isolated agenesis of the corpus collosum will rarely require any additional support once born.

Babies with associated anomalies and severe central nervous system involvement may require airway and breathing support.

Generally, supportive care should be provided. Any seizures will require symptomatic management.

All babies should have a brain MRI. Other postnatal investigations to consider include a metabolic screen, chromosomal analysis and blood glucose monitoring as clinically indicated.

OTHER CONSULTS REQUIRED
Consultations to consider include:
- paediatric neurologist or neurosurgeon depending on the type of malformation;
- metabolic consultation to exclude an underlying metabolic disorder;
- physiotherapy/speech therapy; and
- ophthalmology review.

LONG-TERM FOLLOW-UP
Neurodevelopmental follow-up may be all that is required. Paediatric subspecialty follow-up may be required as determined by the nature of the lesion and clinical presentation. Neuropsychological assessment may be necessary along with cognitive assessment at school age.

ETHICS

For severe cases, the options of termination of pregnancy or postnatal palliative care should be discussed with the parents, particularly if significant associated abnormalities have been identified.

RECURRENCE

The recurrence risk of agenesis of the corpus callosum depends on the aetiology. In agenesis of the corpus callosum associated with chromosomal aneuploidy, the recurrence risk is 1% or the maternal-age related risk for aneuploidy, whichever is greater. Isolated agenesis of the corpus callosum with no known cause is usually sporadic and the recurrence risk is very low. In familial cases, the recurrence risk is approximately 2–3%.

REFERENCE

1. Glass HC, Shaw GM, Ma C, et al. Agenesis of the corpus callosum in California 1983–2003: a population-based study. *Am J Med Genet A.* 2008 Oct 1;146A(19):2495–2500.

Further Reading

Andermann E. Agenesis of the Corpus Callosum. In: Vinken PJ, & Bruyn GW, eds. *Handbook of clinical neurology.* Vol 42. Amsterdam: Elsevier/North Holland Biomedical Press; 1981:6–9.

Bedeschi MD, Bonaglia MC, Grasso R, et al. Agenesis of the Corpus Callosum: Clinical and Genetic study of 63 young patients. *Pediatr Neurol.* 2006;34:186–193.

Blum A, André M, Droulle P, et al. Prenatal diagnosis of the corpus callosum agenesis. The Nancy experience 1982–1989. *Genetic Counseling.* 1990; 38:115–126.

Caddie A. Neurodevelopmental outcome in prenatally diagnosed isolated agenesis of the corpus callosum. *Acta Paediatr.* 2008;97(4):420–424.

Dobyns WB. Absence makes the search grow longer. *Am J Hum Genet.* 1996:58:7–16.

Gupta JK, Lilford RJ. Assessment and management of fetal agenesis of the corpus callosum. *Prenat Diagn.* 1995;15:301–312.

Jeret JS, Seur D, Wisniewski K, Fisch C. Frequency of agenesis of the corpus callosum in the developmentally disabled population as determined by computerised tomography. *Paediatr Neurosci.* 1985–86;12:101–103.

Moutard M-L. Isolated Corpus callosum agenesis. Orphanet Encyclopedia [Internet]. 2001. [Updated September 2003; cited 26 May 2011]. Available from: <http://www.orpha.net/data/patho/Pro/en/IsolatedCorpusCallosumAgenesis-FRenPro447.pdf>.

National Institute of Neurological Disorders and Stroke. Agenesis of the Corpus Callosum Information Page. [Internet]. [updated 7 February 2011; cited 26 May 2011]. Available from: <http://www.ninds.nih.gov/disorders/agenesis/agenesis.htm>.

Nissenkorn A, Michelson M, Ben-Zeev B, et al. Inborn errors of metabolism. A cause of abnormal brain development. *Neurology.* 2001;56:1265–1272.

Sztriha L. Spectrum of corpus callosum agenesis. *Pediatr Neurol.* 2005;32:94–101

Young ID. Genetics of neurodevelopmental abnormalities. In: Levene MI, Lilford RJ, Bennet MJ, et al, eds. *Fetal and Neonatal Neurology and Neurosurgery.* London: Curchill Livingstone; 1995:256.

CHAPTER 48

Ventriculomegaly

Luke A Jardine

Enlargement of the cerebral ventricles can be seen on fetal ultrasound scans from about 14 weeks gestational age. See Figure 48.1. Ventriculomegaly is diagnosed when the width of the atrium of the lateral ventricle is ≥10 mm (which is ≥4 SD above the mean of 7.6 ±5 mm) regardless of gestation.[1]

The degree of enlargement is classified as:

▶ mild—10–12 mm;
▶ moderate—12.1–15 mm; or
▶ severe—>15 mm.[2]

The measurements should be made in the transverse diameter of the lateral ventricle on an axial plane, at the level of the glomus of the choroid plexus.[3]

PREVALENCE
Ventriculomegaly is the most frequently seen fetal brain anomaly. It occurs in approximately 1–22 in 1000 live births.[4]

DIFFERENTIAL DIAGNOSIS
Isolated ventriculomegaly is characterised by the absence of any associated anomalies. The aetiology is generally unknown. It occurs in 0.39–0.87 in 1000 births. The following causes should be considered in the differential diagnosis:

▶ aqueduct of Sylvius stenosis;
▶ foramen of Monro stenosis;
▶ central nervous system tumours (including arachnoid, choroid plexus and posterior fossa cysts);
▶ chromosomal abnormalities (trisomy 13, 18, 21; unbalanced translocation, aneuploidy, triploidy);
▶ infection (including cytomegalovirus, toxoplasmosis, herpes, mumps, enterovirus, human T-lymphotropic virus type 3, parainfluenza virus type 3, rubella, varicella, parvovirus, human immunodeficiency virus (HIV), leishmaniasis);
▶ intraventricular haemorrhage;
▶ holoprosencephaly;
▶ porencephaly;
▶ hydranencephaly; and
▶ X-linked hydrocephalus.

ASSOCIATED ABNORMALITIES
Other abnormalities can be found in 10–76% of cases.[5] The rate of associated abnormalities is often underestimated by fetal ultrasound and

fetal magnetic resonance imaging (MRI). Approximately 10% of cases may not be recognised until after birth.[5]

Associated neurological abnormalities include:

- agenesis of the corpus callosum;
- Chiari malformation;
- Dandy-Walker malformation;
- neuromigrational disorders (e.g., lissencephaly, schizencephaly, septo-optic dysplasia);
- neuronal proliferation disorders (e.g., megalencephaly, microcephaly);
- neural tube defects;
- cerebellar hypoplasia; and
- third ventricle enlargement.

Many chromosomal abnormalities have been reported in association with ventriculomegaly including trisomy, unbalanced translocations, aneuploidy and triploidy.

Syndromes in which ventriculomegaly is associated include:

- Apert syndrome;
- Miller-Dieker syndrome;
- Smith-Lemli-Opitz syndrome;
- Walker-Warburg syndrome;
- Seckel syndrome;
- Cornelia de Lange syndrome;
- Weaver syndrome;
- Neu-Laxova syndrome;
- Aicardi syndrome;
- Acrocallosal syndrome;
- VATER/VACTERL association (vertebral anomalies, anal atresia, cardiovascular anomalies, tracheo-oesophageal fistula, oesophageal atresia, renal and/or radial anomalies, limb defects); and
- CHARGE syndrome (coloboma, central nervous system abnormalities, congenital heart defects, choanal atresia, growth restriction, neurodevelopmental delay, genital and/or urinary tract abnormalities, ear and/or hearing defects).

The following anomalies have also been reported in association with ventriculomegaly:

- cardiac anomalies include coarctation of the aorta, ventriculo-septal defect, atrio-septal defect, double outlet right ventricle and hypoplastic left heart syndrome;[6]
- surgical anomalies include congenital diaphragmatic hernia, intestinal atresia, omphalocele and gastroschisis;[6]
- genitourinary anomalies include ambiguous genitalia, hypospadias, undescended testes, renal dysplasia, renal agenesis, autosomal recessive polycystic kidney disease and bladder exstrophy;[6]
- vertebral malformations;
- limb anomalies including polydactyly, talipes;

- craniosynostosis; and
- facial cleft.[6]

INVESTIGATIONS

A thorough tertiary level antenatal ultrasound scan should be done to identify the possibility of other abnormalities. Fetal magnetic resonance imaging (MRI) should also be considered.

Maternal serology should be done to test for evidence of infections (including cytomegalovirus, toxoplasmosis, herpes, parvovirus, human immunodeficiency virus [HIV]).

Fetal karyotype is recommended.

PROGNOSIS

Not all fetuses will survive to delivery as there is an increased chance of intra-uterine fetal death during pregnancy and delivery (10% for moderately severe ventriculomegaly and 25% for severe).[5]

The prognosis is ultimately determined by the primary aetiology and the presence of associated abnormalities. If the ventriculomegaly is isolated, the chance of normal neurodevelopmental outcome is as follows[2,7,8]

- 90–95% if mild;
- 80–84% if moderate; and
- 10–60% if severe.

The following developmental abnormalities have been reported: gross motor delay, intellectual impairment, hypotonia, cerebral palsy, speech delay, neonatal seizures, visual impairment including nystagmus, visual field defects and blindness and hearing impairment.

Below is a list of factors which may influence prognosis:

- unilateral dilatation appears to have a better prognosis;
- asymmetrical bilateral dilatation (>2 mm difference) in one study was associated with a worse outcome—50% had neurological impairment;[2]
- prenatal progression (increase of >3 mm) is associated with a worse outcome;[2] and
- the presence of associated white matter abnormalities significantly increases the risk of adverse outcome.[7]

MANAGEMENT—ANTENATAL

The options of termination of pregnancy or postnatal palliative care should be discussed with the parents, particularly if significant associated abnormalities have been identified.

If there is significant hydrocephalus, consider elective caesarean section. In view of increased incidence of fetal death, if active management is requested, pregnancy should not be allowed to go post-term.

If there is macrocephaly with severe ventriculomegaly, the ventricles can be drained before delivery. This may decrease the likelihood of a traumatic caesarean section,[9] but will significantly increase the risk of fetal demise.

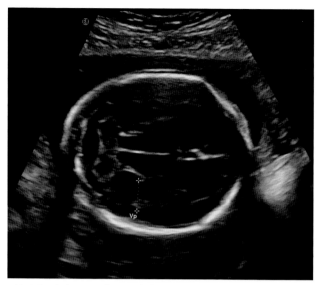

Figure 48.1 Fetal ultrasound scan of the brain at 22 weeks gestational age—the callipers show the width of the atrium of the lateral ventricle which is 11 mm.

If significant abnormalities have been identified and active management is warranted, then delivery should occur at a hospital with an intensive care nursery.

MANAGEMENT—POSTNATAL

The baby should be closely examined for other abnormalities.

A cranial ultrasound scan should be done to establish the degree of ventriculomegaly. If required, neurosurgical review should be arranged.

A magnetic resonance imaging (MRI) scan should be considered to identify other central nervous system abnormalities not previously identified.

Chromosomal studies should be done (if they have not been done antenatally). If a syndrome has been identified, consider parental chromosomes looking for balanced translocation or mosaicism.

A full blood count and film examination is done to determine the platelet count. If the platelet count is low, the parents may need testing the for alloimmune thrombocytopaenia.

Coagulation studies should be done if intraventricular haemorrhage is considered a possible cause.

An ophthalmology assessment and an auditory assessment should be done before hospital discharge.

Long-term neurodevelopmental follow-up by a paediatrician will be required.

RECURRENCE

Referral should be made to a genetic service to appropriately counsel parents about risk in subsequent pregnancies. The recurrence rate will depend upon the family history, environmental history, presence of chromosomal abnormalities and co-existing syndromes. If the hydrocephalus is X-linked then there is a 50% recurrence rate in males.

If the ventriculomegaly is isolated, then the recurrence rate is approximately 4%.

REFERENCES

1. Cardoza JD, Goldstein RB, Filly RA. Exclusion of fetal ventriculomegaly with a single measurement: the width of the lateral ventricular atrium. *Radiology.* 1988;169: 711–714.
2. Gaglioti P, Danelon D, Bontempo S, et al. Fetal cerebral ventriculomegaly: outcome in 176 cases. *Ultrasound in Obstetrics and Gynecology.* 2005;25(4):372–377.
3. ISUOG Guidelines. Sonographic examination of the fetal central nervous system: guidelines for performing the "basic examination" and the "fetal neurosonogram". *Ultrasound Obstetric Gynaecology.* 2007;29:109–116.
4. Ouahba J, Luton D, Vuillard E, et al. Prenatal isolated mild ventriculomegaly: outcome in 167 cases. *BJOG: An International Journal of Obstetrics & Gynaecology.* 2006;113(9):1072–1079.
5. Gaglioti P, Oberto M, Todros T. The significance of fetal ventriculomegaly: etiology, short- and long-term outcomes. *Prenatal Diagnosis.* 2009;29:381–388.
6. Wax JR, Bookman L, Cartin A, et al. Mild Fetal Cerebral Ventriculomegaly: Diagnosis, Clinical Associations, and Outcomes. *Obstetrical and Gynaecological Survey.* 2003;58(6):407–427.
7. Falip C, Blanc N, Maes E, et al. Postnatal clinical and imaging follow-up of infants with prenatal isolated mild ventriculomegaly: a series of 101 cases. *Pediatric Radiology.* 2007;37:981–989.
8. Breeze CG, Alexander PMA, Murdoch EM, et al. Obstetric and neonatal outcomes in severe fetal ventriculomegaly. *Prenatal Diagnosis.* 2007;27:124–129.
9. Kennelly MM, Cooley SM, McParland PJ. Natural history of apparently isolated severe fetal ventriculomegaly: perinatal survival and neurodevelopmental outcome. *Prenatal Diagnosis.* 2009; 29:1135–1140.

CHAPTER 49

Neural Tube Defects

Lisa Copeland, Leisha Callaghan, David Millar, Pieter J Koorts

Neural tube defect is a general term used for the heterogeneous group of disorders of the central nervous system that occur secondary to failure of closure of the neural tube during fetal development (this process should be complete by 23–26 days). Neural tube defects include anencephaly, encephalocoeles, cranial meningocoeles and spinal dysraphism (spina bifida).

Anencephaly results in absence of a major proportion of the brain, skull and scalp—it is uniformly fatal.

An encephalocoele is caused by herniation of the brain and/or meninges through the skull (cranium bifidum). It is the least common form of neural tube defect. Frequently, other malformations occur along with encephalocoele. These are frequently associated with recognised syndromes such as Meckel Gruber syndrome. Hydrocephalus and brain malformations are typically seen associated with encephalocoeles.

Spinal dysraphism or spina bifida encompasses several disorders including:

▶ meningocoele—protrusion of the meninges through a vertebral defect;
▶ myelomeningocoele—protrusion of the spinal cord and meninges through a vertebral defect;
▶ lipo(myelo)meningocoele—a meningocoele or myelomeningocoele that is covered by a deposit of fatty tissue; and
▶ spina bifida occulta—vertebral lesion without protrusion of meninges.

Approximately 80% of cases of spinal dysraphism occur in the lumbar region.

The diagnosis is usually made on antenatal ultrasound scans (see Figure 49.1).

AETIOLOGY / PATHOPHYSIOLOGY / EMBRYOLOGY

The exact causal mechanism for neural tube defects is incompletely understood. However, both genetic and environmental factors have been shown to be important.

Two randomised controlled studies[1,2] established the definitive role of folic acid in the prevention of neural tube defects. Adequate folic acid intake (diet or tablet) is recommended for women planning to become pregnant and in early pregnancy. Folic acid is now added to wheat flour for making bread in Australia. The biological mechanism for reduction of neural tube defect associated with folic acid supplementation remains unknown.

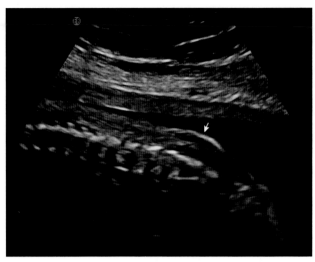

Figure 49.1 Fetal ultrasound at 25 weeks gestational age showing a large lumbosacral meningomyelocoele (arrowed). The upper level of the lesion is at L1.

Gene studies have not elucidated a single gene defect causative of neural tube defects, but there is a definite increased risk in siblings and this is higher in twins. Research is ongoing regarding potential associated genetic enzyme defects.

PREVALENCE

The average prevalence of neural tube defects is 1 in 1000 births, with marked geographical variation. The incidence of neural tube defects is approximately equally divided between spina bifidas and anencephaly/encephalocoeles. The true incidence of neural tube defects is difficult to determine as there is a high rate of spontaneous first trimester abortion and an increasing rate of termination of pregnancy with antenatal diagnosis.

Risk factors include:

▶ genetic risk—there is a higher risk in Australian Aboriginal populations, and a higher risk with a previously affected child (or family history);
▶ chromosomal disorders (e.g., trisomy 18);
▶ valproic acid, folate antagonists (methotrexate, aminopterin) and vitamin A;
▶ maternal diabetes;
▶ maternal obesity; and
▶ maternal hyperthermia.

ASSOCIATED ABNORMALITIES—SPINA BIFIDA

Spina bifida is a complex condition with variable severity dependent upon the type of spina bifida and the level of the lesion. Hydrocephalus is an often associated feature (up to 90%).

The Chiari type 2 malformation occurs in over 90% of cases of myelomeningocoele. The hallmark of the lesion is herniation of the cerebellar vermis and brain stem into the cervical spine. The Chiari type 2 malformation typically presents with hydrocephalus.

Talipes, hip dysplasia and other bony formation anomalies may be seen (particularly affecting the lower limbs). This tends to be associated with the limitation in fetal movement. Scoliosis associated with bony fusion defects may also occur, especially with higher level defects.

There is a higher incidence of renal formation anomalies in children with spina bifida compared to the general population.

CONSEQUENCES

The prognosis of long-term functional outcomes can be considered by the type and level of the lesion (in spina bifida) as well as the presence and severity of the Chiari type 2 malformation.

Children with myelomeningocoeles have increased neurological disability compared with those with meningocoeles. The higher the level of the lesion the worse the functional disability is likely to be.

Children with higher lesions are more likely to have the Chiari type 2 malformation compared with those with lower lesions. Infants with the Chiari type 2 malformation typically present with hydrocephalus. Other signs and symptoms of the Chiari type 2 malformation are stridor, apnoea, bradycardia, facial palsy, a weak high pitched cry, swallowing difficulties and poor feeding, nasal regurgitation, recurrent bouts of aspiration pneumonitis and learning and behavioural difficulties.

Neurogenic bladder and bowel should be expected in all cases of myelomeningocoele; however the presentation is variable.

Scoliosis may become a problem in later life.

Just under half of young adults with spina bifida walk the majority of the time. Many children however will require a wheelchair. The level of the defect has a direct bearing on the ability to walk (with or without aids). Determining the functional level of lesion after birth is important for prognostication. The functional level of lesion does not always correlate with antenatal ultrasound findings making accurate prognosis of ambulatory ability difficult before the baby is born.

Children with thoracic level lesions tend to have lower limb paralysis and therefore are dependent upon a wheelchair for mobility. Children with high lumbar lesions (L1–L3) have capacity for hip flexion with limited knee extension (L3). These children may achieve some capacity for upright mobility with the use of orthotic devices and walking aids. Children with low lumbar lesions (L3–L5) have strong hip flexion with knee extension.

Children with low-lumbar lesions are more likely to achieve independent ambulation using ankle-foot orthoses with many continuing to walk as the primary form of mobility in adulthood. Children with sacral level lesions tend to walk well but may continue to have problems with rocker bottom feet or pes cavus.

Almost all children with spina bifida without hydrocephalus have normal intelligence and cognitive function. Some children with the Chiari type 2 malformation and hydrocephalus may have a degree of cognitive impairment, which can include intellectual impairment, or other more specific difficulties, including issues with executive functioning. Factors which influence this include the presence of a shunt, the number of shunt revisions and infections and associated brain malformations, as well as the level of the lesion.

In children with encephalocoele the site of the lesion and the volume of tissue involved, as well as associated anomalies, affects prognosis. The outcomes vary from favourable to severe developmental disability.

MANAGEMENT—ANTENATAL

The rate of prenatal diagnosis approaches 90% in developed countries with dedicated screening programs. Antenatal management includes counselling for parents regarding potential outcomes and options. Improved ultrasound techniques and fetal magnetic resonance imaging (MRI) have allowed for better determination of the level of lesion and this allows for more accurate antenatal counselling (see Figure 49.2). We recommend counselling from paediatric rehabilitation and neurosurgical teams.

Some centres outside of Australia have advocated fetal repair with lower rates of hydrocephalus postnatally. However, the risk to the mother and infant is higher; a randomised study is currently underway to assess risk versus benefit.

MANAGEMENT—LABOUR

Delivery is preferable at a tertiary centre that has an intensive care nursery and paediatric neurosurgical services. Delivery by caesarean section is usually encouraged; however this is controversial as there is limited supporting evidence. The need for caesarean section is more definite in cases of known hydrocephalus and breech presentations.

MANAGEMENT—IMMEDIATE POSTNATAL CARE
Meningocoeles and Myelomeningocoeles

Exposed tissue should be wrapped with sterile saline soaked material to avoid drying with the neonate nursed in the prone position.

Prophylactic antibiotics are usually used to prevent ventriculitis if delay in closure of neural placode expected.

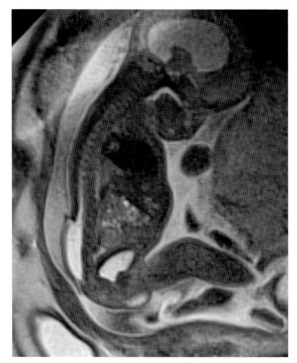

Figure 49.2 Fetal magnetic resonance imaging (MRI) of the same fetus at the same gestation as shown in Figure 49.1.

Surgical closure of the defect within the first 24–72 hours is usually recommended. This does not reverse the neurological dysfunction but prevents infection of the placode which may lead to ventriculitis and meningitis.

Magnetic resonance imaging (MRI) of the brain and spine is typically performed to confirm the level of the lesion and the presence of the Chiari type 2 malformation (it may be done pre or post neural placode closure).

Avoid latex exposure as these infants are exposed to multiple surgical interventions during their lifetime and this often leads to a latex allergy.

Hydrocephalus

A ventriculo-peritoneal shunt may be inserted at time of spinal closure in cases of overt hydrocephalus. Otherwise, management of hydrocephalus is expectant with daily measurement of the head circumference and monitoring for other signs and symptoms of the Chiari type 2 malformation. Those looking after the infant with spina bifida must be aware to observe for signs of hydrocephalus and raised intracranial pressure.

Renal
Renal management should include the involvement of the spina bifida team. Neurogenic bladder should be expected. Urine output should be monitored as urinary retention is commonly seen (especially immediately post neural placode closure). The use of indwelling or clean intermittent catheterisation (latex free) may therefore be needed during this period.

A renal ultrasound is suggested at about 5 days after surgery as a baseline measure. A repeat renal ultrasound, a DMSA (dimercaptosuccinic acid radionucleotide) scan and a micturating cysto-urethrogram (MCU) are recommended at 6 weeks of age. These investigations are performed to detect signs of a high pressure bladder. Video-urodynamic studies may also be used to detect a high pressure system.

Bowel
A neurogenic bowel should be expected. Constipation is common and this may require early initiation of laxatives and/or enemas.

Orthopaedic
The initial clinical examination should include checking for developmental dysplasia of the hips and talipes. Orthopaedic surgeons should be involved if required.

Physiotherapists skilled in the care of children with spina bifida should be involved early. They will assist in the orthopaedic management and skin care. Manual muscle testing will detail the level of the lesion.

Ongoing surveillance for scoliosis is essential.

MANAGEMENT—LONG TERM
Spina bifida is a complex condition with potential effects on many organ systems. As such, coordinated, long-term multidisciplinary medical care is required. This should involve:

- a general paediatrician or a paediatric rehabilitation specialist with a special interest in the care of children with spina bifida;
- a paediatric neurosurgeon;
- a paediatric urologist;
- a paediatric orthopaedic surgeon with special interest in the care of children with spina bifida; and
- physiotherapists, occupational therapists, speech therapists, dieticians, social workers and neuropsychologists.

The paediatric team responsible for ongoing care of the baby should optimally review the baby prior to discharge from hospital.

RECURRENCE

The risk of spina bifida in siblings of affected individuals is 3–4%. This risk nearly triples with each subsequent affected pregnancy. The recurrence risk of neural tube defect is 4.5% with one parent affected and 30% with both parents affected.

ETHICS

Recommendations during antenatal counselling should be based upon known outcomes dependent on the level of the lesion (myelomeningocoele) or the position and extent of the lesion (encephalocoele). As anencephaly is usually fatal, the recommendations are more straightforward.

Consideration of the parents' wishes, and ensuring they are fully informed, is important. Some parents choose termination of pregnancy if given the option early enough.

It is considered that all children born with a neural tube defect should be offered treatment.

REFERENCES

1. MRC Vitamin Study Research Group. Prevention of neural tube defects: results of the Medical Research Council vitamin study. *Lancet*. 1991;338:131–137.
2. Czeizel AE, Dudas I. Prevention of the first occurrence of neural-tube defects by periconceptional vitamin supplementation. *N Engl J Med*. 1992;327:1832–1835.

Further Reading

Boyd PA, Devigan C, Khoshnood B, et al. Survey of prenatal screening policies in Europe for structural malformations and chromosome anomalies, and their impact on detection and termination rates for neural tube defects and Down's syndrome. *BJOG: In J Obstet Gynaecol*. 2008;115(6):689–696.

Cameron M, Moran P. Prenatal screening and diagnosis of neural tube defects. *Prenatal Diagnosis*. 2009;29:402–411.

Fletcher JM, Copeland K, Frederick JA, et al. Spinal lesion level in spina bifida: a source of neural and cognitive heterogeneity. *J Neurosurg (Pediatrics 3)*. 2005;102:268–279.

Iddon JL, Morgan DJ, Loveday C, et al. Neuropsychological profile of young adults with spina bifida with or without hydrocephalus. *J Neurol Neurosurg Psychiatry*. 2004;75:1112–1118.

Josan V, Morokoff A, Maixner W. Ch 4. Epidemiology and Aetiological Factors. In: Ozek MM, Cinalli G, Maixner W, eds. *Spina Bifida*. Milan: Springer; 2008:59–65.

Niazi T, Walker ML. Myelomeningocele and Medical Ethics. In: Ozek MM, Cinalli G, Maixner W, eds. *Spina Bifida*. Milan: Springer; 2008:67–71.

Nussbaum RL, McInnes RR, Willard HF. Genetics of disorders with complex inheritance. In: *Thompson and Thompson Genetics in Medicine*. 6th ed. Philadelphia(PA): WB Saunders; 2001:289.

Thompson D. Postnatal management and outcome for neural tube defects including spina bifida and encephalocoeles. *Prenat Diagn*. 2009;29:412–419.

Food Standards Australia New Zealand. Addition of vitamins and minerals to food. Canberra, ACT: FSANZ; 2010 [accessed 12 September 2011]. Available at: <http://www.foodstandards.gov.au/consumerinformation/fortification/>.

CHAPTER 50

Cerebellar Hypoplasia

Kate Sinclair, Mark Davies

Cerebellar hypoplasia is a neurological condition where the cerebellum has a small volume. This is distinct from cerebellar atrophy where there is evidence of tissue loss after formation. Cerebellar hypoplasia can involve the whole cerebellum, the vermis or, rarely, one hemisphere. It can be acquired or inherited. It can be found alone (i.e., isolated) or as part of a syndrome or more complex malformation.

The normal cerebellum continues to develop beyond term. The diagnosis of cerebellar hypoplasia requires accurate assessment of gestational age. It is difficult to determine whether the cerebellum is pathologically small before 18–20 weeks gestation. Despite detailed fetal magnetic resonance imaging (MRI) showing cerebellar hypoplasia, especially vermian hypoplasia, the cerebellar development may be normal. Conversely, neonates with normal antenatal scans have been shown to have cerebellar abnormalities on postnatal imaging. For these reasons, as well as the fact there are often hidden syndromic associations and unknown biochemical defects, predicting outcome for infants with an antenatal diagnosis of cerebellar hypoplasia is difficult.

The definitive diagnosis will usually not be possible until after the baby is born.

PREVALENCE

There are no firm prevalence figures. Total cerebellar agenesis is extremely rare.

Isolated sporadic cerebellar hypoplasia is found in about 5% of children with developmental delay.

Hypoplasia of the cerebellar vermis is more common than hemispheric hypoplasia.

Focal or unilateral hemispheric hypoplasia is usually related to ischaemia, haemorrhage or infection (e.g., rubella, parvovirus, cytomegalovirus).

DIFFERENTIAL DIAGNOSIS

The differential diagnosis includes cerebellar atrophy. This can only be diagnosed with certainty if a normally grown cerebellum has been seen on previous scans. Clues to the diagnosis of cerebellar atrophy are enlarging cerebellar fissures and intervening sulci; there may be gliosis. This appearance suggests a progressive process as seen in the cerebellums of patients with congenital disorders of glycosylation type 1 (CDG1), ataxia telangiectasia and infantile neuraxonal dystrophy.

ASSOCIATED ABNORMALITIES

Cerebellar hypoplasia can be associated with the following:

▶ hypoplasia of the brainstem (particularly the ventral pons) with cerebellar hypoplasia is known as pontocerebellar hypoplasia;

▶ vermian hypoplasia can be part of the Dandy-Walker malformation when the hypoplastic vermis is accompanied by an enlarged 4th ventricle and elevation of the tentorium;

▶ congenital muscular dystrophies such as:
  • Walker–Warburg syndrome, or
  • muscle-eye-brain disease;

▶ lissencephaly—a heterogeneous group of usually autosomal recessive conditions known as lissencephaly with cerebellar hypoplasia (LCH);

▶ aneuploidy—e.g., Down syndrome, Edwards syndrome, Patau syndrome; and

▶ other rare associated abnormalities including:
  • quadripedal locomotion—a rare familial condition where cerebellar hypoplasia is associated with four-legged ambulation linked to chromosome 17p,
  • microcephaly,
  • pancreatic agenesis,
  • opthalmoplegia,
  • pancytopaenia,
  • pachygyria endosteal osteosis.

INVESTIGATIONS

If cerebellar hypoplasia is diagnosed on fetal ultrasound, fetal magnetic resonance imaging (MRI) should be done after 18 weeks gestation. This should include 3D reconstruction of the cerebellum. Detailed imaging should look for any other supratentorial malformation, hypomyelination or other central nervous system (CNS) anomalies and non-CNS abnormalities. Serial imaging may be useful.

A fetal karyotype should be considered if there are other abnormalities.

If the antenatal findings suggest a specific syndrome or there is an informative family history then specific genetic tests can be done (e.g., muscle-eye-brain disease, lissencephaly with cerebellar hypoplasia, pontocerebellar hypoplasia). However, usually the results are only available after the baby is born so it is often better to decide which tests to do once the full phenotype can be evaluated post-delivery.

If there is focal cerebellar hypoplasia then consider screening for thrombophilia and congenital infections.

CONSEQUENCES

The consequences of cerebellar hypoplasia are variable; from benign to devastating.

Isolated cerebellar hypoplasia is usually non-progressive and the severity of its effects is dependent on the degree of hypoplasia. If development is affected, it commonly includes speech delay, autistic features, ataxia, hypotonia and nystagmus or strabismus.

With isolated inferior vermian hypoplasia, the long-term prognosis is unclear. Most of the cases diagnosed antenatally will have normal development; the remainder can have developmental delay or behavioural problems.

Babies with pontocerebellar hypoplasia (PCH) often have a severe progressive phenotype such as:

▶ pontocerebellar hypoplasia type 1 with degeneration of the anterior horn cells gives mainly profound muscular weakness;
▶ pontocerebellar hypoplasia type 2 with microcephaly, severe feeding difficulties, psychomotor delay and dyskinesia;
▶ congenital disorders of glycosylation type 1 with developmental delay, parkinsonism and ataxia; and
▶ progressive encephalopathy, hypsarrhythmia and optic atrophy (PEHO).

MANAGEMENT—ANTENATAL

The investigations, as above, should initially focus on determining the severity and extent of the cerebellar hypoplasia and other brain abnormalities.

Evaluation by a multidisciplinary team which should include a radiologist, maternal fetal medicine specialist, paediatric neurologist, neonatologist and geneticist is recommended.

The parents should be warned about the significant uncertainty associated with the diagnosis of cerebellar hypoplasia. Many babies who have cerebellar hypoplasia diagnosed antenatally will have normal postnatal scans. Regardless of the ultimate outcome, the diagnosis of cerebellar hypoplasia during the pregnancy has been shown to be extremely stressful for families.

MANAGEMENT—POSTNATAL

Delivery should be planned in a hospital with an intensive care nursery. Resuscitation should proceed as for any baby but the need for intubation and mechanical ventilation increases with increasing severity of the brain abnormalities and other associated abnormalities.

Investigations should include:

▶ magnetic resonance imaging (MRI) of the brain;
▶ evaluation for possible inborn errors of metabolism;
▶ genetic testing as suggested by the specific abnormalities and phenotype; and
▶ screening for thrombophilia and congenital infections in cases of focal cerebellar hypoplasia.

Skin or muscle biopsies may be needed in some cases of pontocerebellar hypoplasia (these are always best done antemortem).

If the antenatal abnormalities are confirmed with postnatal imaging, the baby should be referred to a paediatric neurologist. Long-term follow up will be required by a general and/or developmental paediatrician.

RECURRENCE

This is entirely dependent on family history, associated anomalies and genetic abnormalities. The parents of all cases should have genetic counselling before any subsequent pregnancies.

Further Reading

Barth PG. Pontocerebellar hypoplasia—how many types? *European Journal of Paediatric Neurology*. 2000;4(4):161–162.

Bolduc ME, Limperopoulos C. Neurodevelopmental outcomes in children with cerebellar malformations: a systematic review. *Developmental Medicine & Child Neurology*. 2009;51(4):256–267.

Limperopoulos C, du Plessis AJ. Disorders of cerebellar growth and development. *Current Opinion in Pediatrics*. 2006;18(6):621–627.

Limperopoulos C, Robertson RL, Estroff JA, et al. Diagnosis of inferior vermian hypoplasia by fetal magnetic resonance imaging: potential pitfalls and neurodevelopmental outcome. *American Journal of Obstetrics & Gynecology*. 2006;194(4):1070–1076.

Malinger G, Lev D, Lerman-Sagie T. The fetal cerebellum. Pitfalls in diagnosis and management. *Prenat Diagn*. 2009;29:372–380.

Millen KJ, Gleeson JG. Cerebellar development and disease. *Current Opinion in Neurobiology*. 2008;18(1):12–19.

Poretti A, Prayer D, Boltshauser E. Morphological spectrum of prenatal cerebellar disruptions. *European Journal of Paediatric Neurology*. 2009; 13(5):397–407.

Triulzi F, Parazzini C, Righini A. Magnetic resonance imaging of fetal cerebellar development. *Cerebellum*. 2006;5(3):199–205.

Section 14
Musculoskeletal Problems

CHAPTER 51
Skeletal Dysplasias

Angelika Zankl, Andreas Zankl

Skeletal dysplasias are a group of genetic disorders affecting skeletal development that occur in 1 in 3000–5000 births. More than 400 different skeletal dysplasias are currently recognised. Skeletal dysplasias are usually detected on routine fetal ultrasound scans (preliminary findings may include short limbs, a small or abnormally shaped thorax and/or bones that are short, deformed or missing).

MANAGEMENT—ANTENATAL

Prenatal diagnosis is difficult and requires significant expertise. Whenever possible, an experienced clinical geneticist should be involved. Despite this, it is rarely possible to make a firm clinical diagnosis antenatally and genetic testing options are limited in the prenatal setting.

Assessment of a fetus who is thought to have a skeletal dysplasia should include a determination of whether the skeletal dysplasia is likely to be lethal, either prenatally or in the newborn period. Lethality is usually thought to occur as a result of a small chest circumference and restricted fetal breathing movements—both limit lung growth and cause pulmonary hypoplasia. However, not all babies with skeletal dysplasias with a small thoracic circumference will die immediately after birth.

A chest-to-abdominal circumference ratio of <0.6[1] and a femur length-to-abdominal circumference ratio of <0.16[2] are strongly suggestive of a lethal skeletal dysplasia. Concomitant abnormalities in other organ systems increase morbidity and mortality in these disorders.

Common lethal skeletal dysplasias include osteogenesis imperfecta type 2, thanatophoric dysplasia, achondrogenesis, campomelic dysplasia and short-rib-polydactyly syndrome.

The paragraphs below outline the management for presumed lethal and non-lethal skeletal dysplasias, respectively. However, as outlined above, lethality cannot be predicted with 100% accuracy and this will need to be taken into account when counselling parents.

The family should be referred to a geneticist for genetic counselling as soon as it is known that the fetus has or may have a skeletal dysplasia.

MANAGEMENT OF PATIENTS WITH PRESUMED LETHAL SKELETAL DYSPLASIAS

Counsel the parents about the poor prognosis. The options for management include termination of the pregnancy or continuing. The option of not continuing the pregnancy should be discussed with the obstetric team and the parents. If the pregnancy is allowed to continue, the fetus may die spontaneously *in utero* or be born alive. Discuss with the parents the level of life support to be provided if the infant is born alive. The plans for management immediately after birth should be documented and communicated to the neonatal staff.

Discuss the need for a detailed autopsy. Often only autopsy results can confirm a diagnosis, which is vital for counselling the parents about the recurrence risk in future pregnancies.

If the baby is born alive and the parents do not wish advanced life support, provide comfort care and limit life support as previously agreed upon with parents. This may involve the palliative care team to provide ongoing support for the family. A sample of blood should be collected (e.g., cord blood)—2–5 mL of blood in an EDTA tube—and sent for DNA extraction and storage.

Following the death of either the fetus or the baby, a complete autopsy should be done. This should include:

- a whole body X-ray, or 'babygram';
- clinical photography;
- histology of the bone growth plates; and
- storage of DNA—take a skin biopsy for fibroblast culture and storage.

MANAGEMENT OF PATIENTS WITH PRESUMED NON-LETHAL SKELETAL DYSPLASIAS

Counsel the parents on the likely clinical presentation based on the fetal ultrasound findings and presumed diagnosis. More detail is shown below for the two most common conditions: achondroplasia (see Box 51.1) and osteogenesis imperfecta (see Box 51.2).

Delivery should be planned in a hospital with an intensive care nursery if the fetal ultrasound findings suggest possible complications in the postnatal period (e.g., a small thoracic circumference, associated malformations).

Once the baby is delivered:

- a sample of blood should be collected (e.g., cord blood)—2–5 mL of blood in an EDTA tube—and sent for DNA extraction and storage; and
- arrange a whole body X-ray, or 'babygram'.

Box 51.1 ACHONDROPLASIA

Achondroplasia is the most common form of short-limb dwarfism. It is a single gene disorder with an autosomal dominant mode of inheritance, caused by mutations in the fibroblast growth factor receptor-3 (FGFR3) gene on chromosome 4.[3] The birth prevalence is 1 in 25,000.[4]

Antenatal findings

The disproportionately short limbs typically only become evident after 22 weeks gestation. Other signs include widening of the distal femur, frontal bossing and relative macrocephaly when compared to femur length.

Management of labour and delivery

There are no specific complications to be expected during labour and delivery; however, vaginal delivery may not be readily accomplished due to the relative macrocephaly. In general, there is no need for a referral to a tertiary neonatal care centre.

Postnatal management

Clinical findings include:[5]

- skeletal findings
  - rhizomelic (proximal) and acromelic (hands) limb shortening,
  - trident fingers,
  - large head with prominent forehead,
  - depressed nasal bridge and a flat midface,
  - long narrow trunk,
  - narrow foramen magnum with cervicomedullary junction obstruction,
  - kyphotic deformity of the thoracolumbar junction;
- hypotonia;
- obstructive sleep apnoea; and
- hydrocephalus.

The differential diagnosis includes thanatophoric dysplasia, SADDAN syndrome (severe achondroplasia with developmental delay and acanthosis nigricans), hypochondroplasia and spondyloepiphyseal dysplasia congenita.

In contrast to most other bone dysplasias, genetic testing for achondroplasia is available in most major hospitals. It is relatively inexpensive and has a short turn-around time. It can be done antenatally on a chorionic villous sample or with a postnatal blood test.

The immediate postnatal management focuses on confirming the diagnosis and assessing the newborn for common complications of achondroplasia. A skeletal survey (including an antero-posterior and lateral babygram as well as separate hand films) should be arranged and reviewed by a clinician with expertise in skeletal dysplasias.

Care should be taken in plotting the newborn's measurements (head circumference, length and weight) on achondroplasia-specific growth charts.[6]

All newborns with achondroplasia should have:

- assessment by a paediatric neurologist for symptoms of cervicomedullary junction compression;
- magnetic resonance imaging (MRI) of the brain and cervical spine before discharge;[7]
- polysomnography—this is strongly recommended as infants with achondroplasia are at risk for central sleep apnoea (cervico-medullary junction compression) as well as obstructive sleep apnoea (narrow airways and abnormal skull configuration);[8] and
- referral to a geneticist for genetic counselling before discharge.

Anticipatory guidance

Plot growth on achondroplasia-specific growth charts.

The parents should avoid carrying a child with achondroplasia in curled-up positions and unsupported sitting should be discouraged to avoid the development of a fixed thoracic kyphosis.[9]

Regular audiometric and tympanometric assessments help detect hearing loss early.

Parents and the medical team should be made aware of the anaesthetic risks related to the cervical spine stenosis.

Children with achondroplasia have delayed motor development and possible language related problems, but have an overall normal cognitive development.[10]

Box 51.2   OSTEOGENESIS IMPERFECTA

Osteogenesis imperfecta (OI) is a genetic disorder characterised by increased bone fragility.[11] The disease is caused by abnormalities of type 1 collagen, which is a major constituent of the extracellular matrix of bone. It is traditionally subdivided into four types:[12]

- type 1—the mildest form, is characterised by relatively few fractures and blue sclerae;
- type 2—the most severe form, is almost uniformly lethal;
- type 3—the progressive deforming type, presents with multiple fractures and deformities; and
- type 4—is similar to type 1, with the exception of the characteristic blue sclerae.

All forms of osteogenesis imperfecta can present with prenatal or perinatal fractures.[12]

Approximately 90–95% of cases of osteogenesis imperfecta are caused by mutations in the COL1A1 or COL1A2 genes, which code for the alpha-1 and alpha-2 fibrils that form type 1 collagen.[13] Mutations in either of these genes result in abnormal type 1 collagen. Mutations in COL1A1 and

COL1A2 are usually dominant. Approximately 5–10% of cases of osteogenesis imperfecta are caused by mutations in other genes (LEPRE1, CRTAP, PPIB, FKBP65, SERPINH1, OSX).[14–16] These usually cause a severe form of osteogenesis imperfecta and have an autosomal recessive mode of inheritance.

The incidence of osteogenesis imperfecta is 1 in 30,000 births.

Antenatal findings
Depending on the type of osteogenesis imperfecta, antenatal findings can include decreased echogenicity of all bones, shortening and bowing of long bones, thorax deformities and a thin skull.

The antenatal diagnosis of osteogenesis imperfecta is mainly based on the ultrasonographic findings described above. Genetic testing is commercially available, but not always feasible in the short timeframes required for prenatal diagnosis. Biochemical analysis of collagen synthesis on a chorionic villous sample is quicker but less sensitive and less specific than genetic testing.

Management of labour and delivery
If a severe but nonlethal form of osteogenesis imperfecta is suspected, delivery should be planned in a hospital with an intensive care nursery. The mode of delivery should be based on obstetric considerations and maternal risks; caesarean section does not seem to decrease the risk of fractures.[17]

Postnatal findings
Osteogenesis imperfecta type 1:
- baby is usually average size;
- fractures; and
- blue sclerae.

    Osteogenesis imperfecta type 2:
- small for gestational age;
- large head with minimal or no calvarian mineralisation;
- multiple Wormian bones;
- short and bowed limbs;
- long bone fractures, poor mineralisation;
- small narrow thorax;
- short ribs with possible callus formation from antenatal fractures;
- platyspondyly; and
- fetal death or death in the perinatal period is common, 60% are stillborn, 80% die by 1 month of age.[18]

    Osteogenesis imperfecta type 3:
- skeletal findings similar to type II but milder;
- short stature;
- large head with multiple Wormian bones;
- large anterior fontanelle;
- triangular face shape with bossed, broad forehead;
- tapered, pointed chin;

- long bone fractures, poor mineralisation;
- short and bowed limbs; and
- small narrow thorax.

The differential diagnosis includes different types of osteogenesis imperfecta, thanatophoric dysplasia, infantile hypophosphatasia, campomelic dysplasia.

Postnatal management

A postnatal skeletal survey to identify possible fractures should be done. Fractures can be managed with standard methods.

Pushing, pulling or lifting the infant by the extremities and under the axilla should be avoided. When lifting a newborn with osteogenesis imperfecta one hand should be placed under the head, the other hand under the thorax and buttocks—the goal is an even and wide distribution of pressure on the body. Patting on the back for burping is not recommended. Positions should be changed frequently to prevent cranial deformity.

If the child has limb or spine deformities, the orthopeadic surgeon should be involved. The family should be provided with a letter stating the diagnosis to avoid possible unnecessary concerns about child abuse.

Genetic counselling

The risk of recurrence of osteogenesis imperfecta in future pregnancies is usually low if the parents are unaffected. However there is wide clinical variability and some parents may only be mildly affected. Also, 5–10% of osteogenesis imperfecta, especially severe forms, have an autosomal recessive mode of inheritance with a 25% recurrence risk in future pregnancies. Referral to a clinical geneticist is recommended.

Anticipatory guidance

Ideally, patients with osteogenesis imperfecta should be managed by a multidisciplinary team. Treatment with bisphosphonates in conjunction with specialised nursing, physiotherapy and occupational therapy reduces fracture frequency and significantly improves the quality of life.

Despite this, many patients will require assist devices to stand or walk. Swimming should be encouraged.[19]

It is advisable to refer infants with osteogenesis imperfecta to an orthopaedic specialist for review of possible development of kypho-scoliosis, positional torticollis and hip abduction contractures; these may need surgical intervention.

An endocrinologist should be involved for the consideration of treatment with growth hormone and bisphosphonates.[20,21] Regular audiology and orthodontic assessments should be planned.[22] Pain management should maximise non-pharmacological methods. Intelligence and language development are unaffected and life expectancy is normal in the mild to moderate forms of osteogenesis imperfecta.

REFERENCES

1. Yoshimura S, Masuzaki H, Gotoh H, et al. Ultrasonographic prediction of lethal pulmonary hypoplasia: comparison of eight different ultrasonographic parameters. *Am J Obstet Gynecol.* 1996;175(2):477–483.

2. Rahemtullah A, McGillivray B, Wilson RD. Suspected skeletal dysplasias: femur length to abdominal circumference ratio can be used in ultrasono graphic prediction of fetal outcome. *Am J Obstet Gyneco.* 1997; 177(4):864–869.

3. Shiang R, Thompson LM, Zhu YZ, et al. Mutations in the transmembrane domain of FGFR3 cause the most common genetic form of dwarfism, achondroplasia. *Cell.* 1994;78(2):335–551.

4. Orioli IM, Castilla EE, Scarano G, et al. Effect of paternal age in achondroplasia, thanatophoric dysplasia, and osteogenesis imperfecta. *Am J Med Genet.* 1995;59(2):209–217.

5. Cassidy SB, Allanson JE. *Management of Genetic Syndromes*, 2nd ed. Hoboken: Wiley and Sons; 2005.

6. Horton WA, Rotter JI, Rimoin DL, et al. Standard Growth Curves for achondroplasia. *J Pediatr.* 1978;93(3):435–438.

7. Pauli RM, Horton VK, Glinski LP, et al. Prospective assessment of risks for cervicomedullary-junction compression in infants with achondroplasia. *Am J Hum Genet.* 1995;56(3):732–744.

8. Sisk EA, Heatley DG, Borowski BJ, et al. Obstructive sleep apnea in children with achondroplasia: surgical and anesthetic considerations. *Otolaryngol Head Neck Surg.* 1999;120(2):248–254.

9. Pauli RM, Breed A, Horton VK, et al. Prevention of fixed, angular kyphosis in achondroplasia. *J of Pediatr Orthopedics.* 1997;17(6):726–733.

10. Ireland PJ, Johnson S, Donaghey S, et al. Developmental milestones in infants and young Australasian children with achondroplasia. *Journal of developmental and behavioral pediatrics.* 2010;31(1):41–47.

11. Smith R. Osteogenesis imperfecta: from phenotype to genotype and back again. *Int J Exp Pathol.* 1994;75(4):233–241.

12. Sillence DO, Senn A, Danks DM. Genetic heterogeneity in osteogenesis imperfecta. *J Med Genet.* 1979;16(2):101–116.

13. Byers PH. Collagens: building blocks at the end of the development line. *ClinGenet.* 2000;58(4):270–279.

14. Marini JC, Cabral WA, Barnes AM. Null mutations in LEPRE1 and CRTAP cause severe recessive osteogenesis imperfecta. *Cell Tissue Res.* 2010;339(1):59–70.

15. Alanay Y, Avaygan H, Camacho N, et al. Mutations in the gene encoding the RER protein FKBP65 cause autosomal-recessive osteogenesis imperfecta. *Am J Hum Genet.* 2010;86(4):551–559.

16. Lapunzina P, Aglan M, Temtamy S, et al. Identification of a frameshift mutation in Osterix in a patient with recessive osteogenesis imperfecta. *Am J Hum Genet.* 2010;87(1):110–114.

17. Cubert R, Cheng EY, Mack S, et al. Osteogenesis imperfecta: mode of delivery and neonatal outcome. *Obstetrics & Gynecology.* 2001;97(1):66–69.

18. Monti E, Mottes M, Fraschini P, et al. Current and emerging treatments for the management of osteogenesis imperfecta. *Therapeutics and Clinical Risk Management.* 2010;6:367–381.

19. Van Brussel M, Takken T, Uiterwaal CS, et al. Physical training in children with osteogenesis imperfecta. *J Pediatr.* 2007;152(1):111–116.

20. DiMeglio LA, Ford L, McClintock C, et al. Intravenous pamidronate treatment of children under 36 months of age with osteogenesis imperfecta. *Bone.* 2004;35(5): 1038–1045.
21. Antoniazzi F, Zamboni G, Lauriola S, et al. Early bisphosphonate treatment in infants with severe osteogenesis imperfecta. *J Pediatr.* 2006;149(2):174–179.
22. Imani P, Vijayasekaran S, Lannigan F. Is it necessary to screen for hearing loss in the paediatric population with osteogenesis imperfecta? *Clin Otolaryngol.* 2003;28(3): 199–202.

Further Reading

Forlino A, Cabral WA, Barnes AM, et al. New perspectives on osteogenesis imperfecta. *Nature Reviews Endocrinology.* 2011;7:540–557.

Starr SR, Roberts TT, Fischer PR. Osteogenesis imperfecta: primary care. *Pediatr Rev.* 2010;31(8):e54–e64.

Trotter TL, Hall JG, American Academy of Pediatrics Committee on Genetics. Health Supervision for Children with Achondroplasia. *Pediatrics.* 2005;116(6):771–783.

CHAPTER 52

Talipes Equinovarus (Clubfoot)

Judith Hough, Catherine Bagley, Pieter J Koorts

A clubfoot or congenital talipes equinovarus is a congenital deformity involving either one or both feet. The affected foot appears rotated internally at the ankle and can be classified as either postural or structural. This condition is often diagnosed by visualisation on antenatal scan but in some instances may not be noticed until birth.

EPIDEMIOLOGY

The incidence of clubfoot in the general population is 1 in 1000 deliveries with 25% of affected individuals having a family history of idiopathic clubfoot.[1] If the family already has one affected child, the chance of a second child having clubfoot is 1 in 35.[2] Twin studies report a rate of 33% in monozygotic twins compared to 3% in dizygotic twins.[3]

Clubfoot is more common in males than females by a ratio of 2.5 to1[4] and the defect is more frequently unilateral although it can be bilateral in 40% of cases.

Certain racial groups appear to have an increased incidence of clubfoot such as the Polynesians (6.8 in 1000 in the Polynesian races) as well as populations of the Middle East and the Mediterranean coast of North Africa.[5] In contrast, there is a decreased incidence in the Chinese (0.4 in 1000).

DEFORMITIES

Congenital idiopathic clubfoot is a complex foot deformity involving four main characteristics: cavus and adduction of the forefoot, varus of the heel and equinus of the ankle joint (plantar flexion).[6] Although clubfoot may be an isolated entity, in 20% of cases there will be associated malformations. Therefore detection *in utero* can help to ascertain whether other fetal abnormalities may be present.

CAUSES

The cause of clubfoot is unknown and the aetiology is multifactorial with both environmental and genetic factors playing a role. There is seasonal increase in winter and spring implying viral infection.[7,8] Other environmental factors which may play a role include the possibility of toxins and early amniocentesis (before 11th week).[9] Or it may in fact be a spectrum of genetic disorders.

ASSOCIATED ABNORMALITIES

Clubfoot can be diagnosed antenatally at the 20 weeks gestation fetal abnormality scan. The importance of the antenatal diagnosis of clubfoot deformity is that this finding may serve as a marker for other anomalies. Up to 20% of affected fetuses have lethal conditions because of associated defects. There is a strong association with congenital hip dysplasia.

Clubfoot is a frequent component of neuromuscular disorders, skeletal dysplasias and genetic abnormalities and includes conditions such as neural tube defects (e.g., spina bifida), muscular dystrophy, arthrogryposis multiplex congenita, dwarfism, trisomy 13 and associated cleft palate. It may also be associated with other chromosomal or genetic factors such as Edwards syndrome, Ehlers-Danlos syndrome and some other connective tissue disorders such as Loeys-Dietz syndrome.

The incidence of clubfoot is also higher in conditions that result in oligohydramnios such as renal agenesis and abdominal pregnancies.

ANTENATAL MANAGEMENT

If clubfoot is noted on ultrasound, a thorough ultrasound examination is required to detect any related anomalies.[10] Even if the clubfoot is the only anomaly present in a fetus, antenatal diagnosis allows time for parental counselling about the therapeutic consequences of clubfoot. Other than identification and counselling, no antenatal management of clubfoot is indicated. The parents must be also be aware that not all abnormalities can be detected on an antenatal ultrasound.

False positive results are also a possibility because of a foot's position against the uterine wall. This may account for many postural foot deformities but it is not believed to be the primary cause of clubfoot.

MANAGEMENT—POSTNATAL

Even if there has been an antenatal diagnosis of isolated clubfoot, the diagnosis should be confirmed after birth and careful examination undertaken to exclude other associated conditions. This should include a careful examination for congenital hip dysplasia.

The severity of an isolated clubfoot can range from mild to severe. The differential diagnosis includes postural (self-resolving) intoeing or metatarsus adductus and these need to be identified by an experienced clinician.

The management will depend on the diagnosis.

▶ Postural talipes will self-resolve and simply requires parental education and reassurance.
▶ A clubfoot associated with other conditions will require referral to other specialists and sub-specialists (e.g., paediatric orthopaedic surgeon, paediatric neurologist) depending on the underlying cause. Therapy plans would be established after further investigations and consultation with the multidisciplinary team caring for the child and the family.

Often the management of the clubfoot is similar to that for an isolated clubfoot.

▶ Isolated clubfoot—management detailed below.

Historically, it was thought that the sooner the treatment for congenital clubfoot began the better the outcome. It is now generally accepted that a baby should commence treatment a few weeks post delivery so the mother can recover from the delivery, establish breast feeding and for the family and baby to bond, unencumbered by long leg casts.

MANAGEMENT OF ISOLATED CLUBFOOT

The Ponseti method of management (serial casting to gain initial correction and longer-term night splinting to maintain correction) is now accepted worldwide as the gold standard of treatment and is available in most tertiary paediatric centres. This results in a functional flexible foot which causes very few, if any, long-term problems.

According to the Ponseti protocol, treatment will commence within 2–3 weeks of delivery. Treatment consists of approximately 5 weeks of serial casting. Most feet (80–90%) will require a percutaneous tenotomy at the end of this time. This procedure involves a release (clipping) of the Achilles tendon under local anaesthesia. After recasting for three weeks and allowing for healing, the feet are placed in a foot abduction brace to be worn continually for three months and then for night time and naps for three to four years.

There is a small risk of recurrence which is managed by re-casting and occasionally further soft-tissue surgery in the form of repeat tenotomy or transfer of the tibialis anterior tendon to the lateral side of the foot (30% of reported cases).

CONSEQUENCES

If left untreated, or with sub-optimal treatment, clubfoot can result in significant disability involving pain, stiffness and decreased quality of life. In the hands of experienced clinicians, following accepted guidelines for management, the consequences of clubfoot are mild.

▶ The calf may be smaller and slightly weaker than normal and, if the condition is unilateral, the foot on the affected side will often be a shoe size smaller.

▶ The expected outcome of current accepted management for idiopathic clubfoot is a flexible, functional, pain-free foot which allows the child to lead a normal life.

▶ In some cases, where the treatment has been problematic and has required invasive joint surgery, the outcomes are not as good. In those cases, adults may have stiff painful feet affecting activities of daily living; this may impact on work options.

▶ For clubfoot associated with arthrogryposis or neuromuscular disorders, results are consistently less good, however this will depend on the underlying condition.

OTHER CONSULTS

Discussion with a physiotherapist and/or paediatric orthopaedic surgeon may be helpful.

ETHICS

Isolated clubfoot is a readily treatable condition which usually has an excellent outcome. If it is associated with other more complex conditions, in some cases it may be appropriate to discuss the option of providing comfort care only following delivery. In such cases, some parents may decide that advanced life support is not appropriate.

REFERENCES

1. Lochmiller C, Johnston D, Scott A, et al. Genetic epidemiology study of idiopathic talipes equinovarus. *Am J Med Genet.* 1998;79:90–96.
2. Wynne-Davies R. Family Studies and the Cause of Congenital Club Foot. Talipes Equinovarus, Talipes Calcaneo-Valgus and Metatarsus Varus. *J Bone Joint Surg Br.* 1964;46:445–463.
3. Tachdjan M. *Pediatric Orthopedics.* Philadelphia: Saunders; 1972.
4. Kruse LM, Dobbs MB, Gurnett CA. Polygenic threshold model with sex dimorphism in clubfoot inheritance: the Carter effect. *J Bone Joint Surg Am.* 2008;90:2688–2694.
5. Turco VJ. *Clubfoot.* New York: Churchill-Livingstone; 1981.
6. Lehman WB. *The Clubfoot.* Philadelphia: J.B. Lippincott; 1980.
7. Pryor GA, Villar RN, Ronen A, Scott PM. Seasonal variation in the incidence of congenital talipes equinovarus. *J Bone Joint Surg Br.* 1991;73:632–634.
8. Barker SL, Macnicol MF. Seasonal distribution of idiopathic congenital talipes equinovarus in Scotland. *J Pediatr Orthop B.* 2002;11:129–133.
9. Farrell SA, Summers AM, Dallaire L, et al. Club foot, an adverse outcome of early amniocentesis: disruption or deformation? CEMAT. Canadian Early and Mid-Trimester Amniocentesis Trial. *J Med Genet.* 1999;36:843–846.
10. Chervenak FA, Tortora M, Hobbins JC. Antenatal sonographic diagnosis of clubfoot. *J Ultrasound Med.* 1985;4:49.

CHAPTER 53

Fetal Dyskinesia (Arthrogryposis Multiplex Congenita)

Anita Cairns, Pieter J Koorts

Lack of normal movements can have profound and devastating effects on a fetus. Not only is the underlying cause often a significant problem but the secondary effects of reduced fetal movements can also have a major impact (e.g., joint contractures, pulmonary hypoplasia and polyhydramnios). Any abnormality along the pathway from the brain to the muscles can disturb fetal movements.

DEFINITION
Arthrogryposis multiplex congenita is a descriptive term for a symptom complex of multiple joint contractures that are present at birth. It is the final point in a pathway of reduced or absent fetal movements (fetal dyskinesia). The severity of arthrogryposis is directly proportional to the degree of fetal dyskinesia.

Localised congenital contractures such as talipes equinovarus (TEV) and developmental dysplasia of the hip (DDH) can also be regarded as part of the arthrogryposis spectrum with reduced fetal movements as the underlying mechanism.

Arthrogryposis can be caused by any limitation of fetal movements. It is likely that the abnormality occurs at the end of the first trimester after the peripheral nerves and muscles have formed. This theory is supported by evidence of a reduction in the size and number of anterior horn cells in the spinal cord and/or brain, with evidence of degeneration, rather than a failure of formation, in neurogenic arthrogryposis. Secondary changes occur with replacement of muscle with fat and fibrous tissue.

PREVALENCE
Table 53.1 details the birth rates across the arthrogryposis spectrum.

DIFFERENTIAL DIAGNOSIS
The differential diagnosis of fetal dyskinesia and arthrogryposis multiplex congenita includes any condition that affects the pathway from the brain to muscle. As the differential diagnosis can be extensive (see Table 53.2), separating patients into groups according to the clinical findings may focus investigations and aid in achieving a diagnosis. Such separation into groups is:

Table 53.1 Birth rates across the arthrogryposis spectrum

Abnormality	Prevalence
Arthrogryposis multiplex congenita	1 in 4000 live births
Talipes equinovarus	1 in 300 live births
Developmental dysplasia of the hip	1 in 200 live births

Table 53.2 Differential diagnosis

Causes	Subtypes	Example
Neurogenic—most common aetiology	Central nervous system disorders	Structural brain/spine abnormalities Syndromic diagnoses (e.g., chromosomal anomalies, Pierre Robin syndrome)
	Anterior horn cell disorders	Dysgenesis of anterior horn cells Amyoplasia Spinal muscular atrophy
	Neuropathies	Congenital hypomyelinating neuropathy
Myogenic	Neuromuscular junction	Congenital myasthenic syndrome (DOK7 and RAPSN mutations)
	Congenital muscular dystrophies	Fukayama, Ullrich and merosin deficient congenital muscular dystrophies Congenital myotonic dystrophy
	Congenital myopathies	Nemaline myopathy Central core disease
	Mitochondrial cytopathies	
Connective tissue		Multiple pterygium syndrome Restrictive dermopathy
Limitation of space	Multiple pregnancies	
	Intrauterine abnormalities	Fibroids Amniotic bands Oligohydramnios
Maternal factors	Illnesses	Myasthenia gravis Rubella
	Toxins	Fetal alcohol syndrome Medications
Compromised vascular supply	Maternal	Hypotension Hypoxia
	Fetal	Placental insufficiency

Box 53.1 AMYOPLASIA

Amyoplasia (meaning "no muscle growth") is a specific form of arthrogryposis multiplex congenita and accounts for up to one-third of cases. Clinically, these infants have involvement of the limbs with sparing of the trunk.

The typical appearance is:

- upper limbs have a "waiter's tip" appearance:
  - internal rotation with adduction at the shoulders,
  - extension of the elbow,
  - pronation of the forearm,
  - flexed wrists,
  - camptodactyly (flexion contracture of fingers);
- lower limbs:
  - contractures at the hips often with dislocation,
  - usually flexion of the knee,
  - severe talipes equinovarus;
- associated features:
  - reduced muscle bulk,
  - lack of skin creases at the elbows and knees,
  - dimpling over the joints,
  - pterygia,
  - midline facial haemangioma,
  - mild micrognathia,
  - gastroschisis, and
  - genital abnormalities.

Children with amyoplasia are usually of normal intelligence. As adults, up to 70% are living independently and up to 78% have open employment.

▶ limbs only—e.g., amyoplasia (see Box 53.1), distal arthrogryposis;
▶ limbs and other body areas—e.g., multiple pterygium syndrome, congenital myotonic dystrophy; and
▶ limbs and central nervous system and/or lethal—e.g., fetal akinesia deformation sequence, chromosomal abnormalities.

ASSESSMENT

Assessment of the fetus and neonate with arthrogryposis can provide clues to the underlying aetiology as well as identify the complications of fetal dyskinesia that require treatment. Fetal assessment has two broad aims; firstly to begin the process of determining a cause, and secondly to determine if there are any important secondary effects on the fetus.

Table 53.3 lists appropriate antenatal and postnatal assessments. A definitive diagnosis may not be possible.

ASSOCIATED ABNORMALITIES IN ARTHROGRYPOSIS MULTIPLEX CONGENITA

Reduced fetal movements can cause polyhydramnios due to impaired fetal swallowing.

If fetal breathing movements are affected, this can restrict lung growth. This can result in severe pulmonary hypoplasia.

Other intrauterine abnormalities can include:

- short umbilical cord;
- intrauterine growth restriction;
- osteoporosis; and
- craniofacial abnormalities, including:
  - micrognathia (due to reduced movement of masticatory muscles),
  - cleft palate,
  - hypoplasia of the maxilla.

In the most severe form, fetal akinesia deformation sequence (FADS), fetal or early neonatal death is the usual outcome.

LABOUR AND DELIVERY

The location of delivery should be determined by the expected condition of the baby at birth. In cases of severe arthrogryposis and suspected pulmonary hypoplasia, delivery should be planned at a hospital that has an intensive care nursery.

Breech presentation or unstable lie is significantly more common in babies with arthrogyposis, necessitating delivery by caesarean section.

POSTNATAL MANAGEMENT

Appropriate antenatal counselling should be provided in all cases of arthrogryposis. Given the severity of the underlying condition in some cases, the option of providing comfort care following delivery should be discussed with the parents. Some parents may decide that advanced life support is not appropriate. Whatever course of action is decided upon, the plan for immediate postnatal management should be documented and known by staff attending the delivery. It may be appropriate to provide advanced life support whilst a definitive diagnosis is sought.

Respiratory support including intubation and mechanical ventilation is often required immediately after delivery.

Ongoing care with aggressive physiotherapy and occupational therapy will usually be required. This should include early mobilisation of limbs and possibly splinting of some joints.

Orthopaedic procedures may be required and include tendon or soft tissue release, hip reduction and scoliosis surgery.

Table 53.3 Assessment for fetal dyskinesia and arthrogryposis multiplex congenita

	Prenatal	Postnatal
Clinical assessment	Maternal factors • illness, drugs • history of previous miscarriages, stillbirths, neonatal deaths • examination—signs of neuromuscular disorders (e.g., myotonic dystrophy, myasthenia) • family history—neuromuscular disorders, contractures (including TEV) Pregnancy • pregnancy complications—bleeding, trauma • fetus—growth, movements • liquor volume	Document contractures Detailed neurological examination Dysmorphic features Muscle bulk, connective tissue, skin, fat Associated abnormalities (e.g., dermatoglyphs)
Investigations	Maternal ACh receptor antibodies and anti-MuSK antibodies Antenatal ultrasound • at 12 and 18 weeks gestational age • look for: - TEV or other contractures - reduced fetal movements or inactivity - abnormal positioning of specific joints - increased nuchal translucency - space limitations (e.g., fibroid) • if any abnormality, then needs tertiary scan plus or minus serial scans Amniocentesis and chorionic villus sampling—karyotype, FISH Fetal MRI	Clinical photos X-rays • joint position • long bone fractures • osteoporosis Bloods/urine • creatine kinase • viral cultures/antibodies • metabolic screen Ophthalmology MRI • brain • spine • muscle Genetic testing • karyotype • microarray • specific genetic testing Electromyography/nerve conduction studies Ophthalmology review Muscle ±skin biopsy • histopathology—may be greater abnormality in opposing rather than prime moving muscles (e.g., triceps rather than biceps)[1] • immunohistochemistry • electron microscopy • mitochondrial studies Autopsy if lethal outcome

Key: TEV—Talipes equinovarus, ACh—acetyl choline, MuSK—muscle specific kinase, MRI—magnetic resonance imaging, FISH—fluorescent in situ hybridisation.

OTHER CONSULTS

A multidisciplinary team should be involved with any child with fetal dyskinesia. Other specialists to be consulted antenatally include neurologists and geneticists.

Postnatally the following may also be required: rehabilitation specialists, orthopaedic surgeons, respiratory paediatricians and allied therapists (physiotherapy, occupational therapy, speech therapy).

RECURRENCE

The recurrence rate depends on the underlying aetiology. Amyoplasia occurs sporadically.

Formal genetic counselling should be obtained in all cases.

OUTCOME

The outcome depends on the severity and the underlying aetiology.

Good prognostic factors include:

- increasing strength over time;
- mostly upper limb involvement;
- hip contractures <20 degrees;
- knee contractures <15 degrees;
- plantigrade feet; and
- no central nervous system involvement.

Studies report 40% or more of children walk independently, with up to 85% achieving assisted ambulation.

Further Reading

1. Banker BQ. Arthrogryposis multiplex congenita: spectrum of pathologic changes. *Hum Pathol.* 1986;17(7):656–672.
2. Hall JG, Vincent A. Arthrogryposis. In Jones HR, De Vivo DC, Darras BT, eds. *Neuromuscular disorders of infancy, childhood and adolescence: a clinician's approach.* Philadelphia: Butterworth–Heinemann; 2003:123–142.
3. Moessinger AC. Fetal akinesia deformation sequence: an animal model. *Pediatrics.* 1983;72(6):857–863.
4. Hall JG, Reed SD, Driscoll EP. Part I. Amyoplasia: a common, sporadic condition with congenital contractures. *American journal of medical genetics.* 1983;15(4):571–590.
5. Hall JG. Arthrogryposis multiplex congenita: etiology, genetics, classification, diagnostic approach, and general aspects. *J Pediatr Orthop B.* 1997;6(3):159–166.
6. Jago RH. Arthrogryposis following treatment of maternal tetanus with muscle relaxants. *Arch Dis Child.* 1970;45(240):277–279.
7. Drachman DB, Banker BQ. Arthrogryposis multiplex congenita. Case due to disease of the anterior horn cells. *Arch Neurol.* 1961;5:77–93.
8. Vuopala K, Ignatius J, Herva R. Lethal arthrogryposis with anterior horn cell disease. *Hum Pathol.* 1995;26(1):12–19.
9. Banker BQ. Neuropathologic aspects of arthrogryposis multiplex congenita. *Clin Orthop Relat Res.* 1985;(194):30–43.

10. Witters I, Moerman P, Fryns JP. Fetal akinesia deformation sequence: a study of 30 consecutive in utero diagnoses. *Am J Med Genet.* 2002;113(1):23–28.

11. Gaitanis JN, McMillan HJ, Wu A, et al. Electrophysiologic evidence for anterior horn cell disease in amyoplasia. *Pediatr Neurol.* 2010;43(2):142–147.

12. Hall JG. Pena-Shokeir phenotype (fetal akinesia deformation sequence) revisited. *Birth Defects Res A Clin Mol Teratol.* 2009;85(8):677–694.

13. Makrydimas G, Sotiriadis A, Papapanagiotou G, et al. Fetal akinesia deformation sequence presenting with increased nuchal translucency in the first trimester of pregnancy. *Fetal Diagn Ther.* 2004;19(4):332–335.

14. Nemec SF, Hoftberger R, Nemec U, et al. Fetal akinesia and associated abnormalities on prenatal MRI. *Prenat Diagn.* 2011;31(5):484–490.

15. Sells JM, Jaffe KM, Hall JG. Amyoplasia, the most common type of arthrogryposis: the potential for good outcome. *Pediatrics.* 1996;97(2):225–231.

16. Fassier A, Wicart P, Dubousset J, et al. Arthrogryposis multiplex congenita. Long-term follow-up from birth until skeletal maturity. *J Child Orthop.* 2009;3(5):383–390.

17. Sodergard J, Hakamies-Blomqvist L, Sainio K, et al. Arthrogryposis multiplex congenita: perinatal and electromyographic findings, disability, and psychosocial outcome. *J Pediatr Orthop B.* 1997;6(3):167–171.

CHAPTER 54

Cystic Hygroma

Linda McLaughlin

Cystic hygroma is a congenital malformation of the lymphatic system. Abnormalities of the connections between the lymphatic and venous systems cause accumulation of lymphatic fluid which forms a cystic mass. Cystic hygromas are most often seen in the nuchal region, but they can occur in other locations. They can be septated or simple (non-septated).

Cystic hygromas are diagnosed on antenatal ultrasound scans.

EMBRYOLOGY AND PATHOLOGY

The lymphatic system begins to develop in the fifth week of gestation, with formation of lymphatic sacs. Communications later form between these sacs and also between the lymphatic and venous systems.

Two of the lymphatic sacs (the jugular sacs) are located in the neck region. The jugular sacs form connections with the thoracic ducts and the jugular veins. If this does not occur properly, lymph accumulates in the jugular sacs, causing distension and the formation of a cystic hygroma.

AETIOLOGY

The cause is unknown in the majority of cases. There is an increased risk with chromosomal anomalies, maternal alcohol abuse and parvovirus infection.

PREVALENCE

Cystic hygromas are the most common type of fetal neck mass and they are seen in about 1 in 100 first trimester fetuses. There is a high risk of fetal demise. Many spontaneously resolve. Therefore, cystic hygromas are only seen in about 1 in 6000 live births.

DIFFERENTIAL DIAGNOSIS

The major differential diagnoses include:
◗ cervical meningocoele;
◗ posterior encephalocoele;
◗ cystic teratoma; and
◗ haemangioma.

There is significant overlap between first trimester cystic hygroma and increased nuchal translucency.

Increased nuchal translucency occurs with enlargement of the normal hypoechoic space seen on ultrasound in the posterior neck at 10–14 weeks gestational age. High-resolution ultrasound may show subtle trabeculation. Increased nuchal translucency is less likely than cystic hygroma to persist and/or be associated with adverse fetal outcome.

Cystic hygroma is usually larger in size than increased nuchal translucency and may extend along the length of the fetus (i.e., not restricted to neck region). Septations are usually thick and multiple comprising discrete fluid loculations. A cystic hygroma may resolve to become nuchal thickening alone.

ASSOCIATED ABNORMALITIES

The risk of associated abnormalities is increased with the presence of septation and with larger lesions.

Chromosomal anomalies are present in 50–70% of fetuses with cystic hygroma. The associated syndromes include Down, Turner, Klinefelter, Edwards and Patau syndromes. In the first trimester, trisomy (especially trisomy 21) is the most common aneuploidy. In the second trimester, monosomy X is more common.

Non-chromosomal syndromes associated with cystic hygroma include Noonan, Fryn, multiple pterygium and Roberts syndromes.

Other (non-syndromic) structural anomalies occur in about 30% of fetuses with a septated cystic hygroma in the first trimester. These include:
- hydrops;
- cardiac anomalies;
- diaphragmatic hernia;
- abdominal wall defects;
- skeletal dysplasia; and
- renal anomalies.

ANTENATAL INVESTIGATIONS
Imaging
Routine antenatal ultrasound can detect cystic hygroma from 12 weeks gestational age. If a cystic hygroma is seen, the scan should also carefully assess for associated structural abnormalities, as well as monitor fetal growth and well being throughout pregnancy.

High-resolution transvaginal ultrasound or 3D ultrasound can provide more detail than routine ultrasound.

Fetal echocardiography is recommended at 18–22 weeks gestational age if a cystic hygroma persists.

Fast-spin magnetic resonance imaging (MRI) may clarify the situation if the diagnosis is uncertain. It also helps delineate the extent of the cystic hygroma and its relationship to the surrounding structures.

Combined First Trimester Screening Test

An ultrasound to determine the nuchal translucency thickness and maternal blood for the Triple test (alpha-fetoprotein, unconjugated oestriol and human chorionic gonadotrophin) assesses for the risk of aneuploidy (Table 1.1 in Chapter 1).

Amniocentesis

An amniocentesis will provide cells for a fetal karyotype and FISH (fluorescence in situ hybridisation) testing, particularly to test for abnormalities of chromosomes 13, 18, 21, X and Y.

CONSEQUENCES

The risk of fetal death is substantially increased in fetuses with cystic hygroma. In pregnancies which continue to term, cystic hygromas often resolve (approximately 80%). Where resolution has occurred, there may be some residual redundant skin ("webbed neck").

The outcome for a particular patient depends on:

❯ gestational age at diagnosis:
  • first trimester cystic hygroma—overall, 15–30% have a normal outcome and 75% of euploid patients survive beyond the neonatal period,
  • second trimester cystic hygroma—complications are more likely than with first trimester cystic hygroma and only 10–20% survive to delivery;
❯ presence and nature of associated abnormalities;
❯ karyotype (prognosis is worse in aneuploid fetuses);
❯ nature of cystic hygroma (simple versus septated):
  • a septated cystic hygroma carries a much higher risk of fetal demise,
  • even with the resolution of a cystic hygroma, the outcome is worse with a septated cystic hygroma—after resolution of a simple cystic hygroma in a euploid fetus the most likely outcome is birth of a normal infant, but despite resolution of septated cystic hygromas, about 80% of cases will have significant problems (as listed below); and
❯ lesion size (a large cystic hygroma is generally associated with a worse outcome).

After birth, cystic hygromas rarely resolve spontaneously.

Potential complications of cystic hygromas in infancy and childhood include:

❯ airway compromise;
❯ feeding difficulties;
❯ speech problems;
❯ dental malocclusion;
❯ inadequate oral hygiene with dental caries and periodontal inflammation;
❯ infection;

▶ bleeding into the lesion;
▶ soft tissue malformation and/or hypertrophy;
▶ bony malformation and/or hypertrophy; and
▶ cosmetic problems.

MANAGEMENT—ANTENATAL
Screening for other abnormalities as detailed above is crucial. Fetal magnetic resonance imaging (MRI) is recommended if airway compromise is suspected.

The parents should be counselled by the neonatal team regarding post-partum management. A paediatric ear, nose and throat (ENT) specialist should be involved if there is any possibility of airway compromise.

An ultrasound scan just prior to birth is recommended to reassess the size of the lesion and assess any degree of hydrops and associated pleural effusions and compromised lung growth.

MANAGEMENT—INTRAPARTUM
Delivery by caesarean section is considered if the cystic hygroma is large, as vaginal delivery may not be possible.

Babies with significant lesions should be delivered in a maternity centre with an intensive care nursery.

If the cystic hygroma is obstructing the fetal airway, then the EXIT (*ex utero* intrapartum treatment) procedure may be considered.

MANAGEMENT—IMMEDIATE POSTNATAL
The baby will be assessed for the adequacy of the airway and any compromise managed accordingly. Resuscitation should otherwise proceed as for any neonate.

The baby should be examined carefully for any associated anomalies.

MANAGEMENT—POSTNATAL
Spontaneous decompression or shrinkage of cystic hygromas present at birth is rare.

A paediatric ear, nose and throat (ENT) specialist should be involved for assessment and planning of treatment. Whilst intervention is being planned, close observation is imperative, particularly monitoring for the development of any airway compromise.

Feeding difficulties can occur, leading to failure to thrive.

Avoid trauma to the lesion, as this can precipitate bleeding.

An infected cystic hygroma requires treatment with intravenous antibiotics.

Expectant Management
Expectant management is sometimes used in asymptomatic patients (especially small infants). It may be an interim strategy only, until timing is

optimal for definitive treatment (e.g., allowing growth in order to reduce the technical difficulty of any planned operation).

Medical Treatment

Sclerosants (e.g., OK-432) are sometimes used in the management of cystic hygromas.

Surgical Treatment

Aspiration or incision and drainage of the lesion is occasionally used, but this often needs to be repeated. Fibrosis often results, and this can complicate future surgery. Haemorrhage and infection are other risks.

Surgical resection with complete removal of the cystic hygroma is the aim of treatment although this is impossible in about 60% due to the proximity of neurovascular structures.

Staged procedures should be avoided if possible as fibrosis can make later operations difficult.

Potential complications include damage to adjacent tissues (e.g., nerve palsy, chylothorax, bleeding) and recurrence of the cystic hygroma (if incompletely excised).

Other Treatments

Laser therapy and radiofrequency ablation have been trialled for some variants of cystic hygroma.

RECURRENCE

The recurrence risk for cystic hygroma due to aneuploidy is usually very low.

Cases of cystic hygroma with a normal karyotype can occur as a familial condition with autosomal recessive inheritance (25% recurrence risk).

Further Reading

Acevedo JL, Shah RK, Neville HL, et al. Cystic hygroma. *In eMedicine*. 2009.

Brumfield CG, Wenstrom KD, Davis RO, et al. Second-trimester cystic hygroma: prognosis of septated and nonseptated lesions. *Obstetrics & Gynecology*. 1996;88(6): 979–982.

Malone FD, Ball RH, Nyberg DA, et al. First-trimester cystic hygroma. Prevalence, natural history, and pediatric outcome. *Obstetrics & Gynecology*. 2005;106(2):288–294.

Nyberg DA, McGahan JP, Pretorius DH, et al. *Diagnostic imaging of fetal anomalies*. Lippincott Williams & Wilkins; 2003.

Perkins JA, Manning SC, Tempero RM, et al. Lymphatic malformations: review of current treatment. *Otolaryngology—Head & Neck Surgery*. 2010;142(6):795–803.

Simpson L. *First trimester cystic hygroma and enlarged nuchal translucency*. In: Levine D, Wilkins-Haug L, Barss V, eds. UpToDate Version 18.3. 2010.

Zimmer EZ, Drugan A, Ofir C, et al. Ultrasound imaging of fetal neck anomalies: implications for the risk of aneuploidy and structural anomalies. *Prenatal Diagnosis*. 1997;17(11):1055–1058.

CHAPTER 55

Teratomas—Sacrococcygeal and Neck

Craig A McBride

The word teratoma is derived from the Greek for monster, and it was first used by Virchow in 1869 for a sacrococcygeal mass.

A teratoma is a tumour composed of multiple tissues foreign to the site of origin; classically described as having all three embryonic layers (endoderm, mesoderm and ectoderm). Recent definitions recognise monodermic teratomas.

Tumours generally occur in the midline, with 35–60% being sacrococcygeal teratomas. About 8% of all teratomas are cervical.

AETIOLOGY / PATHOPHYSIOLOGY / EMBRYOLOGY
There are three theories on how teratomas develop:

1. Derivation from totipotent primordial germ cells—Originating from endodermal cells of the yolk sac near the allantois, these cells migrate to the gonadal ridges during weeks 4 and 5 of gestation. Cells that don't reach their target may give rise to midline teratomas anywhere from the brain to the coccygeal area.
2. Originating from remnants in Hensen's node of the primitive streak—In week 3 caudal midline cells in Hensen's node give rise to all three germ layers of the embryo. The primitive streak shortens and disappears by the end of week 3. Persistence would explain the commonest site of a teratoma being sacrococcygeal.
3. Incomplete twinning.

PREVALENCE
Teratomas are the most common neoplasm in newborn infants. The incidence is 1 in 35,000–40,000 live births. There is a 4:1 female to male ratio.

DIFFERENTIAL DIAGNOSIS
These tumours are usually found on early scans.

The differential diagnosis of a sacrococcygeal lesion includes:
- sacrococcygeal teratomas;
- lumbosacral myelomeningocoele;
- lipoma;
- dermoid; and
- other tumours.

The differential diagnosis of a cervical lesion includes:
- teratoma;
- cystic hygroma;
- congenital goitre;
- foregut duplication cyst; and
- pharyngeal pouch anomaly.

ASSOCIATED ABNORMALITIES

Teratomas are usually isolated lesions. They may form part of the Currarino triad (anorectal malformation, sacral anomaly, presacral mass).

Other anomalies reported are:
- urogenital (hypospadias, vesicoureteral reflux, vaginal or uterine duplications);
- congenital dislocation of the hip;
- central nervous system lesions (anencephaly, trigonocephaly, Dandy-Walker malformations, spina bifida, myelomeningocoele);
- Klinefelter syndrome (strongly associated with mediastinal teratoma); and
- rare associations with trisomies 13 and 21, anterior diaphragmatic hernia, congenital heart defects, Beckwith-Wiedemann syndrome, pterygium, cleft lip and palate, Proteus syndrome, Schinzel-Giedion syndrome.

Other anomalies relate to the physical effects of the tumour itself, such as pulmonary hypoplasia (cervical tumour) and urinary obstruction (sacrococcygeal teratomas).

CONSEQUENCES

In recent series, overall survival of those with antenatally diagnosed sacrococcygeal teratomas approaches 80%, and of liveborn infants it approaches 95%.

Vascular steal and increased metabolic demand from the (highly vascular) tumour can lead to high output cardiac failure. This can lead to polyhydramnios, cardiomegaly, fetal hydrops and intrauterine death. Mortality approaches 100% if these complications arise prior to 37 weeks gestation.

Mirror syndrome (maternal pre-eclampsia associated with fetal and placental hydrops) has been described in mothers of fetuses with sacrococcygeal teratomas.

There is a 10% risk of malignancy at birth.

The Kasabach-Merritt phenomenon (consumptive coagulopathy and thrombocytopaenia) may ensue, due to high flow through tumour vessels. This in turn may lead to haemorrhage at sites distant from the tumour.

Sacrococcygeal teratomas with a large intrapelvic component may cause urinary or gastrointestinal obstruction. Approximately one-third of patients will have long-term bowel and/or bladder dysfunction following sacrococcygeal teratomas.

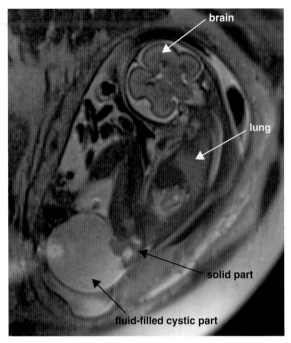

Figure 55.1 Fetal magnetic resonance imaging (MRI) of a large sacrococcygeal teratoma at 24 weeks gestation.

MANAGEMENT—ANTENATAL

Antenatal counselling is mandatory, by specialists (especially neonatologists and paediatric surgeons) with experience in the condition and its long-term follow-up.

Closely follow-up the mother and fetus, to enable early detection of complications.

Regular antenatal Doppler ultrasound scanning can assist in defining:

▶ intracorporeal tumour extension;
▶ haemorrhage into the tumour;
▶ associated anomalies; and
▶ development of hydrops.

Antenatal magnetic resonance imaging (MRI) can better characterise complex lesions and assist peripartum planning. See Figure 55.1.

Depending on the exact problems encountered, a variety of other antenatal interventions may be necessary or considered, including:

▶ amnioreduction;
▶ laser ablation of feeding vessels;
▶ alcohol sclerosis;
▶ cyst drainage;
▶ vesicoamniotic shunt; and
▶ tumour resection.

About 33% of fetuses with cervicofacial teratomas have associated polyhydramnios. The prognosis is poor for fetuses requiring antenatal intervention, with approximately 25% dying *in utero* and a further 25% dying after delivery.

MANAGEMENT—LABOUR / DELIVERY / IMMEDIATE POSTNATAL MANAGEMENT

Delivery should be in a centre with an intensive care nursery and immediate access to neonatologists and paediatric surgeons.

Caesarean section may be offered in the case of high risk lesions to minimise the risk of tumour bleeding during delivery.

Ex-utero Intrapartum Treatment (EXIT) may be necessary for cervical tumours with potential airway compression. EXIT to extracorporeal membrane oxygenation (ECMO) has also been used in some centres. These decisions will be made by the specialists involved.

Blood should be collected soon after birth for full blood count and film examination, a coagulation profile, alpha-fetoprotein (AFP) and beta human chorionic gonadotrophin (β-hCG).

Malignancy at birth is about 10% and increases with age, with incomplete resection and if the coccyx is not resected in the case of sacrococcygeal teratomas. The most common tumour marker used is alpha-fetoprotein, but this is high in neonates and thus its real use is as a marker for recurrence.

OTHER CONSULTS REQUIRED

All require a consult by a neonatologist and a paediatric surgeon.

Others will depend on the site of the lesion and its expected associated problems, but may include:
▶ paediatric otorhinolaryngology for teratomas in and around the airway;
▶ paediatric cardiothoracic surgery for teratomas extending into the central mediastinum; and
▶ paediatric neurosurgery if there is evidence of extension into the spinal canal.

MANAGEMENT—POSTNATAL

Surgical excision is mandatory and ideally performed as soon as the neonate is stable. The surgical approach used for sacrococcygeal teratomas— abdominal (open or laparoscopic), perineal or combined—depends on the size and extent of the tumour. See Figure 55.2. Baby will require intubation

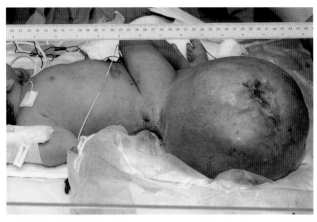

Figure 55.2 Term baby with a large sacrococcygeal teratoma soon after birth (fetal MRI seen in Figure 55.1).

and mechanical ventilation for surgery, and may require prolonged ventilation, especially for cervical teratomas.

Given the possibility of recurrence, and the risk of long-term bladder and/or bowel dysfunction, ongoing follow-up by clinicians experienced in these matters is essential.

RECURRENCE
Recurrence of the tumour in the individual:
▶ In recent series local recurrence rates in sacrococcygeal teratomas range from 4–11%, with half being malignant.
▶ Failure to remove the coccyx in sacrococcygeal teratomas confers a 37% risk of recurrence.
   Recurrence of a teratoma in future siblings:
▶ Increased risk in familial Currarino triad (50% of cases). Mutation of *HLXB9* located at 7q36 is present in 50% of sporadic and 90% of familial cases. There is variable phenotypic expression.

ETHICS
Prognosis is poor with prenatal hydrops, dystocia, tumour rupture, prematurity, very vascular lesions and larger tumours. In such cases, it is important that discussion with the parents about the treatment options after birth should cover the entire spectrum—from active resuscitation and treatment, with an intent to operate, through to the possibility of not initiating resuscitation and instead providing palliative care.

Further Reading

Altman RP, Randolph JG, Lilly JR. Sacrococcygeal teratoma: American Academy of Pediatrics Surgical Section Survey-1973. *J Pediatr Surg.* 1974;9:389–398.

Barksdale Jr EM, Obokhare I. Teratomas in infants and children. *Curr Opin Pediatr.* 2009;21:344–349.

Gabra HO, Jesudason EC, McDowell HP, et al. Sacrococcygeal teratoma—a 25-year experience in a UK regional center. *J Pediatr Surg.* 2006;41:1513–1516.

Ho KO, Soundappan SV, Walker K, et al. Sacrococcygeal teratoma: the 13-year experience of a tertiary paediatric centre. *J Paediatr Child Health.* 2011 May;47(5):287–291.

Lakhoo K. Neonatal teratomas. *Early Hum Dev.* 2010;86:643–647.

Makin EC, Hyett J, Ade-Ajayi N, et al. Outcome of antenatally diagnosed sacrococcygeal teratomas: single-center experience (1993-2004). *J Pediatr Surg.* 2006;41:388–393.

Yoshida A, Maoate K, Blakelock R, et al. Long-term functional outcomes in children with Currarino syndrome. *Pediatr Surg Int.* 2010;26:677–681.

CHAPTER 56
Cleft Lip and Cleft Palate

Linda McLaughlin

A cleft lip occurs when embryonic tissues which form the lip fail to fuse normally during the 4th to 7th weeks of gestation. The cleft can be unilateral, bilateral or median (rare). The extent of the cleft can range from a notch in the vermillion border to a complete lip cleft with involvement of the nostrils and extension into the midface or palate. See Figure 56.1.

An isolated cleft palate occurs due to failure of fusion of the palatal shelves in the midline during the 6th to 9th weeks of gestation. The cleft may involve the soft palate, hard palate or both. The extent of the cleft can range from a mild sub-mucosal cleft or bifid uvula to a complete cleft of the hard and soft palates. See Figure 56.1.

DIAGNOSIS
Cleft lip, with or without a cleft palate, can be diagnosed on ultrasound from 14 weeks gestational age (detection rates increase with increasing gestational age).

An isolated cleft palate is difficult to diagnose on antenatal ultrasound, and may not be detected until after birth.

AETIOLOGY
Genetic and environmental factors interact to cause clefts.

Genetic factors in most cases involve the interaction of multiple genes. Twin studies of clefts have shown that there is approximately 45% concordance in monozygotic twins and about 5% concordance in dizygotic twins.

Various maternal environmental factors that increase the risk of a cleft lip or palate include some medications (including phenytoin, valproate, retinoic acid, methotrexate), excessive vitamin A, cigarette smoking, alcohol intake and obesity. Multivitamin supplements have been associated with a reduced risk of clefts.

Mechanical obstruction from an abnormal tongue position during embryological development (as occurs with micrognathia) can prevent palatal fusion.

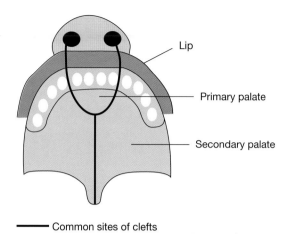

Common sites of clefts

Figure 56.1 An inferior view of the palate and upper gum and lip showing the common sites of cleft lip and cleft palate.

PREVALENCE

Clefts of the lip and/or palate occur in 1 in 700 live births in Australia. Cleft lip, with or without a cleft palate, is most prevalent in Asians and Native Americans, and least prevalent in Negroes (intermediate in Caucasians).

The prevalence of an isolated cleft palate is relatively constant across races (different aetiology).

In general:

▸ cleft lip, with or without a cleft palate (60%), is more common than an isolated cleft palate (40%);
▸ cleft lip, with or without a cleft palate, is more common in males, and an isolated cleft palate is more common in females; and
▸ unilateral cleft lip, with or without a cleft palate, is more common than bilateral cleft lip, with or without a cleft palate.

DIFFERENTIAL DIAGNOSIS

Clefts are seen in more than 300 different syndromes, including:

▸ Van der Woude syndrome;
▸ Pierre Robin syndrome;
▸ Velocardiofacial syndrome; and
▸ Stickler syndrome.

ASSOCIATED ABNORMALITIES

Cleft palate is associated with cleft lip in 85% of cases of bilateral cleft lip and 70% of cases of unilateral cleft lip.

Other abnormalities are associated with clefts in 50% of cases of cleft palate. Other abnormalities also occur in 30% of cases of cleft lip, with or without a cleft palate (in 10% of cases of cleft lip without a cleft palate and 20% of cases of cleft lip with a cleft palate).

Of all cases of cleft lip, with or without a cleft palate, abnormalities are associated in:

▶ 100% of midline cleft lip, with or without a cleft palate;
▶ 25% of bilateral cleft lip, with or without a cleft palate; and
▶ 10% of unilateral cleft lip, with or without a cleft palate.

The associated anomalies usually involve the cardiovascular, skeletal or central nervous systems.

INVESTIGATIONS

Fetal ultrasound should assess the extent of any cleft found. A careful assessment should also be made for other abnormalities (up to 20% of associated defects are not detected on antenatal ultrasound). 3D ultrasound can clarify the extent of a cleft lip, and increase the detection of a cleft palate. It can also be useful for parents to see the extent of the deformity.

Magnetic resonance imaging (MRI) is occasionally used to assess the severity of any cleft and to detect other anomalies.

Amniocentesis for fetal karyotyping should be offered if other abnormalities are present as there is a 40–60% risk of chromosomal anomaly. It may also be considered in cases of an isolated cleft despite a very low risk of chromosomal anomaly; however, associated abnormalities may be present but missed on ultrasound.

POTENTIAL CONSEQUENCES

Any cleft (lip, palate or both) will need surgical repair in infancy and possibly other operations later in childhood. The following occur frequently in babies with a cleft palate:

▶ feeding difficulties;
▶ speech difficulties;
▶ nasal regurgitation;
▶ dental abnormalities; and
▶ recurrent otitis media and conductive hearing loss.

MANAGEMENT—ANTENATAL

Ideally the parents should be counselled by members of the multidisciplinary team that manage clefts in infants. Counselling can also be provided by general paediatricians or a member of the neonatal team.

The parents should be warned that antenatal diagnosis may not accurately assess the severity of any clefts and that associated abnormalities may be missed. Complete assessment will not be possible until after birth.

A genetics review is recommended if there are other abnormalities or if a specific syndrome is suspected.

Support groups (e.g., CleftPALS www.cleftpals.org.au/) are available.

MANAGEMENT—IMMEDIATE POSTNATAL

The baby should be examined thoroughly (before the first feed). This should include:

▶ assessment of the airway—obstruction by the tongue may occur with cleft palate (especially in Pierre Robin deformation sequence);
▶ inspection and palpation of the palate (a sub-mucosal cleft palate may not be visible, but should be suspected if the uvula is bifid);
▶ assessment of the ability to suck; and
▶ looking for associated anomalies.

If possible feeds should be established as soon as possible. With an isolated cleft lip major feeding difficulties are rare. The baby can usually breast feed with appropriate positioning (the support of a lactation consultant may be needed).

Babies with a cleft palate (with or without a cleft lip) often have feeding difficulties with significant delays in establishing feeds. The cleft palate interferes with normal sucking, and usually prevents exclusive breast feeding or bottle feeding with a regular bottle and teat. The mother should be told that breast feeding may still be possible although it will take a lot of extra effort to achieve. Experienced nursing support is invaluable and can provide specialised bottles, teats and other devices.

The time taken to establish feeds is the major influence on length of hospital stay.

MANAGEMENT—LONG TERM

Long-term follow-up is required by a multidisciplinary cleft team. This will include plastic and maxillofacial surgeons, otolaryngologists, speech pathologists, dentists and others.

The major long-term management issues include:

▶ feeding—occasionally an obturator (a prosthetic device which occludes the cleft palate) may be used in some infants to facilitate feeding;
▶ growth and development;
▶ dental/orthodontic care will be required if there is any cleft palate and/or tooth abnormalities;
▶ surgical repair:
  • cleft lip is usually repaired at 3–4 months of age (see Figure 56.2),
  • cleft palate is usually operated on at 6–9 months of age,
  • other operations may be required later in childhood;
▶ detection and treatment of possible complications of cleft palate, including:
  • speech difficulties (may require speech therapy),
  • nasal regurgitation,
  • recurrent otitis media, with or without hearing loss, will require referral to an ear, nose and throat surgeon and audiology (tympanostomy tubes may be needed and are sometimes used prophylactically);

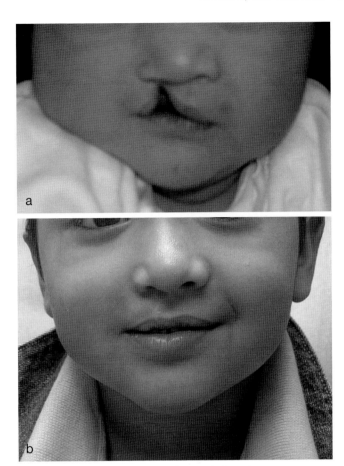

Figure 56.2 A—Unilateral cleft lip; B—after surgical repair.

▶ genetics review, if familial or syndromic clefts are suspected, to counsel regarding recurrence risk; and
▶ potential for psychosocial problems.

RECURRENCE

The recurrence risk depends on:
▶ the type of cleft:
   • in general the risk of a recurrent isolated cleft palate is greater than that for a cleft lip, with or without a cleft palate,

- an isolated sub-mucosal cleft palate or bifid uvula will recur more often than other forms of isolated cleft palate;
- the cleft location:
  - unilateral—2.7% recurrence,
  - bilateral—5.4% recurrence;
- family history;
- associated anomalies (with or without a specific syndrome);
- exposure to potential teratogens;
- sex; and
- racial background.

The following are general estimates of recurrence risk for sporadic, non-syndromic clefts:

If parents are not affected:
- with one affected offspring the recurrence risk is about 4%; and
- with two affected offspring, the recurrence risk is about 10%.

If one parent is affected:
- with no affected offspring the recurrence risk is about 4%; and
- with one affected offspring the recurrence risk is about 14%.

The cleft severity in the baby does not predict the severity of future defects.

Further Reading

Jones KL. *Smith's recognizable patterns of human malformation.* 6th ed. Elsevier; 2006.

Larsen WJ. *Human Embryology.* 3rd ed. Churchill Livingstone; 2001.

Wilkins-Haug L. *Prenatal diagnosis of orofacial clefts.* In: Levine D, Firth H, Barss V, eds. UpToDate Version 18.3 2010.

Merritt L. Understanding the embryology and genetics of cleft lip and palate. *Advances in Neonatal Care.* 2005;5:64.

INDEX

Page numbers followed by "f" indicate figures, "t" indicate tables, and "b" indicate boxes.